365
HEALTH
HINTS

365
HEALTH
HINTS

QUICK,
PRACTICAL WAYS TO
PROTECT YOUR HEALTH,
MAINTAIN YOUR WELL-BEING, AND
FEEL BETTER THAN EVER EVERYDAY

DON R. POWELL, Ph.D.
AND THE AMERICAN INSTITUTE
FOR PREVENTIVE MEDICINE

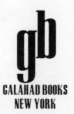

GALAHAD BOOKS
NEW YORK

Notice

To my parents, Bob and Yvette Powell, for all the love and encouragement they have provided and continue to provide. To my sons, Jordan and Brett, two bundles of joy who make me want to be the healthiest I can be. And to my wife, Nancy, for her understanding and support.

Contents

Contents

Foreword

Never before have individuals needed to assume more responsibility for their health care. Traditionally, health care has been disease oriented: People went to the doctor when they were sick. The doctor prescribed a treatment, the patient paid the bill, and that was that. People are now expected to decide when they should or should not see a physician, know the pros and cons of surgery and medical treatments, choose from various types of medical care coverage and health care plans, and modify their lifestyles to prevent illness and disease.

Also, people are living longer. Thanks to preventive medicine and advances in treatment of disease, people can survive heart disease, high blood pressure, diabetes, and other conditions that killed most people just a couple of decades ago. Yet these people are still susceptible to other, less threatening problems. Technology has even improved the odds of surviving accidents and infections. With more and better medical care available, more and more people make up the older segment of the U.S. population. And in turn, people in this age group require a significant amount of medical care.

While being a patient isn't as simple as it used to be, doctors aren't as autonomous as they used to be, either. The way physicians practice medicine is influenced by health care insurers regulating what kind of tests they can order, whom they admit to the hospital, what procedures must be done on an outpatient basis, and how they charge for their services.

Considering the accompanying escalation in health care delivery costs, it's easy to see why medical care has gotten so complicated—and why the medical care consumer is faced with so many decisions.

How can you, the consumer, get the information you need to successfully navigate this maze? You have to learn about the cause, detection, and treatment of serious health problems like heart disease, cancer, infections, and accidents. You also need to know how to alter the course of less serious, nagging, or irritating conditions like back pain or sore throats. You also need to know what you can do to ensure that your diet, sleep habits, sexual practices, work routine, and other aspects of your environment are safe and healthy.

Every day, newspapers, magazines, radio, television, and other sources of information bombard us with assorted facts and theories about what we should and shouldn't do to protect our health. Making sense out of a constant barrage of random information is no easy task. Neither is deciding what's best for you and your family.

365 Health Hints can make health education—and medical decision making—easier for you. It serves as a framework of solid medical information, arranged in a practical format allowing the reader to chart a course toward good health. With this very readable and prevention-oriented book, the individual need not wait until a health problem becomes urgent to take action. Instead, health-conscious individuals can periodically review their diets and living habits and head off trouble before it begins. The 365 tips herein will help readers ask the right questions, find the right answers, and most important, protect their most precious resource—their health.

—Richard N. Matzen, M.D., Chairman
Department of Preventive Medicine
Cleveland Clinic, Cleveland, Ohio

and

Richard S. Lang, M.D., M.P.H., Head
Section of Occupational Medicine
Department of Preventive Medicine
Cleveland Clinic

Preface

Business, fashion, and economics follow trends, and so do health and disease. The past 90 years have seen major changes in how long people live and what they die of. In 1900, the average life expectancy was 47 years, and most people died from typhoid, polio, smallpox, tuberculosis, diphtheria, or pneumonia—diseases caused by viruses or bacteria, both of which no one could control. Either you caught these diseases or you didn't. And if you caught them, there was no effective treatment.

Two medical breakthroughs improved life expectancy dramatically. The first was the development of vaccines to immunize people against many fatal or crippling illnesses. In fact, vaccines have virtually eliminated many diseases that were prevalent up until just a generation ago. For example, you most likely grew up knowing someone who had polio; your children will not. The other significant breakthrough was the discovery of penicillin to treat pneumonia and other often-fatal diseases.

Today the life expectancy for a baby girl is 79 years. For a baby boy, it's 72 years. And the most common causes of death are heart disease, stroke, cancer, emphysema, and cirrhosis of the liver—entirely different diseases from those that afflicted our great-grandparents.

This year alone, nearly one million people, more than all the Americans who died in World War I, World War II, the Korean conflict, and the war in Vietnam combined—will die from cardiovascular disease. Another half million people will suffer a stroke. There will be 500,000 newly diagnosed cases of diabetes. And according to projections, approximately one out of three Americans will eventually develop cancer.

With the possible exception of cancer, microscopic viruses and bacteria don't cause these illnesses. Our lifestyle—what we eat, drink, smoke, and do—is largely to blame. In fact, the Centers for Disease Control maintains that over 50 percent of all deaths in this country are lifestyle related. In other words, we don't "catch" these fatal diseases, we give them to ourselves. Accordingly, the most important medical advances of the past two decades haven't occurred in the laboratory or even the operating room. Rather, better health comes from changes people make in their lives—changes that take place in kitchens, on jogging trails, in cars, and at work. Prevention is an idea whose time has come.

You might say the United States is in the midst of a revolution—a health revolution. More people are taking positive steps to improve their health and well-being now than at any other time in history. Hardly a day passes that you don't see walkers, joggers, or bicyclists on the road. Blood pressure machines crop up in airports and shopping malls. Legislation has banned smoking on many airplane flights, in public buildings, and at work sites. Alcohol consumption is steadily declining by about 2 percent a year. Television commercials tout foods that are low in sodium and fat and high in healthful substances like fiber. Advertisements for health clubs coax you to "get physical." Public service announcements urge kids (and their parents) to "Just say no" to drugs. Medical reports make headlines in newspapers, in magazines, and on the nightly news. Conversation at social gatherings frequently turns to health. And in bookstores, shelf upon shelf is stocked with self-help health titles.

In light of this unprecedented explosion of health information, we asked family, friends, and colleagues how they keep informed about health. All remarked that in some ways, there's almost too much information to assimilate. For most, their days are so jam-packed with family and work obligations that they don't have nearly enough time to read and digest all the information generated. To confound matters, the pertinent information in magazines and books doesn't always jump out at readers. Often you have to read page after page to dig up one nugget of useful information. Even then, much of what's published is not supported by medical fact. Another concern is that many books and magazines focus on treating illness, not preventing it.

One of the most popular health books ever written was Dr. Benjamin Spock's *Guide to Infant and Child Care*. Unfortunately, Dr. Spock's book addresses health issues that pertain only to children. At the American Institute for Preventive Medicine, we felt a need for a book on adult health care that was as thorough and authoritative as Dr. Spock's and was also prevention oriented.

Such were the issues that inspired us to write *365 Health Hints*. We drew on the advice and expertise of an extensive team of health professionals, including physicians, psychologists, nurses, dietitians, exercise physiologists, health educators, public health officials, and safety specialists. And we've made every effort to see that the information is accurate and-up-to date, based on recent medical and behavioral research.

Written in an easy-to-read, tip-a-day format, *365 Health Hints* tells you how you can prevent, detect, or treat dozens of health problems, from everyday complaints like headaches and sore throats to major medical conditions like heart disease and cancer. You'll also find out how to stay healthy in many other ways: losing weight; eating a nutritious diet; reducing stress; preventing home accidents; staying healthy when you travel; exercising wisely; taking care of your teeth; having a happier, healthier sex life; and getting the best medical care for your money. Our goal is to provide short, practical, easy-to-follow tips that will help you take charge of your health and the health of those you love.

Acknowledgments

365 Health Hints took well over a year to complete. Hundreds of colleagues, friends, and family members played a part, and my efforts would have fallen far short if not for their invaluable assistance.

First of all, I want to thank Carole Singer, M.Ed., Program Director of the American Institute for Preventive Medicine, for her help and expertise throughout the project. There is not a better person to work with than Carole. I particularly want to express my gratitude to Andrew J. Ruden, M.D., for his invaluable assistance in both the contribution of medical facts to the text, particularly in chapters 1 and 2, and his review of the entire manuscript for medical accuracy. Elaine Frank, R.D., the Institute's Director of Nutrition Services, also played an important role in the book's development, as did Colleen Christopher, R.N., a senior consultant to the Institute. I am also extremely grateful to Sharon Faelten, my editor at Rodale Press, for her knowledge of writing, candid feedback, and ability to turn what I thought was very good work into something even better.

365 Health Hints went through an extensive review process in order to ensure medical accuracy and present the latest medical and behavioral research. I am indebted to the physicians and other health professionals listed below who reviewed various parts of the manuscript according to their areas of expertise.

Patrick T. Ainslie, D.D.S., M.S., Periodontist, Farmington Hills, Michigan.

Charles B. Arnold, M.D., M.P.H., Medical Director, Medical Relations, Metropolitan Life Insurance Company, New York, New York.

Jeffrey D. Band, M.D., Corporate Epidemiologist, Chief of Infectious Diseases, and Medical Director, InterHealth: Health Care for International Travelers, William Beaumont Hospital, Royal Oak, Michigan.

Judith M. Berman, Chief, Regional Coordination, Michigan State Police, Office of Highway Safety Planning, Lansing, Michigan.

Ronald Berris, D.D.S., Team Dentist, Detroit Pistons basketball team, and Family Dentistry, West Bloomfield, Michigan.

Dennis I. Blender, Ph.D., Psychologist, Grant Thornton Company, Southfield, Michigan.

Joyce Brownson-Booth, M.A., Director of Training, American Institute for Preventive Medicine, Costa Mesa, California.

Elaine Frank, R.D., Director, Nutrition Services, American Institute for Preventive Medicine, Southfield, Michigan, and instructor, Department of Health and Physical Fitness, Henry Ford Community College, Dearborn, Michigan.

Barry A. Franklin, Ph.D., Director, Cardiac Rehabilitation and Exercise Laboratories, William Beaumont Hospital, Royal Oak, Michigan.

Dwight D. Gaal, M.A., Director, Health Promotion, Bon Secours Hospital, Grosse Pointe, Michigan.

Michael R. Garr, Lieutenant/Fire Prevention, Farmington Hills Fire Department, Farmington Hills, Michigan.

Abe Gershonowicz, D.D.S., Family Dentistry, Sterling Heights, Michigan.

William Hettler, M.D., Director, University Health Service, University of Wisconsin, Stevens Point, Wisconsin.

Ronald D. Kerwin, M.D., Clinical Instructor, Department of Dermatology, Wayne State University School of Medicine, and staff physician, Crittenton Hospital, Rochester, Michigan; Huron Valley Hospital, Milford, Michigan; and Sinai Hospital, Detroit, Michigan.

James Kohlenberg, M.D., Internal Medicine, John R. Medical Clinic, Madison Heights, Michigan.

Melvin Korobkin, M.D., Professor of Radiology, University of Michigan Medical School, Ann Arbor, Michigan.

Richard S. Lang, M.D., Head, Section of Occupational Medicine, Department of Preventive Medicine, Cleveland Clinic, Cleveland, Ohio.

Donald B. Levitt, Ph.D., Corporate Health Promotion and Counseling Administrator, Ford Motor Company, Dearborn, Michigan.

James V. McConnell, Ph.D., Professor Emeritus of Psychology, University of Michigan, Ann Arbor, Michigan.

Richard N. Matzen, M.D., Chairman, Department of Preventive Medicine, Cleveland Clinic, Cleveland, Ohio.

Jeffrey A. Meer, M.D., Internal Medicine, Birmingham, Michigan.

Michael P. O'Donnell, M.P.H., M.B.A., Director, Health Promotion and Wellness, William Beaumont Hospital, Royal Oak, Michigan.

Thomas C. Overholt, M.D., Department of Internal Medicine and Pediatrics, Henry Ford Hospital, Detroit, Michigan.

Owen Z. Perlman, M.D., Director, Department of Physical Medicine and Rehabilitation, Catherine McAuley Health Center, Ann Arbor, Michigan.

William H. Rattner, M.D., Adjunct Assistant Professor, Department of Urology, Wayne State University School of Medicine, and Staff Physician, Sinai Hospital, Detroit, Michigan.

Edward J. Roccella, Ph.D., M.P.H., Coordinator, National High Blood Pressure Education Program, Office of Preventive Education and Control, National Heart, Lung, and Blood Institute, Bethesda, Maryland.

F. David Rollo, M.D., Ph.D., Senior Vice President, Medical Affairs, Humana, Inc., Louisville, Kentucky.

Michael Rontal, M.D., F.A.C.S., Clinical Assistant Professor, University of Michigan Medical School and Wayne State University School of Medicine, and Staff Physician, Sinai Hospital, Detroit, Michigan, and William Beaumont Hospital, Royal Oak, Michigan.

Susan Herman Ryskamp, M.S., R.D., Lecturer/Interim Director, Dietetics Program, Department of Nutrition and Food Science, Wayne State University, Detroit, Michigan.

E. A. Shaptini, M.D., Vice President and Medical Director, American Natural Resources Company, Detroit, Michigan.

John S. Shelton, Sergeant, Southfield Police Department, Southfield, Michigan.

William Solomon, M.D., Clinical Instructor, Department of Internal Medicine, Wayne State University School of Medicine, and Medical Director, Jewish Home for the Aged, Detroit, Michigan.

Steven Starr, D.P.M., Director, Birmingham Foot Care, Birmingham, Michigan.

Neill D. Varner, D.O., M.P.H., Medical Director, Saginaw Steering Division, General Motors Corporation, Saginaw, Michigan, member of the UAW-GM Health Promotion Task Force, and Medical Director, Saginaw County Department of Public Health.

George Watkins, Editor in Chief, *EAP Digest,* and President, Performance Resource Press, Troy, Michigan.

Marvin S. Weckstein, M.D., Psychotherapy and Outpatient Psychiatry, Assistant Director of Adult Psychiatry Training, Fairlawn Center, Pontiac, Michigan.

Mark Werner, M.D., Obstetrics and Gynecology, Staff Physician, William Beaumont Hospital, Royal Oak, Michigan.

Above all, this book could not have been completed without the tremendous assistance and support I received from the American Institute for Preventive Medicine, one of North America's leading developers of health promotion programs and materials. The Institute's mission is to improve the public health and quality of life for all people. This book represents one way for that goal to be achieved. Many Institute staff members participated in the development of the book, while others kept the innovative work of the Institute going at full speed while I spent the majority of my time writing. I particularly want to thank Jeanette Karwan, Director, Product Development, for the tremendous job she did in updating the book for the 2nd and 3rd editions. Many thanks, also, go to Susan Jackson, Vice President of Marketing, Elaine Frank, Vice President of Operations, Yael Zoldan, Manager, Graphic Design, and Wendy Fiorentino.

Dr. James V. McConnell deserves special mention. As my academic advisor and mentor, Dr. McConnell was responsible for leading me into the arena of health promotion. In addition, being the positive role model that he is, Jim inspired me to write this book.

My appreciation also goes to Bob and Yvette Powell, Steve Powell, and Edith and Joseph Stein for providing research materials for many hints. And to Anita Diamant, my agent, for placing the book with the great people at Rodale Press.

Finally, I want to thank all the people who have influenced my life and career-family, friends, colleagues, teachers, students, and patients. I have learned from all of you.

CHAPTER

1

Fast Relief for Everyday Health Problems

Most of the tips in this book tell you how to prevent and deal with major illness: how to sharpen your nutritional awareness to prevent heart disease, how to quit smoking to prevent cancer, how to manage stress to prevent high blood pressure and stroke, how to control alcohol intake to prevent cirrhosis and other diseases. Yet many minor health problems can be prevented or treated, too. Heartburn, blemishes, sore throat, back strain, fatigue, nosebleeds, hay fever—pesky problems that may not propel you to an emergency room but are bothersome just the same.

Here, then, are 49 of the most common health problems you're likely to encounter on any given day, arranged from head to toe, with some quick tips on how to prevent or treat them.

◢ Ways to Prevent and/or Relieve a Throbbing Headache

People have been looking for—sometimes *praying* for—relief from headache pain for almost as long as heads have been aching. Back in the Middle Ages, when people thought demons in the brain caused headaches, treatment consisted of boring a small hole in the skull. Fortunately, doctors understand headaches a little bit better today and suggest less drastic remedies.

Not all headaches are alike. *Tension or muscular headaches* are the most common. Unconscious tensing of the face, neck, or scalp muscles produces a dull, relentless ache. You feel the pressure in your forehead, temples, or around the back of the head, where the muscles of your upper back attach. Lack of sleep or the stress of everyday hassles can trigger tension headaches. Doing tedious work or reading frequently causes muscular headaches.

Migraine headaches are more common among women, tend to run in families, and are more debilitating. A migraine usually originates on one side of the head and throbs. Alternative constriction and dilation (narrowing and widening) of blood vessels in the head causes migraines, which are often accompanied by vomiting, nausea, blurred vision, flashing spots, sensitivity to light, and ringing in the ears.

Sinus headaches are characterized by pain over the sinuses of the face, in the area of your upper cheekbones, forehead, and the bridge of your nose. Inflammation and fluid buildup cause the pain, and bending over or touching the affected area seems to aggravate it. Colds, allergies, air pollution, and other respiratory problems can trigger a sinus headache.

For on-the-spot headache relief:

▶ Rest in a quiet, dark room with your eyes closed.

▶ Massage the base of your skull with your thumbs. Work from the ears toward the center of the back of your head. Also, massage both temples gently.

▶ Take hot baths.

▶ Place cold washcloths over your eyes.

▶ Take the recommended dose of aspirin or an aspirin substitute.

▶ Practice a relaxation technique (such as visualizing a serene setting, meditating, or deep breathing, as described in chapter 6, Success over Stress).

To prevent headaches from recurring:

▶ Try to anticipate when pain will strike. Keep a headache journal that records when, where, and why headaches seem to occur.

▶ Note early symptoms and try to abort a headache in its earliest stages.

▶ Exercise regularly. (This seems to keep headaches at bay.)

▶ Avoid foods known to trigger headaches in sensitive people.

Particularly troublesome foods may include:

— Alcoholic beverages, especially red wine

— Bananas (if more than $1/2$ banana per day)

— Caffeine (from coffee, tea, cola soft drinks, or some medications)

— Chocolate

— Citrus fruit (if more than $1/2$ cup per day)

— Cured meats (like frankfurters)

— Food additives (such as monosodium glutamate, or MSG)

— Hard cheeses (like aged cheddar or provolone)

— Nuts and peanut butter

— Onions

— Sour cream

— Vinegar

Note: See a doctor if you have persistent or recurring headaches, or if you are experiencing a migraine-like headache for the first time.

How to Fight a Fever

Elevated temperature isn't always a sign that something's wrong. Although 98.6°F has been considered normal for years, many healthy people walk around with a temperature a degree above or below this.

Body temperature even fluctuates throughout the day—it's usually lowest in the morning and highest in the late afternoon and evening. The type of thermometer you measure your temperature with also makes a difference. Rectal thermometer readings are usually more accurate and read a degree higher than oral thermometers.

Taking your temperature by mouth after you drink a hot liquid like soup or tea can mislead you into thinking you have a fever when you don't. Other factors that can temporarily affect your temperature include:

▶ Wearing too much clothing (if you're overdressed enough to raise your body temperature)

▶ Exercise

▶ Hot, humid weather

► Hormones (increased progesterone levels increase body temperature, so women's basal body temperature increases following ovulation)

If you've ruled out confounding factors and your temperature is higher than 99°F, you might have a fever, If your temperature is higher than 101°F you definitely have a fever.

Call a doctor if a fever:

► Occurs in a child less than 6 months old.

► In a child, exceeds 101°F orally or 102°F rectally and doesn't go down within 48 hours despite efforts to reduce the fever.

► Lasts four to five days in an adult.

► Is accompanied by other symptoms, like stiff neck, persistent sore throat, vomiting, diarrhea, listlessness, rash, cough, or earache.

Adults probably don't have to do anything to treat a fever if they feel okay. But be sure to treat a fever if you don't feel good or if it goes over 104°F (102°F in the elderly).

To cool a fever:

► Drink fruit juice, water, and other replenishing liquids.

► Take a sponge bath with tepid (about 70°F) water. (Sponging with alcohol has no advantage and often makes people feel ill, because of alcohol's pungent odor.)

► Take the appropriate dose of aspirin or acetaminophen for your age every 3 to 4 hours. (*Note:* Don't give aspirin to children under 19 years old, however, if a fever is associated with chicken pox or a flu-like illness. It's been associated with Reye's syndrome, a potentially fatal condition that is discussed in chapter 2, Major Medical Conditions: Prevention, Detection, and Treatment.)

► Get plenty of bed rest.

► Don't bundle up in heavy clothing or several layers of blankets.

► Avoid strenuous exercise.

3 Daily Defense against Dandruff

Dandruff is harmless. But that's no consolation if people call you Commander Whitehead behind your bespeckled back and shoulders.

Dandruff (or seborrheic dermatitis, in medical terms) affects the scalp and eyebrows—areas of the skin where oil glands are most active--leaving them oily and flaky. Unchecked, dandruff can collect around your ears and cascade down your neck and back.

While dandruff seems to run in families, no one knows exactly what causes it. Possible contributing factors include:

► Stress

► Infrequent shampooing

► Oily skin in general

► Extremes in weather (hot and humid or cold and dry conditions)

Whatever the cause of your dandruff, thorough, daily shampooing is the most successful home treatment, To make shampooing more effective:

► Scrub thoroughly to loosen scaly skin, but be gentle, taking care not to scratch or irritate the scalp and increase the risk of infection.

► Use an anti-dandruff shampoo. Over-the-counter shampoos that contain selenium sulfide are often effective for mild cases. More severe dandruff may require a prescription medication containing coal tar or a scalp lotion with cortisone, which is rubbed into the scalp.

4 Eight Ways to Sleep through Insomnia

Do you ever find yourself wide awake long after you go to bed at night? Well, you're not alone. An estimated 40 million Americans are bothered by insomnia. They either have trouble falling asleep at night, wake up in the middle of the night, or wake up too early and can't get back to sleep. And when they're not asleep, insomniacs worry about whether or not they'll be able to sleep.

An occasional sleepless night is, well, nothing to lose sleep over. But if insomnia bothers you for three weeks or longer, it can be a real medical problem.

Many old-fashioned remedies for sleeplessness work--and work well. Next time you find yourself unable to sleep, try these time-tested cures.

► Avoid caffeine in all forms after lunchtime. (Coffee, tea, chocolate, colas, and some other soft drinks contain this stimulant, as do certain over-the-counter and prescription drugs; check the labels for content.) This is the *last* thing a wide-awake insomniac needs.

- Don't nap during the day, no matter how groggy you feel. (Naps decrease the quality of nighttime sleep.)

- Take a nice, long, hot bath before bedtime. (This soothes and unwinds tense muscles, leaving you relaxed enough to fall alseep.)

- Read a book or do some repetitive, tedious activity, like needlework. Try not to watch television or listen to the radio. These kinds of distractions may hold your attention and keep you awake.

- Make your bedroom as comfortable as possible. Create a quiet, dark atmosphere. Use clean, fresh sheets and pillows, and keep the room temperature comfortable (neither too warm nor too cool).

- Ban worry from the bedroom. Don't allow yourself to rehash the mistakes of the day as you toss and turn. You're off duty now. The idea is to associate your bed with sleep.

- Develop a regular bedtime routine. Locking or checking doors and windows, brushing your teeth, and reading before you turn in every night primes you for sleep.

- Count those sheep! Counting slowly is a soothing, hypnotic activity. By picturing repetitive, monotonous images, you may bore yourself to sleep.

If, after three weeks, you still have trouble sleeping despite your efforts, see a doctor to rule out any medical or psychiatric problems that may be at fault.

5 Surefire Relief for Pinkeye

It's early morning and you're just about to open your eyes to start another day. But wait, what's this? Your eyelids are stuck together. You rub the crust from your lashes, look in the mirror, and find yourself face to face with eyes that are swollen, itchy, and red, and produce a clear (or yellowish) discharge. You've got conjunctivitis, or pinkeye.

Pinkeye is an inflammation of the conjunctiva, the underside of both the upper and lower eyelids and the covering of the white portion of the eye.

Some causes (and corresponding solutions) include:

► Allergic reaction to airborne pollens, dust, mold spores, and animal dander, or direct contact with chlorinated water or cosmetics. If you can't avoid the allergens, antihistamines can help. So can eye drops containing a vasoconstrictive agent or steroid. (Steroid preparations require a prescription.)

► Bacterial conjunctivitis, characterized by a puslike discharge. Warm compresses, along with an antibiotic ointment or drops prescribed by your physician, can help. When treated properly, bacterial conjunctivitis will clear up in two to three days.

► Viral conjunctivitis as a complication of a cold or flu. Viral conjuntivitis produces less discharge but more tearing than bacterial conjunctivitis. Antibiotics don't work, and viral conjunctivitis can take 14 to 21 days to clear up.

Here are some ways to relieve the symptoms of pinkeye:

► Don't touch the eye area with your fingers. If you must wipe your eyes, use tissues.

► With your eyes closed, apply a washcloth soaked in warm (not hot) water to the affected eye three or four times a day for at least 5 minutes at a time. (These soaks also help to dissolve the crusty residue of pinkeye.)

► Use over-the-counter eye drops. They may soothe irritation and help relieve itching.

► Avoid wearing eye makeup until the infection has completely cleared up. (And never share makeup with others.)

► Don't cover or patch the eye; this can promote the growth of infectious organisms.

► Don't wear contact lenses while your eyes are infected.

► Wash your hands often and use your own towels. Pinkeye is very contagious and can be spread from one person to another by contaminated fingers, washcloths, or towels.

► See a doctor if there is no improvement in two or three days or your eyes become painful or sensitive to light.

6 What to Do for a Sty

A sty is a small boil or bacterial infection in a tiny gland of the eyelash follicle. If the oil-producing glands on the upper or lower rim of the eyelid become infected, they become swollen and painful. A sty is minuscule at first, but it can blossom into a bright red, painful sore.

Some early symptoms include:

▶ A gritty feeling in the eye

▶ Redness on the rim of the eyelid

▶ Swelling

▶ Sensitivity to touch

Eventually, a "baby" sty will come to a head and appear yellow, due to accumulation of pus. Generally, the tip will face outward, and the sty will rupture and drain on its own. In the meantime, however, you can relieve the discomfort by following these steps.

▶ Apply warm (not hot), wet compresses to the affected area three or four times a day for 5 to 10 minutes at a time.

▶ Avoid situations that expose your eyes to excessive dust or dirt.

▶ Don't poke or squeeze the infected area, no matter how tempted you may be to pop the sty.

Most sties respond well to home treatment and don't require further treatment. If the sty doesn't drain within a day or two, see your physician, who may need to remove the troublesome eyelash or prescribe antibiotic drops for the eye.

7 Help for "Computer Eyes"

Office workers have their share of occupational hazards. People who frequently use video display terminals (VDTs) often complain of eyestrain, pain and stiffness in their backs and shoulders, and stress.

Video display terminals don't emit dangerous rays. But prolonged use, improper positioning of the VDT, improper lighting, poor posture, and tight deadlines are responsible for the discomfort associated with using them.

By making some simple adjustments, office workers can protect themselves from the physical problems associated with using VDTs.

To prevent eyestrain:

▸ Reduce glare by keeping the VDT away from a window, turning off or shielding overhead lights, and using a glare-reducing filter over the screen.

▸ Place your paperwork close enough that you don't have to keep refocusing when switching from the screen to the paper. You might want to use a paper holder.

▸ Place the screen so that your line of sight is 10 to 15 degrees (about one-third of a 45-degree angle) below horizontal.

▸ Clean dust off the screen frequently.

▸ Blink frequently to keep your eyes from getting dry.

▸ Inform your eye specialist that you use a VDT. Glasses and contacts worn for other activities may not be effective for work on a VDT. (Bifocals may create difficulties when using a VDT because the near vision part of the lens is good for looking down, as when you read, but not straight ahead, as you do when looking at a video display screen. So you may need single-vision lenses for VDT work.)

▸ If the image on the VDT screen is blurred, dull, or flickers, have it serviced right away.

To prevent muscle tension when you work at a VDT:

▸ Use a chair that supports your back and can be easily adjusted to a height that's comfortable for you.

▸ Get up and go for a short walk every 1 to 2 hours.

▸ Periodically throughout the day, perform stretching exercises of the neck, shoulder, and lower back.

— Rotate your head in a circular motion, first clockwise, then counterclockwise.

— Shrug your shoulders up, down, backward, and forward.

— While standing or sitting, bend at the waist, leaning first to the left, then to the right.

▸ How to Quiet the Ringing in Your Ears

Imagine hearing an unrelenting noise in your head, its volume ranging from a ring to a roar. This maddening noise, called tinnitus, victimizes nearly 36 million Americans, most of them older adults. Seven million people are so seriously bothered by tinnitus that living a normal life is impossible. No mere distraction, tinnitus can interfere with work, sleep, and ordinary communication with others.

Like a toothache, tinnitus isn't a disease in itself but a symptom of another problem. Ear wax blocking the ear canals, food allergies, reactions to medications, middle-ear infection, blood vessel abnormalities in the brain, auditory nerve abnormality (due to exposure to loud noise), diabetes, and (rarely) brain tumors can cause tinnitus. And sometimes, tinnitus is due to advancing age. It often accompanies loss of hearing. Occasionally, tinnitus is temporary and will not lead to deafness. (For proper diagnosis, consult an ear, nose, and throat specialist.)

What can you do to relieve tinnitus?

▶ For mild cases, play the radio or a white noise tape (white noise is a low, constant sound) in the background to help mask the tinnitus.

▶ Ask your doctor about a recently developed tinnitus masker, which looks like a hearing aid. Worn on the ear, it makes a subtle noise that masks the tinnitus without interfering with hearing and speech.

▶ Biofeedback or other relaxation techniques can help you calm down and concentrate, shifting your attention away from the tinnitus.

▶ Exercise regularly to promote good blood circulation.

How to Stop a Nosebleed

Nosebleeds are usually a childhood problem, a scary but minor bout with broken blood vessels just inside the nose. They're caused by a cold, frequent nose blowing and picking, allergies, a dry environment that parches the membrane linings, or a punch or other blow to the nose.

But not all nosebleeds are simply a nuisance. Some are serious—such as bleeding from deep within the nose (called a posterior nosebleed) that's profuse and hard to stop. This type usually afflicts the elderly and it's most commonly caused by:

▶ Atherosclerosis (hardening) of nasal blood vessels

▶ High blood pressure

▶ Anticoagulant drugs

▶ Primary bleeding disorders (like hemophilia)

▶ Tumor in the nose

A doctor should always treat a posterior nosebleed. In fact, any nosebleed that can't be stopped after 10 to 15 minutes or occurs again and again calls for medical attention. It may require cauterization of the bleeding vessel or nasal packing. (Cauterization destroys tissue by burning it with heat, chemicals, or electricity.)

Although there are lots of ideas about how to treat minor nosebleeds, the following procedure is recommended by the American Academy of Otolaryngology—Head and Neck Surgery.

1. Sit with your head leaning forward.

2. Pinch the nostrils shut, using your thumb and forefinger in such a way that the nasal septum (the nose's midsection) is being gently squeezed.

3. Hold for 15 uninterrupted minutes, breathing through your mouth.

4. At the same time, apply cold compresses (such as ice in a soft cloth) to the area around the nose.

5. For the next 24 hours, make sure your head is elevated above the level of your heart.

6. Also, wait 24 hours before blowing your nose, lifting heavy objects, or exercising strenuously.

10 Declare War on Cold Sores

Nothing is more vexing than a cold sore that appears right on the edge of your lip for all to see. Yet you don't feel much better when they crop up inside your mouth. They hurt and are difficult to treat.

Once a cold sore strikes, it tends to return again and again. This is because the virus herpes simplex I that usually causes cold sores can go underground after the initial attack and lurk in the body for months or years, triggering sporadic flare-ups. Menstrual periods, fevers, colds, dental work, eczema, sun exposure, and stress can trigger repeat performances.

The first visible sign of a cold sore is usually a cluster of small fluid-filled blisters that form a red ring. As the blisters heal, they dry up, and usually disappear within two weeks.

You can take steps to either prevent or treat cold sores. For prevention:

▶ Do your best to manage emotional and physical stress.

▶ Limit exposure to the sun. (Apply zinc oxide or a sun block to lips or other susceptible areas if you expect to spend time outdoors.)

▶ Avoid contact with anyone who has an active cold sore.

▶ Wash your hands frequently while the virus is active, to prevent it from spreading.

To relieve cold sores:

▶ Apply ice for 1 hour within a day of the sore's first appearance.

▶ Drink cool beverages to soothe the pain.

▶ Don't scratch or pick at the sore.

▶ Take a nonprescription pain reliever like aspirin or acetaminophen to relieve cold sore pain.

▶ If the sore is severe, your doctor may prescribe a medication called acyclovir (brand name Zovirax) to both treat and prevent cold sores.

11 A Secret Weapon against Bad Breath

Few other bodily afflictions are more embarrassing than bad breath (halitosis). But it isn't really a problem, it's a symptom of a wide range of possible conditions.

Knowing what your bad breath smells like is a good clue to its cause—and the first step toward getting rid of it. A sweet, fruity odor can indicate undiagnosed diabetes, for example. An ammonia-like scent may signal kidney failure. Fishy-smelling breath is common in people with liver failure. Mouth sores, the flu, and illnesses like lung infections can also result in bad breath.

Diet, of course, is a far more common and less serious cause of bad breath. Garlic and onions have bad reputations, and rightly so: Pungent foods contain volatile oils that eventually reach the lungs (and the air you exhale) via the bloodstream. But few people realize that a high-protein diet can induce bad breath, too.

Probably the most frequent causes of bad breath, though, are either gum disease or poor oral hygiene. Here's why:

▶   Gum disease permits odor-causing bacteria to collect in the spaces between your teeth. (If you have gum disease, you'll know it: The gums bleed and are usually swollen.)

▶   Poor oral hygiene is just a polite way of saying you haven't been brushing, flossing, and visiting the dentist as often as you should. Food particles allowed to remain in the mouth decay and give off a strong odor.

Since mouth odor could be a symptom of a health problem, don't try to rinse it away. See your doctor to uncover the real cause. If bad breath isn't due to anything serious, take the following steps to remedy it.

▶   Brush your teeth more often.

▶   Floss your teeth after meals, to clean spaces your toothbrush can't reach.

▶   Gently brush your tongue to rid the surface of a stagnant coating of bacteria or food that can build up and give off unpleasant odors.

▶   Don't smoke.

▶   Use a mouthwash or rinse until bad breath gets under control.

▶   Visit your dentist to have your teeth professionally cleaned every six months.

For more tips on caring for your mouth, see chapter 15, Dental Health: Beautiful Teeth for Life.

12 Soothing Remedies for Laryngitis

Disc jockeys get laryngitis. So do actors, politicians, and others who talk for hours. But ordinary people who overuse their voices get laryngitis, too. Perhaps you cheer too loud and too often at a basketball game. Or perhaps you lose your voice for no apparent reason.

Air pollution—spending an evening in a smoky room, for example—can also irritate the larynx (voice box) and cause laryngitis. Infections, too, can inflame the larynx. When your larynx is irritated or inflamed, your voice becomes hoarse, husky, and weak. Sometimes, laryngitis is painless, but you may experience a sore throat, a tickling sensation in the back of the throat, fever or dry cough, or have trouble swallowing.

Smoking, drinking alcohol, breathing cold air, and continuing to use already-distressed vocal cords all aggravate the situation. Conversely, resting your voice will usually allow acute laryngitis to heal within a couple of days. If laryngitis persists for more than a week or is accompanied by other symptoms, such as fever or coughing up blood or yellow-green sputum, consult your doctor for treatment.

Otherwise, home treatment for laryngitis is simple.

▶ Don't talk if you don't need to. Use a note pad and pencil to communicate.

▶ If you must speak, do so softly, but don't whisper. Whispering is more stressful than speaking in soft tones.

▶ Use a cool mist humidifier to moisturize the air in rooms where you expect to spend a lot of time (like the bedroom).

▶ Drink plenty of warm liquids like tea.

▶ Take a hot shower or steam bath.

▶ Don't smoke, and avoid smoky environments.

▶ Suck on over-the-counter throat lozenges. (Do not give to children under age 5.)

▶ Take aspirin to relieve discomfort, if necessary.

13 A Cure for Hiccups

Hiccups are simple enough to explain: Your diaphragm (the major muscle involved in breathing) goes into spasm. Hiccups are generally harmless and don't last very long. Luckily, there's no shortage of hiccup cures, and better still, most of them work (although some baffle medical science). A study reported in the *New England Journal of Medicine* found that 1 teaspoon of ordinary table sugar, swallowed dry, cured hiccups immediately in 19 out of 20 people (some of whom had been hiccuping for as long as six weeks).

Other popular folk remedies worth trying include:

▶ Hold your tongue with your thumb and index finger and gently pull it forward.

▶ With your neck bent backward, hold your breath for a count of ten. Exhale immediately and drink a glass of water.

▶ Breathe into and out of a paper (not plastic) bag.

▶ Swallow a small amount of finely cracked ice.

▶ Massage the back of the roof of your mouth with a cotton swab.

▶ Eat dry bread slowly.

▶ Drink a glass of water rapidly.

Frequently occurring or prolonged hiccups may indicate other health problems, like stomach distension or a heart attack, both of which call for immediate medical care.

14 How to Soothe a Sore Throat

Sore throats range from a mere scratch to pain so severe that swallowing nothing more than saliva is uncomfortable. The cause of all this misery can be either a virus or bacteria. Viral sore throats are the more common of the two and don't respond to antibiotics; bacterial ones do. So it's important to know what kind of bug is roughing up your throat.

Bacterial sore throats are most often caused by streptococcus (strep throat) and usually bring a high fever, headaches, or swollen, enlarged neck glands with them. Viral sore throats generally don't. But even doctors have trouble diagnosing a sore throat based on symptoms alone. (A child with a bacterial sore throat may have no other symptoms, for example.) And if left untreated, serious complications, including abscesses, kidney inflammation, or rheumatic heart disease, could arise from a strep throat. So your doctor may take a throat culture. If strep, or other bacteria are the culprits, he or she will prescribe an antibiotic.

You can take some steps to relieve sore throat discomfort.

▶ Gargle every few hours with a solution of ¼ teaspoon of salt dissolved in half a glass of warm water.

▶ Drink plenty of warm beverages, such as tea (with or without honey) and soup.

▶ Use a vaporizer or humidifier in the room where you spend most of your time.

▶ Don't smoke.

▶ Avoid eating spicy foods.

▶ Suck on a piece of hard candy or medicated lozenge every so often. (Do not give to children under age 5.)

▶ Take aspirin or acetaminophen for the pain or fever (or both).
(*Note:* Children age 19 or younger, however, shouldn't take
aspirin for chicken pox or flu-like symptoms because of its
association with Reye's syndrome, a potentially fatal condition
that is discussed in chapter 2, Major Medical Conditions: Prevention, Detection, and Treatment.)

15 Twelve Ways to Banish a Blemish

Just when teenagers begin to find the opposite sex appealing and self-
image becomes important, Mother Nature plays a dirty trick on them: acne.
Whiteheads, blackheads, and reddened, raised, painful pimples sprout on
the shoulders, back, neck, and—the ultimate curse—the face. For some,
acne—or the scars it can leave-persist into adulthood.

Contrary to myth, acne is not caused by:

▶ Greasy foods

▶ Chocolate

▶ Frustrated sex drive

Acne results from normal changes in hormones during adolescence.
This prompts the sebaceous glands to produce oils. Surface oil doesn't
cause acne, though. The culprit is oil in the ducts below the skin's surface.
When oil ducts in hair follicles become clogged, bacteria on the skin
surface can mix with excess oil and cause acne bumps and blemishes.
(Acne that reappears later in life is often a milder version of teenage acne.)

Factors that can contribute to acne include:

▶ Changes in hormone levels preceding a woman's menstrual
period or during pregnancy.

▶ Rich moisturizing lotions or heavy or greasy makeup.

▶ Emotional stress.

▶ Foods containing high levels of iodine, such as kelp, beef liver,
broccoli, asparagus, and white onions.

▶ Nutritional supplements containing iodine.

▶ Exposure to airborne particles from cooking oils, tar, or creosote
(often used as a wood preservative).

▶ Putting pressure on the face by sleeping on one side of the face or resting your head in your hands.

▶ Taking drugs such as birth control pills, systemic steroids, anticonvulsive medications, and lithium (used to treat some forms of depression).

Time is the only real cure for acne, but you can try various ways to minimize blemishes and pimples.

▶ Keep the skin clean by washing several times a day with ordinary soap and water. Using a washcloth, gently massage soap lather into the skin for a minute or two. Rinse well. (Astringents, degreasing pads, and granular face scrubs may also be beneficial.)

▶ Use a fresh washcloth every day. (Bacteria thrive in a damp washcloth, reinfecting your pores if you use it again.)

▶ Ask your dermatologist to recommend a special soap formulated to help acne.

▶ Don't squeeze, scratch, or poke at pimples. This can cause infection or scarring (or both).

▶ Use an over-the-counter acne-drying medication containing benzoyl peroxide. Follow the manufacturer's directions. (Note: Some people are allergic to benzoyl peroxide, so you should test it first by applying a small amount to your hand.)

▶ Wash well immediately after strenuous exercise, to clear away sweat and pore-clogging chemicals.

▶ Shampoo your hair at least twice a week to eliminate buildup of oils that can contribute to acne on your forehead, neck, and shoulders.

▶ Keep hair off your face to keep it free of scalp oil.

▶ If you're a man, soften your beard with a warm towel before shaving, to lessen skin irritation. Shave along the natural grain of the beard, not against it.

▶ Limit time spent in the sun.

▶ Avoid sunlamps.

▶ Avoid greasy or oil-based creams, lotions, and makeups.

Consult a dermatologist if your skin doesn't improve or if you have a severe case of acne.

16 Effective Home Remedies
for the Common Cold

While you read this, approximately 30 million Americans are coughing, sneezing, and blowing their noses. What's wrong with all these people? They've got the most common illness known--the common cold. And if you're feeling lucky because you don't have a cold right now, the odds are three out of four that you'll get one during the coming year.

Colds are caused by many different viruses, and even if you develop immunity to one type of cold virus, more are lurking everywhere, waiting to attack. That's part of the reason we get colds so often (an average of three to four a year, every year).

You probably don't need a book to tell you what a cold feels like. It generally begins with sneezing, a clear-mucused runny nose, and a slight fever (rarely exceeding 101°F), and goes on to develop into a sore throat, and dry cough. The symptoms usually last three to seven days.

Colds are transmitted by the spread of mucus on the hands of someone who has a cold. You touch towels or money, someone else picks them up and thus catches your germs. Cold viruses also travel from one person to another via coughs and sneezes. To avoid spreading your cold to others:

▶ Wash your hands often.

▶ Use a handkerchief or disposable tissues when you sneeze, cough, or blow your nose.

▶ Avoid touching other people and their belongings as much as possible.

Much the same strategy helps to prevent catching a cold.

Unfortunately, no pills or vaccination exists to fight the common cold. None of the hundreds of cold remedies on the market today either cure a cold or shorten the siege. At best, they relieve some of the symptoms--a worthwhile goal. Here are some hints for fighting a cold.

▶ Rest in bed if you're running a fever.

▶ Drink lots of hot or cold beverages. They help to break up accumulated secretions in the respiratory tract and may also discourage complications like bronchitis from developing.

▶ Take a pain reliever for muscle aches and pains. (*Note:* Aspirin should not be given to children under 19 years of age

who have chicken pox or flu-like symptoms, however, because of
its association with Reye's syndrome, a potentially fatal condition that is discussed in chapter 2, Major Medical Conditions:
Prevention, Detection, and Treatment.)

▶ Soothe a sore throat by gargling with warm salt water, drinking
tea with honey and lemon, or sucking on over-the-counter throat
lozenges.

▶ Breathe air from a steam vaporizer or a cool mist humidifier, to
help quiet a cough.

▶ Eat chicken soup. It helps to clear out mucus.

▶ Check with your doctor about using zinc lozenges. They may
shorten the duration of a cold and ease cold symptoms.

17 Relief for Sinus Misery

You've seen the guy in the television commercial who seems to have
the worst cold in the world. He's really suffering—he's got a stuffy nose,
headache, cough, and pressure inside his head, and he can't sleep. Then we
find out he doesn't have a cold at all—he's got a sinus infection.

Healthy sinuses are lined with a moist, mucus-producing membrane,
and they normally drain nearly a quart of mucus daily, humidifying the air
you breathe in the process. If the sinuses become infected, swollen, and
inflamed—say, following a cold—they can't drain properly, and you're
miserable. (Your chances of developing a sinus infection increase if you
have hay fever, if you smoke, or if you have a nasal deformity.) Symptoms
include:

▶ Head congestion

▶ Nasal congestion and discharge (usually yellowish green)

▶ Pain and tenderness over the facial sinuses. Pain in the upper jaw.

▶ Recurrent headache that changes with head position and disappears shortly after getting out of bed

▶ Fever

A cool mist humidifier can help relieve sinus misery. Super-moist air
helps to thin out the thick sinus secretions and loosen the mucus that has
accumulated while your sinuses were out of order. Warm compresses

placed over the sinus area relieve discomfort still further. Other measures that can help include:

► Drinking plenty of fluids to keep secretions thin and flowing.

► Taking a pain reliever.

► Using over-the-counter oral decongestants. (*Note*: Use nose drops cautiously, if at all. Repeated use of nasal decongestants creates a dependency—your nasal passages "forget" how to work on their own and you have to continue using drops to keep nasal passages clear. So never use them for more than three days. And to avoid picking up germs, never borrow nose drops from others.)

If your symptoms persist despite home remedies, see a doctor. Sinus complications can be serious. You may need a prescription antibiotic and decongestant to clear the infection. (Severe cases may require surgery to drain the sinuses.)

18 Seven Ways to Fight Off the Flu

"Oh, it's just a touch of the flu," some say, as if they had nothing more than a cold. Yet each year, 20,000 people die from pneumonia and other complications of the influenza virus, or flu.

Cold and flu symptoms resemble each other, but they differ in intensity. A cold generally starts out with some minor sniffling and sneezing, but the flu hits you all at once; you're fine one hour and in bed the next. A cold rarely moves into the lungs; the flu can cause pneumonia. You may be able to drag yourself to work with a cold, but with a flu you'll be too ill to leave your bed.

If the following symptoms come on suddenly and intensely, you probably have the flu.

► Dry cough

► Sore throat

► Severe headache

► General muscle aches or backache

► Extreme fatigue

► Chills

► Fever up to 104°F

▶ Pain when you move your eyes, or a burning sensation in the
eyes

The most telling symptoms in that list are fatigue and muscle aches--
these are normally absent with a cold.

No cure exists for the flu—as with a cold, the virus has to run its course.
The goal, then, is to minimize discomfort and prevent complications.
Generally, you can treat the flu on your own. (If you have trouble
breathing, a persistent cough, or cough up yellow-green sputum, however,
call a doctor; you may be developing pneumonia.) Try these tips to
minimize discomfort:

▶ Get plenty of rest.

▶ Drink plenty of hot (but not scalding) liquids. They'll soothe
your throat, relieve nasal congestion, and replace bodily fluids
lost through perspiration caused by fever.

▶ Gargle with tepid, strong tea or warm salt water.

▶ Suck on lozenges or hard candies to lubricate your throat. (Don't
give to children under age 5.)

▶ Don't suppress a cough that produces phlegm or sputum-it helps
rid the respiratory tract of mucus. (In other words, avoid cough
suppressant medicines.) If mucus is bloody, yellow, or green,
contact your physician for advice.

▶ Avoid drinking milk or eating cheese and other dairy products for
a couple of days—they can thicken mucus secretions, making
them difficult to expel.

▶ Wash your hands frequently, especially after blowing your nose
and before handling food. (This also helps you avoid spreading
the flu virus to others.)

▶ Take a regular dose of aspirin or aspirin substitute. (Note: Aspirin
should not be given to children under 19 years old, however,
when they have chicken pox or flu-like symptoms, as it has been
linked to an increased risk of Reye's syndrome, a potentially fatal
condition that is discussed in chapter 2, Major Medical Conditions: Prevention, Detection, and Treatment.)

If the symptoms persist despite self-care efforts, see a doctor. He or
she may prescribe an antiviral medicine that can speed relief of symptoms.
(To avoid getting the flu in the first place, medical authorities also
recommend an influenza vaccination before each flu season for people
over age 65 or anyone with a chronic medical illness that would
compromise their ability to fight off the flu on their own.)

19 What You Don't Know about Asthma Can Hurt You

About ten million Americans suffer the wheezing, chest tightness, and breathing difficulty that typifies asthma, which is what doctors call an episodic disease—acute attacks alternate with symptom-free periods. Asthma is a physical problem, not an emotional one (although stress, anxiety, or frustration can cause asthma to worsen), and it can be severe enough to disrupt people's lives.

What makes asthma different from other respiratory problems? Simply stated, the muscles within the small air passages of the lungs go into spasm and narrow the airways, causing wheezing and breathing difficulties. A variety of triggers can set off asthma attacks.

► Breathing an allergen like pollen, mold, animal dander, or particles of dust or smoke

► Eating certain foods or taking certain drugs

► Experiencing emotional distress

► Exercising too hard

► Having bronchitis or an upper respiratory tract infection

Asthma attacks range from mild to severe, and treatment varies accordingly. Generally, asthma is too complex to treat with over-the-counter preparations. A doctor should monitor your condition and, if necessary, prescribe appropriate medications.

Asthmatics can do a number of things to help themselves, though.

► Always drink plenty of liquids (2 to 3 quarts a day) to keep secretions loose.

► Figure out what triggers your asthma, and eliminate allergens or irritants at home and at work.

► Make a special effort to keep your bedroom allergen-free.

► Sleep with a synthetic pillow, not a feather one.

► Don't smoke, and avoid exposure to air pollutants.

► Wear a scarf around your mouth and nose when walking or exercising in cold winter air to warm the air before it can reach sensitive airways.

► Discontinue vigorous exercise immediately if you start to wheeze.

▶ Avoid foods and medications that contain sulfites, used as preservatives and found chiefly in shellfish and wine.

▶ Sit up during an asthma attack; don't lie down.

▶ Always keep your asthma medication close by to abort an attack as early as possible.

▶ Be cautious about using aspirin—some asthmatics are allergic to it. Use acetaminophen instead.

If you consult a doctor for help in controlling your asthma, he or she may prescribe any of the following:

▶ Bronchodilators, either in oral, inhaled, or aerosol form, which open airways to make breathing easier.

▶ Steroids, either in oral or aerosol form, to counteract an allergic reaction and when other medicines are not successful for your asthma.

▶ Cromolyn sodium to be inhaled before an anticipated attack as a preventive measure for asthma that's triggered by allergic reactions or exercise. (Once an attack is under way, this drug is ineffective.)

▶ Peak flow meter to monitor your asthma at home.

20 Don't Let Hay Fever Ruin Your Life

Despite its name, hay fever has nothing to do with hay or fever. A nineteenth-century physician coined the term because he began to sneeze every time he entered a hay barn. But hay fever is, in fact, a reaction of the upper respiratory tract to anything to which you may be allergic; the medical term for hay fever is allergic rhinitis. Symptoms include watery eyes, runny nose, congestion, and sneezing. Although hay fever is most common in spring and fall, some people suffer all year, The best way to control this problem is to minimize your exposure to allergens. Here are a few tips.

▶ Delegate outdoor chores. Mowing the lawn or raking leaves is a potential disaster if you're allergic to the pollen of grains, trees, or weeds (especially ragweed), or to molds.

▶ Keep windows and doors shut and stay inside when the pollen count or humidity is high. (Early morning is particularly bother-some for some.)

▶ Install air conditioning or air purifiers for added relief, particularly in your bedroom. (Be sure to clean the units frequently.)

▶ Keep your surroundings as free of dust, mold, or pollen as possible. Of the three, dust is hardest to avoid—it's everywhere. So:

— Dust your home frequently and vacuum often.

— Wash area rugs.

— Avoid stuffed animals—they're dust collectors.

▶ Avoid household pets (or keep them outside the house).

▶ Don't hang sheets and blankets outside to dry. (Pollen can collect on them.)

If avoiding hay fever triggers gives you little or no relief, consider trying antihistamines, decongestants, nasal sprays, or eye drops.

▶ Antihistamines block the release of histamine, a substance the body automatically produces in response to an allergen. Histamine is responsible for many allergic symptoms. For best results, take the antihistamine 30 minutes before going outside. (*Note*: Over-the-counter antihistamines are more likely to cause drowsiness than prescription ones.)

▶ Decongestants reduce nasal blockage by narrowing blood vessels. (Don't use a nasal spray for more than three days at a time—you may become dependent on them.)

Your doctor may prescribe other medications, such as cromolyn sodium or steroids. If nothing else works, your doctor may recommend immunotherapy (allergy shots). Skin tests are used to determine which allergens bother you, and then you receive injections of small amounts of the allergen to "desensitize" you to it. These injections contain only a minuscule amount of allergen.

21 Bounce Back from Bronchitis

If you've ever had a cough that felt as though it started down in your toes, or if you've ever had uncontrollable coughing fits, you may have had bronchitis.

Bronchitis can be either acute or chronic, depending on how long it lasts and how serious the damage.

Acute bronchitis is generally caused by an infectious agent (like a virus or bacteria) or an environmental pollutant (like tobacco smoke) that attacks the mucous membranes within the windpipe or air passages in your respiratory tract, leaving them red and inflamed. Acute bronchitis often develops in the wake of a sinus infection, cold, or other respiratory infection, and can last anywhere from three days to three weeks. Coughing is often the first sign of bronchitis, and it may be accompanied by chills, low-grade fever, sore throat, and muscle aches.

Treatment includes:

► Breathing air from a steam vaporizer

► Bronchodilators (Prescription drugs that open up the bronchial passages)

► Antibiotics

► Aspirin or acetaminophen (for fever and aches)

► Bed rest

► Drinking plenty of liquids

► Not smoking

As you feel better, you can gradually resume your normal activities. But be patient. Full recovery from acute bronchitis can take up to four weeks. (If acute symptoms last longer than a week or get worse, see a doctor. You may be developing pneumonia.)

In chronic bronchitis the airways produce too much mucus, enough to cause a daily cough that brings up the mucus, for as long as three months or more, for more than two years in a row. Many people—most of them men—develop emphysema (destruction of the air sacs) along with chronic bronchitis. Because chronic bronchitis results in abnormal air exchange in the lung and causes permanent damage to the respiratory tract, it's much more serious than acute bronchitis.

Signs of chronic bronchitis are:

► Shortness of breath upon exertion (in early stages)

► Shortness of breath at rest (in later stages)

► A cough that produces thick, yellowish phlegm

People living in heavily industrialized urban areas and exposed to air pollution, workers exposed to metallic dust or fibers, and people who smoke are most susceptible to chronic bronchitis. In fact, cigarette smoking is the most common cause of chronic bronchitis. So quitting is essential and may bring complete relief.

Here are some other helpful steps.

► Reduce your exposure to air pollution. (Use air conditioning, air filters, and a mouth filter if you have to.) If you develop bronchitis easily, stay indoors during episodes of heavy air pollution.

► Use cough suppressants sparingly. Instead, use expectorants, bronchodilators, and antibiotics (under a doctor's supervision of course).

If you have any symptoms of bronchitis lasting longer than a week, see your physician.

22 How to Take the Heat out of Heartburn

Ah, another big, wonderful Sunday breakfast! A few cups of coffee with your ham-and-cheese omelet, and you'll lie down for a relaxing afternoon on the couch. Nothing could ruin that perfect scenario, right? Nothing but a painful burning sensation in your chest, known only too well as heartburn. (The name is a misnomer, since heartburn occurs in the esophagus, just behind the heart, and in no way involves the heart.)

What causes this irritation? Gastric acids from the stomach splash back up into the lower portion of the esophagus, causing pain. The digestive acids don't harm the stomach, thanks to its protective coating, but the esophagus has no such armor, so you feel discomfort.

The most common heartburn triggers are:

► Taking aspirin, ibuprofen, naproxen sodium, arthritis medicine, or cortisone
► Eating heavy meals or eating too fast
► Eating foods like chocolate, garlic, onions, or peppermint, tomatoes, or citrus fruits
► Smoking or lying down after eating
► Drinking coffee (regular or decaffeinated)
► Drinking alcohol
► Hiatal hernia, a bulging of the upper part of the stomach through the diaphragm
► Being very overweight
► Pregnancy

Treatment consists of avoiding as many contributing factors as possible, plus the following:

► Sit straight while you eat. Stand up or walk around after you eat.

▶ If heartburn bothers you at night, raise the head of the bed slightly.

▶ Lose weight if you are overweight.

▶ Avoid wearing tight fitting garments around the abdomen.

▶ Eat small meals. Don't eat for 2 to 3 hours before bedtime.

▶ Don't smoke. It promotes heartburn.

▶ If you do take aspirin, ibuprofen, naproxen sodium, or arthritis medicines, take them with food.

If other treatments fail:

▶ Take an antacid. They coat your stomach and neutralize acids. For example, take 1 to 2 tablespoons of a non-absorbable liquid antacid such as magnesium hydroxide every 2 to 4 hours or ones that come in tablet form such as Tums.

▶ If antacids don't bring relief, take an over-the-counter acid controller, (examples-Pepcid AC and Tagamet HB). These not only relieve heartburn, but can prevent it. *(Note: Read the label before taking an antacid or acid controller. If you have questions, check with your doctor.)*

▶ Don't take baking soda. It may neutralize stomach acid at first, but when its effects wear off, the acid comes back to a greater degree causing severe gastric acid rebound.

23 Freedom from Constipation

Constipation—hard, small stools, passed infrequently—can be very uncomfortable, but it usually doesn't signal disease or a serious problem. The "cure" for constipation consists of correcting the sort of dietary habits that make bowel habits irregular.

▶ Eat plenty of fresh fruits and vegetables. They serve as natural stool softeners, thanks in part to their fiber content. Some fiber absorbs water like a sponge, turning hard stool into large, soft, easy-to-pass masses.

▶ Eat other foods high in fiber, like whole-grain breads and cereals, and bran.

▶ Drink plenty of water and other liquids, to give the fiber plenty of water to absorb.

▶ Get plenty of exercise, to help your bowels move things along.

▶ Don't resist the urge to eliminate or put off a trip to the bathroom.

▶ Keep in mind that drugs such as antacids and iron supplements can be binding, and stay away from them if you get constipated easily.

▶ If necessary, you may need an over-the-counter stool softener. Ask your doctor.

Try these measures before you consider resorting to laxatives. If you rely on laxatives for a prolonged time, your body loses its natural elimination reflex—the bowel can't evacuate as well on its own. Long-term use of stimulant laxatives can also lead to a mineral imbalance.

Enemas can relieve a serious case of constipation. But don't use them regularly.

If you're still constipated no matter what you try, ask your doctor for advice. Constipation can be the side effect of certain medications (including diuretics) or result from a medical problem (such as hemorrhoids, anal fissures, or an underactive thyroid gland) or problems with the large intestine (such as a tumor or diverticular disease).

24 Put a Stop to Diarrhea

Diarrhea is roughly the opposite of constipation—frequent, loose bowel movements. Almost everyone experiences diarrhea once in a while, but it's rarely serious and doesn't last more than a day or two. But oh, the agony! Stomach cramps or frequent (and inconvenient) bowel movements can make life miserable.

Diarrhea can result from various problems, including:

▶ Infection (by parasites, bacteria, or a virus)

▶ Drinking contaminated water or eating contaminated food while traveling in foreign countries. A variety of infectious organisms can cause "traveler's diarrhea." (See Tips 294 and 295 in chapter 13, The Healthy Traveler)

▶ Food poisoning

▶ Allergic reactions in the gastrointestinal tract

▶ Emotional upset

▶ Overuse of laxatives

► Certain drugs, including some antibiotics (like tetracycline, cleocin, and ampicillin)

► Diverticulitis (inflammation of tiny sacs protruding from the intestines)

► Inflammatory bowel disease (primarily ulcerative colitis and Crohn's disease)

With more fluid than usual being flushed out of your body, dehydration is a potential problem, especially with infants and children, who have less fluid to spare than adults. So the first course of action is to drink plenty of clear fluids, like ginger ale, broth, bouillon, herb tea, or just plain water. Even sucking on ice chips helps.

Other steps to control diarrhea include:

► Eat little or no solid food for the first few days. (Jell-O is okay; it counts as a clear liquid.)

► When diarrhea is waning, follow a B.R.A.T. diet: bananas, rice, applesauce, and toast. These foods tend to be constipating, and should be the first things you eat after a bout of diarrhea.

► Once the diarrhea has subsided, eat small amounts of semisoft foods, like cooked potatoes. Stay away from protein and dairy products.

► Don't eat high-fiber foods like whole-grain bread and bran cereal.

► Avoid eating raw fruits and vegetables, fried foods, and sweets, or drinking coffee, all of which are hard on your digestive tract.

► Limit physical activity until bowel activity returns to normal.

► Try Kaopectate or other nonprescription remedy containing bismuth. (Follow package directions to the letter.)

If diarrhea doesn't let up within 48 to 72 hours, or if you notice blood in your stool, contact your doctor for advice.

25 What to Do about Flatulence

Flatulence may be perfectly natural and something that everyone gets, but if you have more than your share, it's a major annoyance.

Where does all that gas come from, anyway? Often, it comes from swallowing air. It's also generated by intestinal bacteria that produce carbon dioxide and hydrogen (both odorless, by the way) in the course of proteins in the food you eat. The problem is minute quantities of other, more pungent gases that gives flatus its characteristic odor. Eating certain foods, like peas, beans, and certain grains produces noticeably more gas than eating other foods.

Common sense says to avoid swallowing air and to eliminate foods that are considered notorious gas-producers (or eat them in small amounts). Well-known offenders include:

► Apples

► Apricots

► Beans (dried, cooked)

► Bran

► Broccoli

► Brussels sprouts

► Cabbage

► Cauliflower

► Dairy products (for persons allergic to lactose)

► Eggplant

► Eggs

► Nuts

► Onions

► Popcorn

► Prunes

► Raisins

The medication simethicone may help reduce flatulence by dispersing gas pockets (and preventing more from forming). It has no known side effects. Simethicone is available by prescription as well as over the counter (OTC) under the brand name Mylicon. Other OTC products, Bean-O and Phazyme 95, may help curb gas caused by eating foods such as baked beans.

Gas may signal a variety of other problems worth looking into.

► Lactose intolerance (inability to properly digest milk, cheese, and other dairy products). (See Tip 113 in chapter 4, Eating for Better Health.)

► Bacterial overgrowth in the intestines (often caused by certain antibiotics).

► Abnormal muscle contraction in the colon.

26 Say Good-Bye to Urinary Tract Infections

Approximately one out of every five women will experience a urinary tract infection (UTI) during her life. Some will experience many. Men get UTIs too, but not as frequently.

Your urinary tract is made up of your kidneys, bladder, ureters (tubes that connect the kidneys to the bladder), and urethra (the tube through which urine is passed). In most urinary tract infections, bacteria enter the urethra, travel to the bladder, multiply, and travel to other parts of the urinary tract (including the kidney).

In women, bacteria gain easy entry to the urethra as it is massaged during intercourse and can cause a bladder infection. Waiting too long before urinating following sexual intercourse will increase the chance of infection, because bacteria that enter the urethra have an opportunity to move farther up the urinary tract. Women who use a diaphragm for birth control are twice as likely to get a urinary tract infection. Pregnancy and postmenopausal changes make you more prone to UTIs, as do congenital abnormalities (urinary tract defects you were born with), any obstructions in the flow of urine (like a kidney stone or enlarged prostate), or having a history of urinary tract infections.

Surprisingly, UTIs may show no symptoms. But usually, if you've got one, you know it. Symptoms strike suddenly, without warning, and include:

- A strong desire to urinate
- Urinating more often than usual
- A sharp pain or burning sensation in the urethra while urinating
- Blood in the urine
- Feeling that the bladder is still full after you've urinated
- Soreness in the abdomen, back or sides (if the infection involves the kidneys)
- Chills, fever, nausea, and vomiting (in more serious cases, where the infection involves the kidneys)

If you wait too long to get treatment, the consequences can be serious. Consult a physician if you experience any of the symptoms that are mentioned above. By testing a sample of your urine under a microscope and sending it out to be cultured, your doctor can diagnose your problem.

UTIs are treated with antibiotics. Take all the medication you're prescribed, as directed, even if the symptoms disappear.

Here are some things you can do to keep from getting UTIs:

▶ If you're a woman, wipe from front to back after using the toilet to keep bacteria away from the urethral opening.

▶ Drink plenty of fluids to flush bacteria out of your system.

▶ Empty your bladder as soon as you feel the urge, to give bacteria as little time to multiply as possible.

▶ Empty your bladder as soon as you can after intercourse, even if you don't feel the urge.

▶ Wear cotton underwear, to allow air to circulate freely and discourage the kind of warm, moist environment in which bacteria thrive.

▶ Avoid taking bubble baths if you're prone to UTIs.

27 How to Muzzle Frostbite

Frostbite looks like a serious heat burn, but it's actually body tissue that's frozen and, in severe cases, dead. Most often, frostbite affects the toes, fingers, earlobes, chin, and tip of the nose--unprotected extremities that freeze quickly. Danger signs are pain (initially), swelling, white skin, then numbness and eventually loss of function and absence of pain. Blisters may also develop.

Sheer cold causes frostbite, but wind chill speeds up heat loss and increases the risk. Depending on how long you're exposed and how cold or windy it is, frostbite can set in very slowly—or very quickly, before you know what's happening.

The old wives' tale that says you should treat frostbite by rubbing the area with snow or soaking it in cold water is wrong. This treatment is ineffective and dangerous. Instead:

▶ Warm the affected area by soaking in a tub of warm water (101°F to 104°F) and an antiseptic solution.

▶ Stop when the affected area becomes red, not when sensation returns. (This should take about 45 minutes. If done too rapidly, thawing can be painful and blisters may develop.)

▶ Keep the exposed area elevated.

▶ Never massage a frostbitten area.

▶ Protect the exposed area from the cold. It is more sensitive to re-injury.

If you suspect frostbite, you should go to an emergency room, since there is a risk of permanent damage. Also, you may need a tetanus shot.

Needless to say, frostbite is something you should prevent rather than treat. Here are some ways to keep warm if you expect to spend any length of time in the cold.

► Layer your clothing. Many layers of thin clothing are warmer than one bulky layer—the air spaces trap body warmth close to the skin, insulating the body against cold. Wear two or three pairs of socks instead of one heavy pair, for example, and wear roomy shoes.

► Avoid drinking alcohol or smoking cigarettes. Alcohol causes blood to lose heat rapidly, and smoking slows down blood circulation to the extremities.

► Stay indoors as much as possible during periods of extremely low temperatures and high wind.

► When you are outside, shield your face, etc., from the wind.

28 Ten Ways to Get Rid of Winter Itch

Oh, that winter itch! Your skin feels as rough and dry as sandpaper. If your skin is chapped, cracked, and inflamed during the coldest months of the year, take heart. Relief is a simple matter of water conservation.

The basic problem is lack of moisture. Anything that steals moisture from the skin will result in dryness and chapping. The drier the air, the more rapidly moisture evaporates. (In winter, heated indoor air tends to be dry.) Also, soap and excessive bathing or showering strips the skin of its natural oils, compounding the problem. Add it up, and the dehydrated cells begin to shrink and separate like caked mud in a dry lake bed, and a network of painful cracks appear on your skin.

Dry skin affects everyone, but older people have it worse, because oil production gradually declines with age.

Since you can't change the weather or your age, try these suggestions if you want to prevent winter itch.

► Avoid bathing or showering more than once a day.

► Alternate bath or shower days with sponge baths.

▶ Use mild soap, and lather as little as possible. (Deodorant soaps are hard on the skin. Select a moisturizing soap instead.)

▶ Don't apply soap directly to the skin. Soap up a washcloth instead.

▶ Add a bath oil to bathwater.

▶ Pat your skin dry with a towel instead of rubbing it dry, and apply a moisturizer immediately.

▶ Apply lubricating skin cream or lotion several times a day on your hands, elbows, or other areas frequently affected. These provide moisture to hydrate the skin and oil to lock in moisture. Petroleum-based creams work well. (Try to avoid scented products.) Apply a moisturizer after bathing, at bedtime, and in the morning. Start early in the dry-skin season, before skin becomes chapped or severely cracked.

▶ Avoid immersing your hands in hot water and strong dishwashing detergents. Wear rubber gloves.

▶ Lower the setting on your heating thermostat so you're comfortable, but not toasty.

▶ Use a humidifier to add moisture to the air in a room, or have a humidifier connected to your furnace. Also, avoid sitting too close to fireplace heat—it's drying.

29 A Simple Remedy for Prickly Heat

Feeling hot and sticky is bad enough. A visible sign of discomfort only makes it worse. Such is the case with prickly heat (also known as heat rash), identified by clusters of small blisters that itch and appear where you perspire the heaviest—the armpits, neck, back, or creases in the elbows (but never the face).

Hot, humid weather, sensitive skin, and overweight all aggravate prickly heat. Here are some simple ways to find relief.

▶ Wear loose, lightweight clothing.

▶ Dust the affected area with cornstarch.

▶ Take cool baths to reduce itching.

▶ Avoid hot, humid environments and stay in air-conditioned surroundings, if possible.

The key to managing prickly heat is to avoid sweating by staying in a cool environment. The rash will disappear in a couple of days.

30 Leaflets Three, Let Poison Ivy Be

A walk through the woods can include encounters with birds, small animals, and beautiful foliage. But if you encounter poison ivy along the way, you may walk away with an itchy rash as a souvenir of your nature trek.

The problem is caused by urushiol, a resin exuded by poison ivy, poison oak, and other related plants. Strictly speaking, urushiol is an allergen, not a poison—not everyone reacts to it. If you're allergic to the resin and either touch the plant directly or come in contact with clothing or pets that have been exposed to it, you'll develop a rash of itchy, oozing blisters, sometimes accompanied by swelling.

Being able to recognize these poisonous plants is the key to avoiding them and the rash they trigger. And the old adage, "Leaflets three, let it be" holds true. But if it's too late, and you have an accidental brush with the plant, here's what to do.

> Remove and wash all clothes and shoes that have been contaminated. If an article isn't washable, isolate it in a ventilated area for three weeks.

> Bathe with soap and water, then apply rubbing alcohol to the exposed skin with cotton balls. Rinse with water afterward.

> A rash may still develop two or three days after contact with the resin. If that happens, apply calamine lotion.

> Taking an oral antihistamine, such as diphenhydramine (brand name Benadryl), should relieve itching.

> If weeping blisters develop, cover them with gauze and keep them wet, with a solution of 1 tablespoon baking soda in 1 quart of water. (The fluid in blisters will not cause the rash to spread.)

> If symptoms grow worse, the rash spreads to the mouth, eyes, or genitals, or you have had severe reactions to poison ivy (or poison oak) in the past, consult a physician. To control the rash, he or she will probably prescribe steroids, to be taken orally or applied topically.

31 You Can Head Off Hives

No one ever forgets the times they broke out in hives—just before a big date as a teen, or after eating a terrific lobster dinner. Well, if you remember episodes like those, you're not alone. According to estimates, nearly 20 percent of Americans will endure at least one bout with hives some time in their lives.

Hives, or urticaria, are red, raised, itchy welts. They appear, sometimes in clusters, on the face, trunk of the body, and, less frequently, on the scalp, hands, or feet. Like the Cheshire cat in *Alice's Adventures in Wonderland*, hives can change shape, fade, then rapidly reappear. A single hive lasts less than 24 hours, but after an attack new ones may crop up for up to six weeks.

Hives can be (but aren't always) an allergic response to something you touched, inhaled, or swallowed. Some common causes of hives include:

▶ Medications such as aspirin, sulfa, and penicillin

▶ Animal dander (especially from cats)

▶ Cold temperatures

▶ Emotional or physical stress (including exercise)

▶ Foods (especially chocolate, nuts, shellfish, or tomatoes)

▶ Infections

▶ Inhalants (especially pollen, mold spores, or airborne chemicals)

▶ Insect bites

▶ Rubbing or putting pressure on the skin

▶ Malignant or connective tissue disease

Sometimes, there's no identifiable cause of hives. But if you *can* identify the triggers (try keeping a diary), you may be able to prevent future outbreaks. That's important, because while most hives simply itch and don't usually cause other problems, the swelling associated with a serious case of hives can be deadly. If the tongue and throat swell shut, you can't breathe; if your heart, respiratory system, or digestive system becomes involved and you don't get treatment, it can be fatal.

Here are some tips for a case of ordinary, nonthreatening hives.

▶ Avoid hot baths or showers. Heat worsens most rashes and makes them itch more.

▶ Apply cold compresses or take a tepid bath.

▶ Wear loose-fitting clothing, to prevent unnecessarily rubbing the skin and provoking more hives.

▶ Relax as much as possible. Studies have shown that relaxation therapy and even hypnosis help ease the itching and discomfort of hives.

▶ Ask your doctor to recommend an antihistamine. Antihistamines can help relieve itching and suppress hives. (Keep in mind that antihistamines cause drowsiness and may make it dangerous for you to drive or perform other tasks requiring alertness.)

▶ Avoid taking aspirin; it tends to aggravate hives.

32 Treatments for Warts

Warts are ugly—but harmless. They're benign tumors that are caused by a virus, and they're only slightly contagious.

Common warts have a rounded, rough surface and most often crop up on your hands. Sometimes, they're just slightly darker than your skin. Occasionally, a constellation of warts develops around a central wart.

Unlike common warts, *plantar warts* almost always appear on the soles of the feet—and they hurt. Because you can't avoid putting pressure on this kind of wart when you stand or walk, the only way to relieve pain is to wear a protective pad or have the wart removed.

Like other warts, plantar warts are slightly contagious and can be spread wherever communal bathing occurs—like locker rooms. So the only way to prevent plantar warts is to avoid walking barefoot in those areas. And, obviously, don't touch anyone else's feet if they have plantar warts.

If you're lucky, warts will disappear by themselves. But they generally require some sort of treatment. Chemicals such as salicylic acid or lactic acid are popular over-the-counter treatments (and are available in higher concentrations by prescription). Follow directions to the letter if you decide to apply one of these products; if they're not used correctly, they can damage normal skin.

Your doctor can remove warts safely using one of the following methods.

▶ Liquid nitrogen (cryotherapy) can freeze warts.

▶ Surgical removal, under local anesthesia, may be recommended (but is not generally used for plantar warts)

▶ Laser surgery is a relatively new and effective option.

▶ Electrosurgery is *not* usually recommended, because of the risk of scarring.

33 Nine Ways to Take the Itch out of Eczema

Eczema (atopic dermatitis) is a chronic skin condition that usually appears on the scalp, face, neck, or creases of the elbows, wrists, and knees. The symptoms are small blisters and crusty scales on the skin surface, often accompanied by inflammation. Children and adults alike may be affected, and the condition often runs in families. Asthma is often associated with this skin condition.

A variety of irritants or allergens can aggravate eczema, including:

▶ Wearing wool fabric

▶ Sweating

▶ Stress

▶ Exposure to extreme weather conditions (especially high heat and humidity)

▶ Eating foods such as eggs, milk, seafood, or wheat products

▶ Contact with cosmetics, dyes, medicines, deodorants, skin lotions, permanent press fabrics, and other allergens

Eczema is quite unpredictable. Usually, it's at its worst in childhood and gradually lets up as you get older. Sometimes it completely disappears for good. Still, eczema can be a lifetime problem, and although you can't cure it, you can manage it. Here's how:

▶ Bathe less frequently (perhaps sponge bathing in between tub baths) and add oil to the bathwater. Or take quick showers.

▶ Use tepid (not hot) water when bathing or showering.

▶ Use a mild soap or no soap at all on the areas of eczema.

▶ Avoid contact with wool clothing or blankets.

▶ After bathing, moisturize your skin with a light, nongreasy, unscented lotion.

▶ Don't overdress or promote perspiration in any way.

▶ Wear rubber gloves dusted on the inside with talcum powder or cornstarch when doing household chores. Or try cotton-lined latex gloves.

▶ Avoid any foods, chemicals, cosmetics, or other allergens that worsen the condition.

▶ And above all, don't scratch! Scratching eczema only makes it worse. You'll break the skin, allowing bacteria to infect the skin. (If that happens, consult a doctor.) So hands off!

34 What to Do If You Get Shingles

Some of the clearest memories people have of childhood involve bouts with infectious illnesses—measles, mumps, chicken pox. One of these infections—chicken pox—may reappear in a different form during adulthood and cause havoc for a second time. Shingles (herpes zoster) is a skin disorder triggered by the chicken pox virus that you first encountered as a child. (The adult form does not appear to be contagious, but infants and people whose immunity is low should not be exposed to it.)

The risk of getting shingles increases with age, with most cases developing in people over the age of 50. The risk of developing shingles is also higher in those whose infection-fighting system is below par or who have cancer.

Symptoms of shingles include:

▶ Pain, itching, or tingling sensation (before the rash appears).

▶ A rash of painful red blisters, which later crust over. Most often, the rash appears on the torso or side of the face, and sometimes affects the eye. (Invariably, only one side of the face or body is affected.)

▶ Though rare, fever and general weakness sometimes occur.

After the crusts fall off (usually within three weeks), pain can persist in the area of the rash. While no treatment exists for this pain other than analgesics, it usually disappears on its own after one to six months.

The following steps may relieve an active outbreak of shingles.

▶ Keep sores open to the air. Don't bandage them or wear restrictive clothing.

▶ Wash blisters, but never scrub them.

▶ Apply cool compresses, calamine lotion, or baking soda to alleviate the symptoms.

Shingles require medical attention, especially if an eye is affected. Your doctor may prescribe an analgesic to reduce pain or an antibiotic if the blisters become infected. You may also need other medications, like antihistamines, antiviral drugs, or possibly steroids.

35 Protect Yourself against Insect Stings

Warm weather months invariably include days at the beach, picnics in the backyard—and run-ins with bees or wasps. How can you avoid getting stung?

▶ Keep foods and drink containers tightly covered. (Bees love sweet foods like soft drinks.)

▶ Avoid sweet-smelling colognes. Wear insect repellent instead.

▶ Avoid looking like a flower. Choose white or neutral colors that won't attract bees.

▶ Wear snug clothing that covers your arms and legs, and don't go barefoot.

If these preventive strategies fail and you get stung anyway, heed the following advice.

▶ Gently scrape out the stinger as soon as possible.

▶ Don't pull or squeeze the stinger. It contains venom, and you'll end up re-stinging yourself (This applies to bees only; yellow jackets, wasps, and hornets don't lose their stingers.)

▶ Clean the sting area with soapy water.

▶ Apply a cold compress to the sting immediately. Hold it on the site for 15 to 20 minutes. Don't put ice directly on the skin.

▶ Apply a paste made of meat tenderizer (like Ac'cent) to the sting area. It seems to break down the protein in the venom.

▶ Take a painreliever for the pain, and/or an antihistamine for the itching and swelling (provided you don't have to avoid these drugs for medical reasons).

▶ If you're stung in the mouth or tongue, get medical help fast—swelling could close off your airway.

Symptoms of bee and wasp stings vary, depending on where you're stung and how sensitive you are to the sting. The most common symptoms are limited areas of pain and swelling, with redness and itching.

People who are allergic may have a severe reaction known as anaphylaxis (even if they've never had an allergic reaction to a sting before). The symptoms of a severe anaphylactic reaction include generalized swelling, wheezing, difficult breathing, a severe drop in blood pressure, and sometimes coma and death. Needless to say, this is a medical emergency, so if you start to have a serious reaction to a sting, get medical help immediately.

If you've ever had an allergic reaction to an insect sting in the past, you should carry an emergency medical kit containing epinephrine (a drug you inject to stop the body-wide reaction), an antihistamine, and an inhaler that contains adrenaline. Also, people who've had severe reactions to bee or wasp stings should ask their doctor about allergy shots.

36 What Your Fingernails Reveal about Your Health

You may see your hands hundreds of times a day, but do you ever examine them? Probably not. Yet taking a closer look-especially at your fingernails-may not be a bad idea. They're a good indicator of overall health.

Spoon-shaped nails, for example, may simply be an inherited trait-or they can be a clue to a thyroid deficiency or iron deficiency anemia. Nails that have no "moon," or white crescent at the base, and are thin and brittle might indicate an underactive thyroid. Still other changes-like brittleness or pitting-may be signs of other nutritional deficiencies or injury to the nail bed. While no one can diagnose a health problem on the basis of nail irregularities only, the table on page 42 may tip you off to possible health problems. (Consult your doctor if you see any significant changes in your nails.)

Barring any medical explanation for nail problems, the following tips can help your nails look healthier and more attractive.

▶ Eat a well-balanced diet that includes plenty of fresh fruits and vegetables, whole grains, lean meats, and low-fat dairy products.

▶ Wear gloves when you do household chores or hobbies, to avoid contact with detergents or harsh chemicals that can dry or damage nails.

▶ Clean nails with a nail brush, especially if you garden or work with messy materials.

▶ Clip cuticles and rough skin, to prevent tears.

▶ File nails in one direction only, using an emery board, not a metal nail file.

▶ Don't use your nails as tools, to remove staples and so forth.

▶ If you polish your nails, use polish remover sparingly.

Nail Symptoms and What They Mean

Problem	Possible Causes
Brittleness	Frequent immersion in hot water; generally poor health; impaired circulation; possible deficiency of vitamins A, C, or B_6, niacin, calcium, or iron; thyroid deficiency
Clubbing	Chronic lung disease, or lung cancer; congenital heart disease; congenital or hereditary defect
Pitting (may be normal)	Eczema, psoriasis, trauma
Ridges	Emphysema, heredity, kidney failure, old age, rheumatoid arthritis, trauma
Separation (when nail plate lifts off nail bed)	Allergy to nail lacquer and hardeners, fungal infection, iron deficiency anemia, pregnancy, psoriasis, trauma
Splitting at top edge	Immersion in water for long periods, nail polish removers
Spoon shaped	Thyroid deficiency; iron deficiency anemia

SOURCE: *HealthyLife® for Women* (Southfield, Mich.: American Institute for Preventive Medicine, 1986).

37 Free Yourself from Fatigue

Despite the fact that modern technology makes daily life less physically taxing than ever, doctors say that more people than ever complain of fatigue. How can you break out of the web of unrelenting fatigue?

First, ask yourself why you're tired. Are physical or emotional factors responsible for the way you feel? Fatigue brought on by physical causes is generally worse in the evening and is typically relieved by sleep. Emotional fatigue is the opposite: It's usually worse in the morning and lets up toward evening.

Possible physical causes of fatigue include:

▶ Poor eating or sleeping habits

▶ An imbalance in blood levels of electrolytes (sodium, potassium, and other minerals)

▶ Living or working in hot, humid conditions

▶ Anemia

▶ Prolonged effects of the flu or a bad cold

▶ Other underlying infectious diseases such as mononucleosis, or Epstein-Barr virus

▶ A number of endocrine disorders, such as an underactive thyroid gland, or neurologic disorders

Possible emotional causes to consider include:

▶ Burnout (wearing yourself out by trying to do too much)

▶ Boredom (extreme monotony or lack of interest in daily routines)

▶ Change (facing a major life crisis or decision, like divorce or retirement)

▶ Depression

Depending on the reasons for your fatigue, the following strategies may help restore your energy levels.

Eat a better diet. Both extreme overeating and crash dieting can tax the body and lead to exhaustion. Skipping an important meal like breakfast or indulging in rich, sugary snacks are practically guaranteed to leave some people pooped. On the other hand, iron-rich foods, whole-grain breads and cereals, and raw fruits and vegetables contain the nutrients your body needs to maintain your energy level.

Get more exercise. Expending more energy can actually give you more energy, especially if you work at a sedentary job. Exercise also acts as a tranquilizer, counteracting emotionally induced anxiety or weariness. If you're feeling sluggish, try taking a brisk walk in the fresh air. It can renew your energy instantly.

Cool off. Working or playing in hot weather can drag you down. So can living or working in a warm, poorly ventilated environment. The answer: Rest in a cool, dry atmosphere as often as you can, drink plenty of liquids—and open a window.

Other, more specific tips for dealing with possible physical causes for fatigue are covered in chapter 2, Major Medical Conditions: Prevention, Detection, and Treatment.

Rest and relax. You don't need a book to tell you that if you haven't been sleeping too well, getting a good night's sleep (or two) can put the spring back in your stride. But did you know that daily relaxation breaks can also restore your energy? Schedule your work to allow relaxation breaks, then practice deep breathing or meditation. (Various relaxation techniques are described in detail in chapter 6, Success over Stress.)

Change your routine. Nothing makes you feel stale faster than a repetitive, predictable routine. So try to do something novel and interesting once a day (or more). If, on the other hand, you're on the go too much, set aside some time for peace and quiet. (Other, more specific tips for dealing with burnout, boredom, change, and depression appear in chapter 6, Success over Stress.)

If you suffer unrelenting or unexplainable fatigue for more than two weeks, see your doctor. Any one of dozens of medical conditions may be to blame.

38 How to Correct Common Anemia

If someone says you look anemic, glance at yourself in a mirror. Are you pale, tired, listless, and weak—and look it? Maybe you are anemic. But what does that mean?

Strictly speaking, anemia refers to a deficiency of either red blood cells or the amount of hemoglobin (oxygen-carrying protein) in the red blood cells circulating in your blood vessels.

Iron deficiency anemia is the most common form of anemia. In the United States, 20 percent of all women of childbearing age have iron deficiency anemia (compared to 2 percent of adult men). The primary cause is blood lost during menstruation. But eating too few iron-rich foods—or not adequately absorbing iron—can compound the problem. (The recommended daily allowance for iron ranges from 6-30 milligrams. Yet one government source found that females between 12 and 50 years old—those at highest risk for iron deficiency anemia—get about half that much.) Pregnancy, breast-feeding a baby, and blood loss from the gastrointestinal tract (either due to ulcers or cancer) can also deplete iron stores,

Folic acid deficiency anemia occurs when folic acid levels are low, usually due to inadequate dietary intake or faulty absorption. (The need for this vitamin more than doubles during pregnancy.)

Other, less common forms of anemia include pernicious anemia (inability of the body to properly absorb vitamin B12), sickle cell anemia (an inherited disorder discussed in Tip 75 in chapter 2, Major Medical Conditions: Prevention, Detection, and Treatment), and thalassemia anemia (also inherited).

The first step in treating iron deficiency anemia is to pinpoint the cause. If it's due to a poor diet, you're in luck: Iron deficiency anemia is not only the most common form of anemia, it's the easiest to correct if it's due to being female or taking in inadequate amounts of certain foods. Folic acid vitamin supplements may also be necessary. Your doctor may recommend that you:

➤ Eat more food sources of iron. Concentrate on green, leafy vegetables, red meat, beef liver, poultry, fish, wheat germ, oysters, fruit, and iron-fortified cereal.

➤ Boost your iron absorption. (Foods high in vitamin C--like citrus fruit, tomatoes, and strawberries--help your body absorb iron from food. And red meat not only supplies a goodly amount of iron, it also increases absorption of iron from other food sources.)

➤ Don't drink a lot of tea—it contains tannins, substances that can inhibit iron absorption. (Herbal tea is okay, though.)

➤ Take an iron supplement. (Consult your physician before taking an iron supplement and for proper dosage.) While iron is best absorbed when taken on an empty stomach, it can upset your stomach. Taking iron with meals is less upsetting to the stomach.

39 What to Do for Fainting

Just before fainting, you may feel a sense of dread, followed by the sense that everything around you is swaying. And you may see spots before your eyes. Then you go into a cold sweat, your face turns pale, and you topple over.

A fainting victim may pass out for several seconds or up to ½ hour. The cause is a sudden reduction of blood flow to the brain. That reduction can be caused by emotional stress; physical pain; a sudden change in body position, like standing up too quickly (postural hypotension); abnormal heart rhythm; stroke; or heart attack.

Here are some dos and don'ts to remember if someone faints.

Do:

► Catch the person before he or she falls.

► Place the person in a horizontal position, with the head below the level of the heart and the legs raised to promote blood flow to the brain. (If a potential fainting victim can lie down right away, he or she may not lose consciousness.)

► Turn the victim's head to the side, so the tongue doesn't fall back into the throat.

► Loosen any tight clothing.

► Apply cold, moist towels to the person's face and neck.

► Keep the victim warm, especially if the surroundings are chilly.

Here's what you *shouldn't* do.

► Don't slap or shake anyone who's just fainted.

► Don't try to give the person anything to drink, not even water.

► Don't allow the person who's fainted to get up until the sense of physical weakness passes, and then be watchful for a few minutes to be sure he or she doesn't faint again.

If you're prone to fainting spells, ask yourself why. Common faints (not linked to disease) tend to take place in a warm, crowded room, or when your stomach is empty, or when you're in pain, or after an injury. Poor physical condition can leave you more prone to fainting.

If you get dizzy or feel the room is spinning when you stand up or after you have been standing in one position for too long, you're experiencing postural hypotension. To prevent this from happening, try to take your time standing up from a sitting or lying position (count to 60), and don't stand still for long periods of time. Also, check your medications. Blood pressure drugs increase the risk of postural hypotension, and your medication may have to be changed. Or you can wear elastic stockings to increase blood flow from the extremities and help prevent fainting.

40 Help for Your Aching Back

Most backaches are caused by muscular strain of the lower back. The goal of treatment is twofold: Relieve the pain and promote healing. Talk to your doctor about these options.

Medication. Aspirin and other painkillers can relieve back pain temporarily, but can't correct back problems. Aspirin or one of the many nonsteroidal anti-inflammatory agents, such as ibuprofen, can reduce inflammation and dull the sensation of pain. (Taking aspirin with antacids or in a buffered form can reduce the stomach upset associated with it.) Muscle relaxants or analgesics containing codeine may be prescribed.

Activity. Continue your regular activities as much as you can. Rest the back if you must, but don't rest in bed more than 2-3 days, even if your back hurts a lot. Your back muscles can get weak if you don't use them or if you stay in bed longer than 3 days. To make the most of rest:

► Get comfortable when you are lying, standing, and sitting. For example, when you lie on your back, keep your upper back flat, but your hips and knees bent. Keep your feet flat on the bed. Tip your hips down and up until you find the best spot.

► Put a pillow under your knees or lie on your side with your knees bent. This will take pressure off your lower back.

► When you get up from bed, move slowly, roll on your side, and swing your legs to the floor. Push off the bed with your arms.

Cold treatment. Injury to the back can cause blood vessels to tear, producing a bruise. Cold inhibits bruising and swelling and numbs pain, so cold packs (like crushed ice wrapped in a towel) can help. Apply for 5–10 minutes on and 5–10 minutes off, several times a day. For best results, lie on your back with your knees bent and place the ice pack under your lower back. Start right after a back strain occurs and continue for 48 hours.

Heat treatment. Unlike cold, heat increases blood flow to the troublesome area, which promotes healing. But you shouldn't apply heat until 48 or more hours after back symptoms start; if heat is used sooner, the increased blood flow can add to swelling and inflammation.

You can choose from moist heating pads, hot-water bottles, hot compresses, hot tubs, hot baths, or hot showers. Alternate 10-minute periods of gentle heat with 10-minute periods without heat, several times a day. Be careful not to overdo it, or you'll burn yourself.

Massage. Massage won't cure a backache, but it will increase blood flow to tight muscles and loosen them.

Braces or corsets. These support the back and protect the spine by restricting movement, serving as a substitute for strong back muscles. Don't rely on them to correct a weak back.

Spinal manipulation. A chiropractor or physical therapist uses the hands to "adjust" the spine. Check with your doctor about this option.

Once the acute pain passes, exercise programs designed to strengthen abdominal and back muscles are helpful. Also, don't sit for prolonged periods of time—it puts extra strain on the lower back. And make sure you sleep on a firm mattress. Never sleep on your stomach; sleep on your back or side, with your knees bent.

For most people, the above strategies will relieve lower back pain due to muscle strain from overexertion. If the pain lasts for more than five to seven days, however, or if the pain is moving down either or both buttocks into your thighs, or your legs are numb, or you notice a change in bowel or bladder habits, get medical attention. You may have a herniated spinal disk. (To prevent back pain in the first place by using proper lifting techniques, see Tip 43.) Not all back pain is due to a muscle strain or a disk problem. A person may experience back pain from a tumor (rarely) or a compression fracture from osteoporosis (occasionally).

41 How to Describe Your Pain— And Get Relief

Pain is a useful tool--one you wouldn't want to be without. It lets you know when a tooth is infected, a leg is broken, or you've touched something hot enough to burn your skin. But sometimes the fact that you're in pain isn't enough to help your doctor determine what's wrong. You have to explain what kind of pain you have--throbbing or sharp, constant or intermittent, mild or intense.

Keeping a pain diary or journal can help identify the causes of difficult-to-explain pain or measure improvement if you're being treated for a painful condition. Record the following kinds of information.

▶ When did you first notice the pain?

▶ How often do you feel pain, and when does it occur?

▶ Do you associate the pain with some activity?

▶ Does it move from one spot to another?

▶ How long does pain last?

▶ Does aspirin relieve the pain?

▶ What do you do to try to relieve the pain? Does it work?

▶ Is the pain associated with any other symptoms (like nausea or fatigue)?

To describe your pain more precisely, consult the table below, which gives some terms useful for describing pain and a scale to rate its intensity.

Rate Your Pain

Instructions: Using the Pain Intensity Scale, assign a number to each term that best describes your pain and its intensity.

Pain Intensity Scale

Mild: 1, Uncomfortable: 2, Distressing: 3, Horrible: 4

Description of Pain

___ Aching	___ Penetrating	___ Splitting
___ Agonizing	___ Piercing	___ Squeezing
___ Annoying	___ Pinching	___ Stabbing
___ Beating	___ Pounding	___ Stinging
___ Burning	___ Pressing	___ Suffocating
___ Cramping	___ Pricking	___ Taut
___ Crushing	___ Pulsing	___ Tearing
___ Cutting	___ Radiating	___ Tender
___ Dull	___ Scalding	___ Throbbing
___ Gnawing	___ Sharp	___ Tight
___ Hurting	___ Shooting	___ Tingling
___ Intense	___ Sore	___ Wrenching
___ Nagging		

SOURCE: Adapted from "The McGill Questionnaire," by Ronald Melzack, Ph.D., published with permission in "How to Talk to Your Doctor about Acute Pain" (Wilmington, Del.: Du Pont Pharmaceuticals, 1987).

42 Twenty Questions to Diagnose Back Problems

A number of things can cause back trouble. This simple questionnaire can help provide important clues to what's at the root of your back problem. Answer as many questions as you can and take a copy of this section to your doctor when your back needs medical attention.

1. Do you have a history of back problems? _____

2. What is the major complaint? _____

3. When did the pain, stiffness, or symptoms begin? _____

_____

4. Did it begin gradually or suddenly? _____

5. Were you sick in any way when it began? _____

6. Do these symptoms disturb or prevent sleep (awaken you with pain)?

_____

7. Is this the first experience of this kind? _____

8. Is the pain unrelenting? _____

9. Is the pain intermittent? _____

10. Is the pain sharp, dull, burning, aching, cramping, or shooting? __

_____

11. What do you suspect the problem was caused by? Check all that apply.

_____ injury

_____ overweight

_____ poor posture

_____ stress/tension

_____ menstruation

_____ illness

_____ pregnancy

_____ overexertion

_____ other (explain) _____

12. When does the problem annoy you the most? Check all that apply.

_____ at work

_____ when lifting

_____ when in bed

_____ when bending

_____ when stressed

_____ when fatigued

_____ when coughing or sneezing

_____ when sitting

_____ when standing

_____ when driving

_____ when carrying

_____ in the morning

_____ in the afternoon

_____ in the evening

_____ other (explain) _____

13. Does the pain radiate or move in a particular direction? If yes, explain. _____

14. Do you experience muscle spasms? _____

15. Do you sleep on a soft mattress or a hard one? _____

16. Have you been under nervous or emotional strain lately? _____

17. Is there any redness, tenderness, or swelling? _____

18. Is there a daily pattern to the pain? _____

19. What helps relieve the pain? Check all that apply.

_____ heat

_____ ice packs

_____ exercise

_____ bed rest

_____ hot baths

_____ · muscle relaxants

_____ massage

_____ brace

_____ walking

_____ painkillers

_____ nothing

_____ haven't tried anything

20. Are there any other factors that the doctor should be aware of?

---

43 The Dos and Don'ts of Lifting

It's all too familiar: You go to lift an object of some kind, and bam, out of nowhere, the pain hits.

Want to avoid hurting your back? Follow the dos and don'ts of proper lifting.

First, the don'ts.

▶ Don't lift a load that's too heavy.

▶ Don't bend at the waist to pick up objects.

▶ Don't arch your back when lifting or carrying anything.

▶ Don't twist your spine when holding an object. Instead, turn your whole body, head to toe, in the direction you're headed.

▶ Don't lift heavy objects over your head.

▶ Don't lift quickly or with a jerking movement.

▶ Don't lift unbalanced loads (namely, a light load in one arm and a heavy one in the other). Divide the weight evenly.

▶ Don't try to lift an object (like a child) with one arm while holding on to something else (like a grocery bag) with the other. Put one down or lift both objects simultaneously.

▶ Don't lift anything heavy if your footing isn't secure or if you're wearing high heels.

▶ Don't lift with your feet too close together. Stand with your feet shoulder-width apart, for stability.

▶ Don't lift if you're experiencing pain.

▶ Don't lift if you have a history of back trouble.

To lift without strain, do:

▶ Wear good support shoes, not sandals or high heels.

▶ Plant your feet squarely and stand close to the object you plan to lift.

▶ Bend at the knees and assume a crouching position.

▶ Keep your back as straight as possible.

▶ Pull in your abdominal muscles and tuck in your buttocks.

▶ Rely on the leg muscles to bear the weight.

▶ Hold the object very close to your body.

▶ Keep your knees bent as you lift.

▶ Lift slowly and gradually.

▶ Get help if the object is too heavy or large for one person to handle.

▶ Consider using a dolly or other device to move a heavy object.

44 Put Your Tennis Elbow on Ice

If you're a tennis player with a hard, single-handed backhand shot, you can end up with a painful condition called epicondylitis—more popularly known as tennis elbow. Pain originates in the outer portion of the elbow and works its way down the forearm. Tennis players who are new to the game or use their forearms instead of the force of their whole bodies to swing the racket are most vulnerable. A backhand stroke strains the elbow more than a forehand shot. Other factors that contribute to the problem include:

▶ Using a racket that's too heavy.

▶ Using a racket that's too tightly strung.

▶ Using played out, deflated balls.

▶ Using improper grip.

▶ Trying to put spin on the ball with improper wrist action.

▶ Using a one-handed backhand shot instead of assisting with your other hand.

Continuing to use the arm aggravates the situation. Even several weeks of rest won't prevent repeat episodes. The best game plan is to rest, then strengthen your forearm muscles and get coaching to improve your skill level.

To relieve tennis elbow pain:

▶ Apply ice for the first two or three days.

▶ Take aspirin (if there are no medical reasons not to).

If you still have pain after three weeks, see a doctor. You may need a steroid injection in the elbow or an x-ray to make sure nothing is seriously wrong.

To prevent repeat bouts of tennis elbow:

▶ Wait until the pain is gone and your grip strength is normal before resuming play.

▶ Wear an elastic or neoprene support bandage while playing or during flare-ups.

▶ To strengthen your forearm muscles, lift small, 3- to 5-pound weights by alternately flexing and extending your wrists with the palms facing down and your forearms resting on a flat surface. Start with 10 repetitions and work up to 40, three or four times a week.

45 Nine Ways to Relieve Varicose Veins

Varicose veins are unsightly and uncomfortable. Veins bulge, throb, and feel heavy. The lower legs suffer the most, and sometimes your ankles may swell.

To relieve varicose veins:

▶ Don't cross your legs when sitting.

▶ Keep your weight down.

▶ Avoid standing for prolonged periods of time. If your job requires you to stand, alternate your weight from one leg to the other every few minutes.

▶ Wear elastic support socks that go up to (but do not cover) the knee.

▶ Don't wear clothing or undergarments that are tight or constrict your waist, groin, or legs.

▶ Eat high-fiber foods like bran cereals, beans, whole grain breads, and fresh fruits and vegetables. Drink at least 8 glasses of water a day. These things promote regularity.

▶ To prevent swelling, cut your salt intake.

▶ Exercise regularly. Walking is a good choice.

Exercise your legs. (From a sitting position, rotate your feet at the ankles, turning them first clockwise, then counterclockwise, using a circular motion. Next, extend your legs forward and point your toes to the ceiling, then the floor. Then, lift your feet off the floor and gently bend your legs back and forth at the knees.)

▶ Elevate your legs when resting.

Varicose veins aren't usually serious. If a rash or sores develop on the leg, contact your doctor. (See the discussion of phlebitis in Tip 71 in chapter 2, Major Medical Conditions: Prevention, Detection, and Treatment.)

46 Wipe Out Athlete's Foot

It smells bad. It's itchy. It's persistent. It's contagious. And it attacks the skin between the toes (usually the third and fourth). The name of this odious creature? Fungus of the foot, better known as athlete's foot.

People usually contract athlete's foot from walking barefoot over wet floors around swimming pools, locker rooms, and public showers that are contaminated with the fungus, which feasts on moisture. If you get athlete's foot:

▶ Wash your feet twice a day, especially between your toes, and dry the area thoroughly.

▶ Apply an over-the-counter antifungal powder or spray between your toes and to the inside of your socks and shoes.

▶ Wear clean socks made of cotton or wool. (Natural fibers absorb moisture.)

▶ Wear shoes that provide some ventilation, like sandals or canvas loafers, whenever you can.

▶ Alternate shoes daily to allow each pair to air out between wearings.

If this regimen doesn't work, you may need a prescription medication from your doctor or a podiatrist.

Note: People with diabetes need to monitor athlete's foot very carefully for possible bacterial infection and must get medical advice promptly if a problem arises. Diabetics' feet and nails need special care.

47 Winning Remedies for Corns and Calluses

All too often, corns and calluses are the price we pay for neglecting our feet.

Corns and calluses are very much alike—they just differ in where they occur. Corns show up on the bony area on top of the toes, while calluses occur on the ball or heel of the foot or the big toe. Both result from bad walking habits, bone deformities, or repeated rubbing or friction from poorly fitting footwear.

Corns feel hard to the touch, are tender, and have a roundish appearance. A small, clear spot called a hen's eye may form in the center. Never pick at corns or use a knife, razor blade, or any other sharp tool to cut off corns. Also, never use strong medications—you may injure your skin or trigger an infection. Instead:

▶ Get rid of shoes that fit poorly, especially if they squeeze your toes together.

▶ Soak your feet in warm water to soften the corn.

▶ Cover the corn with a protective, nonmedicated pad, usually available in drugstores. (A piece of foam rubber or moleskin will do in a pinch.)

▶ If the outer layers of a corn have peeled away, apply a nonprescription liquid of 5 to 10 percent salicylic acid and cover the area with a small bandage.

If you have continuing pain, consult a podiatrist or your family doctor, who will scrape away the hardened tissue and peel away the corn with stronger solutions. (Sometimes warts lie underneath corns and need to be treated, too.)

Calluses are flat, painless thickenings of the skin. Never try to get rid of a callus by cutting it with a sharp tool. Instead:

▶ Soak your feet in warm water to soften the callus, and dry gently.

▶ Rub the callus gently with a pumice stone.

▶ Cover calluses with protective pads, available in drugstores.

▶ Check for poorly fitting shoes or other sources of pressure that may lead to calluses.

Note: Anyone with diabetes or circulatory problems should seek medical attention for foot problems of any kind. Their risk of infection is higher than average.

48 How to Deal with Ingrown Toenails

An ingrown toenail can make a big, burly guy wince and hobble like a wounded puppy. A toenail that digs into surrounding skin (usually on the big toe) can cause pain, tenderness, redness, and possibly infection.

Possible causes include:

▶ Jamming your toes by making sudden stops, especially while playing sports like tennis or basketball.

▶ Wearing tight-fitting shoes.

▶ Clipping toenails too far back, so that the corners penetrate the skin as they grow out.

▶ Being born with wider-than-average toenails.

Home remedies for a painful ingrown toenail include these steps.

▶ Soak your foot in hot, soapy water three to four times a day.

▶ Gently lift the nail away from the reddened skin at the outer corners, with the tip of a nail file.

▶ Place a small piece of cotton soaked in an antiseptic just under the outer corners, if possible.

▶ Repeat the previous three steps daily until the nail begins to grow correctly and pressure is relieved. (Wear roomy shoes during this period.)

If the toenail edges become red and tender, fill with pus, or otherwise appear infected, see a doctor.

If home treatment fails to work, a physician or podiatrist may have to surgically remove the troublesome portion of the nail, or possibly the entire nail.

To prevent ingrown toenails, cut nails straight across. Don't cut the nails shorter at the sides than in the middle.

Note: Anyone who has diabetes or circulatory problems needs to be very careful to avoid infections of the feet. Trim nails carefully, or have them trimmed by a medical professional, to avoid nicking the skin or fostering an ingrown nail.

49 Warming Up Cold Hands and Feet

Some people wear mittens and heavy socks all year round, even in warm weather, indoors and out. Their hands and feet are always cold.

Supersensitivity to cold may be due to Raynaud's disease. Or the problem may occur in the wake of frostbite, during work that uses vibrating equipment (like a jackhammer), as a result of taking certain medications, or because of an underlying disease affecting blood flow in the tiny blood vessels of the skin. Stress may also increase sensitivity to cold in the hands or feet. Symptoms to look for are:

▶ Fingers or toes turning pale white or blue, then red, in response to cold.

▶ Tingling or numbness.

▶ Pain during the white phase of discoloration.

If wearing gloves and wool socks and staying indoors where it's warm is a nuisance or doesn't help, try these other warm-up tips.

▶ Don't smoke (it impairs circulation).

▶ Avoid caffeine (it constricts blood vessels).

▶ Avoid handling cold objects. (Use ice tongs to pick up ice cubes, for instance.)

▶ With fingers outstretched, swing your arms in large circles, like a baseball pitcher warming up for a game. This may increase blood flow to the fingers. (Skip this tip if you have bursitis or back problems.)

▶ Wiggle your toes; it may help keep them warm as a result of increased blood flow.

▶ Practice a relaxation technique, such as biofeedback (described in Tip 160 in chapter 6, Success over Stress).

CHAPTER

2

Major Medical Conditions: Prevention, Detection, and Treatment

Ask someone what they fear most, and if they think for a few seconds, they'll probably tell you that they dread the prospect of developing a major illness, like heart disease, stroke, or cancer. And in the scheme of things, it's easy to see why personal illness is more stressful than getting fired from your job or suffering a financial collapse.

Yet if you're like most people, you probably don't spend a lot of time worrying about major illness—how you'll survive, how you'll pay the bills, how your family will manage, or whether or not you'll be able to get around the way you're accustomed to. Mostly, you just keep your fingers crossed or pray you'll never have to deal with debilitating medical problems.

A little thought now—and some simple preventive action—can help head off major diseases, though. At the very least, detecting a problem early can save you lots of time, money, and pain—perhaps even save your life. And if you do develop a major medical condition, knowing something about your treatment options can help you minimize its negative impact on your health, your lifestyle, and your finances. (Needless to say, professional medical advice is not only useful and wise at every stage of disease, it's often essential. Consult your doctor if you develop a problem.)

This chapter gives capsule descriptions of 28 major medical conditions and explains what you can do about them. Think of this section as a map to guide you through the medical maze that can confront you if you develop a health problem.

50 Alzheimer's Disease: Making Up for Poor Memory

Mysterious and frustrating, Alzheimer's afflicts nearly four million Americans, about 10 percent of the over-65 population, and 45 percent of those 85 years or older. (In rare instances, it strikes earlier than 65.)

No one knows what causes Alzheimer's disease. Some research hints that a virus is the culprit. Nevertheless, the end result is the death of brain cells that control intellect—the way your brain receives and processes information.

Symptoms of Alzheimer's include:

- Brief attention span
- Decreased bowel or bladder control (rarely)
- Depression
- Disorientation
- Forgetfulness (especially about recent events)
- Inability to handle minor tasks, or to speak clearly
- Irritability, hostile behavior, or paranoia
- Lack of spontaneity
- Mental deterioration
- Neglecting to perform routine tasks

If someone you care about shows signs of Alzheimer's disease, see that they get medical attention to confirm (or rule out) the diagnosis. Not everything that looks like Alzheimer's is Alzheimer's. Brain tumors, blood clots in the brain, severe vitamin B_{12} deficiency, hypothyroidism, and some drug side effects can mimic Alzheimer's disease. (Unlike Alzheimer's, these problems can be treated.)

Two prescription medicines (Cognex and Aricept), if given in the early stages of the disease, may help with memory in some persons. Sometimes medications to treat depression, paranoia, and agitation can minimize symptoms, but will not necessarily improve memory.

It's especially helpful to put structure in the life of someone who's in the early stages of Alzheimer's. Some suggestions include:

▶ Maintain daily routines.

▶ Post reminders on an oversized and prominently displayed calendar.

▶ Make "to do" lists of daily tasks for the person with Alzheimer's to complete, and ask him or her to check them off as they're completed.

▶ Put things in their proper places after use, to help the person with Alzheimer's find things when he or she needs them.

▶ Post safety reminders (like "turn off the stove") at appropriate places throughout the house.

Also, see that the person with Alzheimer's eats well-balanced meals, goes for walks with family members, and otherwise continues to be as active as possible. Alzheimer's victims should wear medical identification tags.

51 Angina: What It Tells You about Your Heart

The symptoms of angina are:

▶ Squeezing pressure or heaviness or mild ache in the chest.

▶ A feeling that you're choking or shortness of breath.

▶ A feeling of aching in the chest muscles, jaw, one or both arms, neck and/or back.

▶ A sensation of heaviness, tingling, or numbness (most commonly in the left arm).

▶ Discomfort similar to indigestion.

Many people who experience angina for the first time fear they're having a heart attack. Here's why angina and heart attack are mistaken for each other.

▶ Both can be caused by a buildup of fatty plaque (atherosclerosis) in the heart arteries, blocking or slowing delivery of blood to the heart.

▶ In both, the pain can be felt in the chest, arms, shoulders, and/or neck.

► Both may be brought on by extreme physical exertion.

► Both are most prevalent in men who are 50 and older and women who are past menopause.

But there is key difference. A heart attack leaves damaged or injured heart muscle in its wake; angina does not. Rather, anginal pain is a warning sign of a potential heart attack. The discomfort indicates that the heart isn't receiving enough blood.

A doctor can generally diagnose angina as stable or unstable based on: your description of the painful episode; tests such as a stress test (a measurement of heart function taken while you exercise on a treadmill); and observation for a day in the hospital. Unstable angina, a symptom of coronary artery disease, requires immediate attention

Exertion or physical work, especially if it strains the muscles of the chest or arms, is associated with an angina attack. So is walking rapidly uphill and emotional shock.

High blood pressure, obesity, diabetes, high cholesterol, smoking, or a family history of atherosclerotic heart disease increase the odds of angina episodes. (See Tip 57 for a description of heart attack signs.) If you've experienced angina, the following steps can head off further attacks.

► Consult your physician. He or she will probably prescribe nitroglycerin or another medication to temporarily dilate, or widen, the coronary arteries. Nitroglycerin takes effect within a minute or two. A low-dose daily aspirin may also be prescribed.

► Don't smoke. Nicotine in cigarettes constricts the arteries and prevents proper blood flow.

► Avoid large, heavy meals; eat lighter meals throughout the day.

► Rest after eating, or engage in some quiet activity.

► Minimize exposure to cold, windy weather.

► Lower your cholesterol level, if high. Follow a low-fat, low-saturated fat diet. Take lipid-lowering medicines if prescribed.

► Avoid sudden physical exertion such as running to catch a bus.

52 Arthritis: Easy Exercise for Creaky Joints

Arthritis robs some 40 million Americans of their freedom of movement by breaking down the protective cartilage in the joints. By destroying cartilage, arthritis results in pain and decreased movement.

The following can be warning signs of arthritis. If any of these symptoms are present, consult your doctor.

▶ Stiffness

▶ Swelling in one or more joints

▶ Deep, aching pain in a joint

▶ Any pain associated with movement of a joint

▶ Tenderness or redness in afflicted joints

▶ Fever, weight loss, or fatigue that accompanies joint pain

Many forms of arthritis exist. Three of the most common are osteoarthritis, rheumatoid arthritis, and ankylosing spondylitis.

Osteoarthritis is a painful degeneration of the cartilage in the weight-bearing and frequently used joints. As far as researchers can tell, this kind of arthritis is typically brought on by genetics and wear and tear on the joints. It can also follow an injury to the joint. Osteoarthritis often affects older people and is the most common type of arthritis. Brief pain and stiffness at the beginning of the day are typical.

Rheumatoid arthritis (RA) is caused by a chronic inflammation of the fingers, wrists, ankles, elbows, and knees, causing pain, swelling, and tenderness. Morning stiffness lasting longer than an hour is very common. RA affects women more often than men, striking in their thirties and forties.

Ankylosing spondylitis generally affects young men between the ages of 15 and 45 and is characterized by a stiff backbone, accompanied by low back pain.

If your doctor does diagnose arthritis, he or she may prescribe medication (usually aspirin or a nonsteroidal anti-inflammatory drug), rest, heat or cold treatment, and some physical therapy or exercise, depending on what kind of arthritis you have. The goal is to reduce pain and improve joint mobility.

Among those treatments, exercise is perhaps the most important, whether it be some form of stretching, isometrics, or simple endurance exercise. Exercise seems to provide both physical relief and psychological benefits. For example, it prevents the muscles from shrinking, while inactivity encourages both loss of muscle tone and bone deterioration. Too much exercise, however, will cause more pain in those with rheumatoid arthritis. So if you have arthritis, consult your physician, a physical therapist, or a physiatrist (a doctor who specializes in rehabilitative treatment) to assist you in developing an exercise program.

One form of exercise that's effective and soothing is hydrotherapy, or movement done in water. It allows freedom of movement and puts less stress on the joints because nearly all of the body weight is supported by the water. Doctors highly recommend swimming, too.

But remember, hydrotherapy—or any form of exercise—should never produce pain. One message that can't be emphasized enough is "Go easy." If you begin to hurt, stop and rest or apply ice packs.

The following exercise suggestions may provide relief.

▶ Choose exercise routines that use all affected joints.

▶ Keep movements gradual, slow, and gentle.

▶ If a joint is inflamed, don't exercise it.

▶ Don't overdo it. Allow yourself sufficient rest.

▶ Concentrate on freedom of movement, especially in the water, and be patient.

53 Cancer: Look for Clues That Can Save Your Life

What do cancer and lightning have in common? The answer: Most people think they come out of the blue—either they strike you down, or (if you're lucky) they don't. But that's where the similarity ends. Far more people die from cancer than get hit by lightning—it's the second leading cause of death in the United States (heart disease is first). Current estimates say that 1 in 3 of all Americans will develop some kind of cancer in their lifetimes, the most common forms being cancer of the skin, prostate, breast, lungs, colon and rectum, urinary tract, and uterus.

Of course, that means 2 in 3 of us won't get cancer. Luck is only part of the explanation. Cancer-free people may be doing something right— like not smoking, eating the right foods, drinking little or no alcohol, or protecting themselves from workplace chemicals. Cigarette smoking is estimated to be responsible for 90 percent of all lung cancer deaths. Diet is thought to be a factor in 35 percent of all cancers. And other lifestyle factors that increase the risk of cancer include alcohol use, work-related exposure to dangerous chemicals, and exposure to radiation. (But whether or not you practice preventive measures against cancer, it's a good idea to be alert to early possible signs of the disease. If you can detect cancer early and get proper treatment, your chances for survival increase considerably.)

Check with your doctor if you notice any of the following symptoms.

▶ Any change in bladder or bowel habits

▶ A lump or thickening in the breast (or anywhere else)

▶ Unusual vaginal bleeding or rectal discharge or bleeding

▶ Persistent hoarseness or nagging cough

▶ A sore throat that won't go away

▶ Noticeable change in a wart or mole

▶ Indigestion or difficulty swallowing

54 Cataracts: New Ways to Restore Vision

Imagine a thick cloud covering the lens of one or both eyes and you'll have a pretty good idea of what it's like to have cataracts. Vision dims, even in broad daylight. Nighttime vision is glazed. Sometimes you see double, and your eyes are sensitive to light. Your pupils may appear milky white. (Fortunately, cataracts are painless.)

Other symptoms to be alert for:

▶ Cloudy, fuzzy, foggy, or filmy vision

▶ Colors are dull and more difficult to distinguish.

▶ Glare from lights becomes bothersome, especially at night.

▶ Glasses that were worn for close work are no longer needed. (This phenomenon is referred to as "second sight.")

The most common cause of cataracts is the aging process. But overexposure to ultraviolet (UV) light, specific damage to an eye, and some diseases, such as diabetes, can lead to cataracts. If the vision loss caused by a cataract is only slight, surgery may not be needed. A change in your glasses, stronger bifocals, or the use of magnifying lenses, and taking measures to reduce glare may help improve your vision and be enough for treatment.

Modern cataract surgery is safe and effective in restoring vision. Ninety-five percent of operations are successful. For the most part, surgery can be done on an outpatient basis or involve no more than an overnight hospital stay.

A person who has cataract surgery usually gets an artificial lens at the same time. A plastic disc called an intraocular lens is placed in the lens capsule inside the eye. Other choices are contact lenses and cataract glasses. Your doctor will help you to decide which choice is best for you.

55 Chronic Fatigue Syndrome: The Way Up from Down

Until about 1983, doctors knew next to nothing about chronic fatigue syndrome. Some researchers used to think it was caused by the Epstein-Barr virus. Others suggest its cause could be a virus that has not yet been found. Most experts now lean toward a theory of multiple causes. The person affected complains of :

- Fatigue for at least six months
- Sore throat
- Swollen glands
- Low-grade fever
- Headaches
- Depression
- Muscle aches
- Mild weight loss
- Short-term memory problems, confusion, difficulty thinking, inability to concentrate
- Sleep disturbances (insomnia or hypersomnia)

These symptoms could signal a number of health conditions. Chronic fatigue syndrome can be diagnosed only after other illnesses, such as HIV/ AIDS, tuberculosis, autoimmune diseases, such as lupus, or psychiatric illnesses have been ruled out. As yet, no specific laboratory tests can diagnose the syndrome.

For some, the symptoms are so debilitating that a normal working life is impossible. Yet others experience only a vague sense of feeling ill. In some cases, symptoms never let up, while in others they come and go.

Until more is known, people with chronic fatigue syndrome are encouraged to do the following:

► Get plenty of rest.

► Learn to manage stress.

► Take good care of their general health.

► Try to lead as normal a life as possible.

► Join a support group of others who have this problem.

Medicine to relieve pain and fever, such as acetaminophen, aspirin or ibuprofen, may be helpful. A low dose of an anti-depressant may also be prescribed. A gradual exercise program, if tolerated, may also be beneficial.

56 Cirrhosis: Be Kind to Your Liver

The liver is probably the most versatile organ you've got. It performs many tasks, including:

► Producing bile (a substance that aids digestion of fats)

► Producing blood proteins

► Helping blood clot

► Metabolizing cholesterol

► Maintaining normal blood sugar levels

► Forming and storing glycogen (the body's short-term energy source)

► Manufacturing more than 1,000 enzymes necessary for various bodily functions

► Detoxifying substances such as alcohol and many drugs

The liver is equipped to handle a certain amount of alcohol without much difficulty. But drink too much alcohol, too often, for too long, and the vital tissues in the liver break down. Fatty deposits accumulate and scarring occurs. This sad state of affairs is known as cirrhosis. It's most commonly found in men over 45, yet the number of women developing cirrhosis is steadily increasing.

To make matters worse, people who drink too much generally have poor nutritional habits. Since alcohol replaces food, essential vitamins and minerals are missing from the diet. So malnutrition aggravates cirrhosis.

While alcohol abuse is the most common cause of cirrhosis, hepatitis, taking certain drugs, or exposure to certain chemicals can also produce this condition.

Doctors recognize the following as signs of advanced cirrhosis.

▶ Enlarged liver

▶ Yellowish eyes and skin, and tea-colored urine (indicating jaundice)

▶ Bleeding from the gastrointestinal tract

▶ Itching

▶ Hair loss

▶ Swelling in the legs and stomach (indicating fluid accumulation)

▶ Tendency to bruise easily

▶ Mental confusion

Cirrhosis can be life threatening, so get medical attention if you suspect your drinking habits may have gotten out of hand or you have any of the above symptoms. And needless to say, you (or anyone you suspect of having cirrhosis) should abstain from alcohol.

57 Coronary Heart Disease: Eight Ways to Avoid the Deadliest Health Problem

Every day, about 4,000 Americans have heart attacks—one every 20 seconds. And each year, nearly 600,000 people die of coronary artery disease, making it the nation's number one killer. Fortunately, heart disease claims fewer and fewer lives each year, thanks to growing public awareness of the benefits of exercise and good nutrition and recent advances in medical treatment of heart disease.

To avoid heart disease, the American Heart Association suggests the following steps:

▶ Have your blood pressure checked regularly. High blood pressure can foster the build-up of fatty deposits in the blood vessels, called atherosclerosis. To control high blood pressure, follow your doctor's advice. (Weight control and low-sodium diets help to control high blood pressure.)

▶ If you smoke, quit. Nicotine constricts blood flow to the heart, decreases oxygen supply to the heart, and seems to play a significant role in the development of coronary artery disease.

▶ Ask your doctor to check you for diabetes, which is associated with atherosclerosis. Follow his or her advice if you have diabetes.

▶ Maintain a normal body weight. (People who are obese are more prone to atherosclerosis, high blood pressure, and diabetes, and therefore coronary heart disease.)

▶ Eat a diet low in saturated fats and cholesterol. (Saturated fats occur in meats, dairy products, hydrogenated vegetable oils and some tropical oils, like coconut and palm kernel oils.) High-saturated fat, high-cholesterol diets contribute to the fatty sludge that accumulates inside artery walls.

▶ Get some form of aerobic exercise at least three times a week for 20 minutes at a time. Sitting around hour after hour, day after day, week in and week out with no regular physical activity may cause circulation problems later in life and contributes to atherosclerosis. (See chapter 3, Get Fit, Stay Fit, for tips on walking, bicycling, and other kinds of aerobic exercise.) Consult your doctor before starting any new exercise program.

▶ Reduce the harmful effects of stress by practicing relaxation techniques and improving your outlook on daily events. Stress has been linked to elevated blood pressure, among other health problems. (See chapter 6, Success over Stress.)

▶ Get regular medical checkups.

You should also know the signs of a heart attack so you can get immediate medical attention if necessary, before it's too late. They are:

▶ Chest discomfort or pressure lasting several minutes or longer

▶ Discomfort or pressure that spreads to the shoulder, neck, arm, and jaw

▶ Nausea or vomiting associated with chest pain

▶ A cold sweat

▶ Difficult breathing

▶ Faintness or dizziness

▶ Stomach upset

▶ A sense of impending disaster

If you think you're having a heart attack, get to a hospital as quickly as possible.

58 Crohn's Disease: Help for an Inflammatory Bowel Disorder

The lower section of your small intestine is called the ileum. It's connected to your colon. When the ileum (and sometimes the colon) becomes chronically inflamed, the condition is called Crohn's disease. Early symptoms include:

▶ Cramps and pain on the lower right side of the abdomen, generally occurring just after eating

▶ Diarrhea (usually without blood)

▶ Slight fever

▶ Nausea

▶ Loss of appetite and weight

▶ Inflammation of the anus

▶ Joint pains

▶ Fatigue

As gastrointestinal disorders go, Crohn's disease is what you might call a young person's problem, generally striking between the ages of 15 and 35.

It tends to run in families and is more common among Caucasians, especially Europeans and people of Jewish heritage. (Doctors also suspect environmental factors may be partially to blame.) The number of people who have Crohn's disease has doubled over the past 20 years, but no one knows why.

Crohn's disease is quite unpredictable: It comes and goes, triggering attacks off and on for months or years. Nevertheless, treatment is fairly successful and consists of medications—usually antidiarrheal drugs, anti-inflammatory agents and vitamin supplements, sometimes steroids, and possibly antibiotics, should infection occur. Doctors recommend bed rest, especially during severe attacks, use of a heating pad to relieve abdominal cramps, and drinking as many liquids as possible to prevent dehydration.

(About 70 percent of those with Crohn's disease undergo surgery. But it's usually not a cure: Crohn's tends to recur in another portion of the intestine.)

Certain foods like milk, eggs, or wheat may irritate the intestines, and avoiding these foods in all forms seems to help control flare-ups (although it doesn't cure the condition). Avoid drinking alcohol—it, too, irritates your system. As for other dietary measures, a diet high in vitamins, protein, and carbohydrates and low in fiber is standard treatment.

Note: Crohn's disease can mimic other intestinal diseases and can only be diagnosed by a physician. If you experience any of the symptoms described, get medical attention.

59 Diabetes: Warnings and Ways to Reduce Your Risk

Since the discovery of insulin in 1921, managing diabetes has become more effective than ever. Today, with care, most diabetics can lead productive lives.

Normally, your body changes sugars and starch into glucose (a simple sugar), which serves as fuel. When diabetes develops, the amount of glucose in the blood may become dangerously high because insulin (the substance that controls glucose levels) is in short supply. Diabetics either don't produce enough insulin or their bodies don't respond to the insulin as they should; that's why they have to take insulin by injection or another medication by mouth to help the body secrete more of its own insulin.

To help you recognize the warning signs of diabetes, the American Diabetes Association uses the acronyms DIABETES and CAUTION.

Watch for the onset of the following symptoms.

Drowsiness

Itching

A family history of diabetes

Blurred vision

Excessive weight

Tingling, numbness, or pain in extremities

Easy fatigue

Skin infection, slow healing of cuts and scratches, especially on the feet

Other signs are:

Constant urination

Abnormal thirst

Unusual hunger

The rapid loss of weight

Irritability

Obvious weakness and fatigue

Nausea and vomiting

You don't necessarily have to experience all of these warning signs to be diabetic; only one or two may be present. Some people show no warning signs whatsoever and find out they're diabetic after a routine blood test. So if you have a family history of diabetes, you should have a glucose test at least once a year. Being overweight increases your risk significantly. A diet high in sugar and low in fiber may increase your risk as well.

There are two forms of diabetes.

Type 1 diabetes is more severe and usually shows up before the age of 40. Insulin injections are essential.

Type 2 diabetes is less severe and affects people who are older and overweight. Often, a change in diet alone will control the problem.

Also, doctors emphasize exercise as an effective way to manage diabetes. Studies seem to support the idea that activity helps the body use insulin more efficiently. So by watching your weight, controlling your eating habits, and exercising, you can reduce your risks.

60 Diverticulosis: Take Action If You Have the Symptoms

No one is sure why, but sometimes small saclike pockets protrude from the intestinal wall, a condition called diverticulosis. Increased pressure within the intestines seems to be responsible. The pockets (called diverticuli) can fill with intestinal waste, causing tenderness, cramps, and abdominal pain, usually on the lower left side of the abdomen. Sometimes the pouches become inflamed, in which case the condition is called diverticulitis. In most cases, though, diverticulosis causes no discomfort; inflammation or bleeding is rare.

Diverticular disease can't be cured, but you can reduce the discomfort and prevent complications. Add more fiber to your diet with fresh fruits, vegetables, and whole-grain foods. These pass through the system quickly, decreasing pressure in the intestines. Avoid seeds and foods with seeds, like figs; seeds are easily trapped in the troublesome pouches.

If you have diverticulosis and experience the following symptoms, get medical treatment.

▶ Blood in the stool

▶ Fever

▶ Chills

▶ Increased lower abdominal pain made worse when you have a bowel movement

61 Emphysema: Make Breathing Easier

Can you imagine what it would feel like to breathe with a plastic bag over your head? That's exactly what emphysema feels like. Over one million Americans are forced to lead restricted lives because they have this chronic lung condition. The air sacs (alveoli) in the lungs are destroyed, and the lung loses its elasticity, along with its ability to take in oxygen. Genetic factors are responsible for 3 to 5 percent of all cases of emphysema, and occupational and environmental exposure to irritants can also cause the disease. But the vast majority of people with emphysema are cigarette smokers aged 50 or older. In fact, emphysema is sometimes called the smoker's disease because of its strong link with cigarettes.

Emphysema takes a number of years to develop, and early symptoms can be easily missed. Symptoms to look out for include:

▶ Coughing

▶ Producing excess sputum

▶ Breathing through pursed lips

▶ Shortness of breath on exertion

▶ Wheezing

▶ Fatigue

▶ Slight body build with marked weight loss and barrel chest

A doctor can diagnose emphysema based on your medical history, a physical exam, a chest x-ray, and a lung function test (spirometry). By the time emphysema is detected, however, anywhere from 50 to 70 percent of your lung tissue may already be destroyed. At that point, your doctor may recommend the following:

▶ A program to help you stop smoking.

▶ Avoidance of dust, fumes, pollutants, and other irritating inhalants.

▶ Physical therapy to help loosen mucus in your lungs.

▶ Daily exercise.

▶ A diet that includes adequate amounts of all essential nutrients.

▶ Prescription medication, including a bronchodilator, steroids, and antibiotics.

▶ Annual flu vaccinations.

▶ Pneumonia vaccination.

Emphysema is irreversible, however, so prevention is the only real way to avoid permanent damage.

62 Gallstones: What They Feel Like, What You Can Do

Have you been feeling bloated and gassy for the past couple of months, especially after eating fried or other fatty foods? Do you suffer bouts of pain in the upper right side of your abdomen that last up to several hours?

Symptoms like that could be caused by stones in the gallbladder. Over 16 million Americans (most of them women) have gallstones. For some, gallstones cause no symptoms. In others, stones cause severe pain or require surgery.

In industrialized countries, the most common type of gallstone consists of cholesterol, the same fat that tends to clog coronary arteries in many people. Doctors aren't sure why gallstones form, but some people are clearly more susceptible than others. Factors that invite gallstones to form include:

▶ A family history of gallbladder disease

▶ Obesity

▶ Middle age

▶ Being female

▶ Pregnancy

▶ Taking estrogen

▶ Diabetes

▶ Eating a diet high in cholesterol-rich foods

▶ Diseases of the small intestine

Treatments for gallstones range from medications (to dissolve the stones), surgery (to remove the gallbladder), or a low-fat diet (to reduce contractions of the gallbladder, thus limiting pain, and possibly keeping more stones from forming). A new treatment involves the use of guided sound waves to dissolve stones.

Dietary measures to discourage stones from forming include the following:

▶ Eat fiber-rich foods such as whole grains, fresh fruits, and vegetables.

▶ Eat less fat.

▶ Avoid refined carbohydrates and foods high in sugar.

63 Glaucoma: You Can Keep Your Sight for Life

Even if you can read an eye chart with 20/20 vision, you may have chronic glaucoma. This is a progressive eye disease that gradually (and often painlessly) robs you of your peripheral vision by damaging the optic nerve. And unless it's treated, your central vision may decline, too.

Glaucoma tends to run in families and is one of the most common eye disorders in people over the age of 60. Some facts to know:

▶ Glaucoma is caused by a dangerous buildup of fluid pressure within the eyeball. (If fluid builds up rapidly, it will cause redness and pain. This form of glaucoma is a medical emergency.)

▶ Glaucoma can cause extensive damage before you notice any symptoms, like blurred vision or seeing rings of color around lights.

▶ Glaucoma can be triggered or aggravated by some medicines, like antihistamines and antispasmodics.

You may not be able to prevent glaucoma, but you may be able to prevent the blindness that may result from glaucoma. Ask to be tested for glaucoma whenever you get a regular vision checkup. It's a simple and painless procedure. If pressure inside the eyeball is high, an eye specialist (ophthalmologist) will probably give you eyedrops and perhaps oral medication. If this fails to control pressure, a couple of options exist.

Ultrasound uses sound waves to reduce the pressure in the eye and is usually performed as a short, outpatient procedure.

Laser beam surgery and other surgical procedures can widen the drainage channels within the eye, relieving fluid buildup.

64 Gout: Relief at Last

If you wake up in the middle of the night with excruciating pain in your big toe, you could have gout. Or perhaps your instep, heel, ankle, or knee hurts. How about your wrists and elbows? Your joints can become so inflamed that even rubbing against the bed sheet can be torture. You may even experience fever and chills.

So goes a classic attack of gout—a form of arthritis most common in men in their fifties, caused by increased blood levels of uric acid, produced by the breakdown of protein in the body. When blood levels of uric acid rise above a critical level, thousands of hard, tiny uric acid crystals collect in the joints. These crystals act like tiny, hot, jagged shards of glass, resulting in pain and inflammation. Crystals can collect in the tendons and cartilage, in the kidneys (as kidney stones), and in the fatty tissues beneath the skin.

A gout attack can last several hours to a few days and can be triggered by:

► Mild trauma or blow to the joint.

► Drinking alcohol (beer and wine more so than distilled alcohol).

► Eating a diet rich in red meat (especially organ meats such as liver, kidney, or tongue).

► Eating sardines or anchovies.

► Taking certain drugs, such as diuretics.

Never assume you have gout without consulting a physician. Many conditions can mimic an acute attack of gout (including infection, injury, or rheumatoid arthritis), and only a doctor can accurately diagnose your problem.

If you do have gout, treatment will depend on why your uric acid levels are high. Your doctor can conduct a simple test to determine whether your kidneys aren't clearing uric acid from the blood the way they should, or whether your body simply produces too much uric acid.

Your first goal, then, is to relieve the acute gout attack. Your second goal is to normalize the uric acid levels to prevent a recurrence.

▶ For immediate relief, your doctor will prescribe colchicine or a nonsteroidal anti-inflammatory drug and tell you to rest the affected joint.

▶ For long-term relief, your doctor will probably recommend that you lose excess weight, limit your intake of alcohol and red meat, drink lots of liquids, and take medication (if necessary).

65 High Blood Pressure: Get It Down, Keep It Down

High blood pressure isn't like a toothache, a bruise, or constipation. Nothing hurts, looks discolored, or fails to work. Usually, people with high blood pressure experience no discomfort or outward signs of trouble. Yet high blood pressure (hypertension) is a killer—a silent killer. Directly or indirectly, high blood pressure accounts for nearly a million deaths a year. Uncontrolled, high blood pressure increases the odds that you'll have a heart attack, a stroke, or kidney failure.

And many who have high blood pressure don't know it. Worse yet, nine out of ten people who know their blood pressures are unhealthfully high are doing nothing to try to control it. And for 95 percent of those affected, there is no known cause.

The amazing part is, blood pressure is one of the easiest health problems to control.

Have your blood pressure checked more than once on several occasions. If your blood pressure is generally pretty good and suddenly registers high, don't be alarmed. Anxiety and other strong emotions, physical exertion, drinking a large amount of coffee, or digesting a recently consumed meal can temporarily elevate normal blood pressure with no lasting effects. If, after several readings, your doctor is convinced you do indeed have high blood pressure, follow his or her advice. Here's a multipoint plan to control high blood pressure.

▶ If you're overweight, lose weight.

▶ Don't smoke.

▶ Limit alcohol to two drinks or less a day.

▶ Eat a low-salt diet and use salt substitutes if your physician says it's okay.

▶ Get regular exercise at least three times a week.

▶ Learn to handle stress by practicing relaxation techniques and rethinking stressful situations. (See chapter 6, Success over Stress, for more details.)

▶ Take any prescribed blood pressure medicine as directed. Don't skip your pills because you feel fine.

▶ If you're a woman, talk to your doctor about oral contraceptives and blood pressure. Many other birth control methods are available.

▶ Avoid over-the-counter cold remedies containing the ingredient phenylpropanolamine. It can raise blood pressure. Talk to your physician or pharmacist.

How's Your Blood Pressure?

Blood pressure is normally measured with a blood pressure cuff placed on the arm. The numbers on the gauge measure your blood pressure in millimeters of mercury (mmHg). The first (higher) number measures the systolic pressure. This is the maximum pressure exerted against the arterial walls while the heart is beating. The second (lower) number records the diastolic pressure, the pressure between heartbeats, when the heart is resting. The results are then recorded as systolic/diastolic pressure (120/80, for example). The term *hypertension* means high blood pressure.

The accompanying table gives the normal and abnormal ranges for both systolic and diastolic blood pressures for adults age 18 or older. To accurately determine your blood pressure, an average of two or more readings should be taken on two or more separate occasions. The risk of stroke, heart attack, and kidney disease increases when blood pressure is in the mild to severe range. So have your blood pressure checked at least once a year, and follow your physician's advice if it is abnormal.

66 Kidney Stones: A New, Painless Solution

John awoke from a deep sleep. An agonizing pain radiated down the side of his abdomen and into his groin. Three years earlier, he'd experienced the same pain when he developed a kidney stone from either too much calcium or uric acid in his urine. At that time, a surgeon had removed the stone. This time, his doctor planned to use a new procedure known as lithotripsy to dissolve the stone.

Lithotripsy causes little or no pain. John will recover more quickly, and it costs less than surgery. Lithotripsy is usually performed as an outpatient procedure in which the patient sits on a special chair and is submerged up to his or her shoulders in a tub of warm water. Harmless

Blood Pressure in Adults

Range (mmHg)	Classification*
Diastolic Blood Pressure	
84 or less	Normal blood pressure
85–89	High normal blood pressure
90–104	Mild hypertension
105–114	Moderate hypertension
115 or greater	Severe hypertension
Systolic Blood Pressure *(when diastolic pressure is less than 90)*	
139 or less	Normal blood pressure
140–159	Borderline systolic hypertension
160 or greater	Systolic hypertension

SOURCE: Adapted from the *Report of the Joint National Committee on Detection, Evaluation, and Treatment of High Blood Pressure* (Washington, D.C.: Department of Health and Human Services, 1988).

*Diastolic blood pressure of 90 or above is more critical than the systolic blood pressure when diagnosing hypertension.

shock waves are directed to the areas where the stone is located, and they break it into fragments. After the treatment, the patient drinks lots of water to flush the stone fragments from his or her system.

Kidney stones can and do recur, though. If you're prone to developing stones, heed these guidelines:

▶ Save any stones you pass, so your doctor can have them analyzed. (Treatment varies with the type of stones you form.)

▶ Follow your doctor's dietary advice. If you tend to form calcium stones, he or she will probably advise you not to take calcium in excess. If you form uric acid stones, your doctor may recommend that you eat less protein and alkalinize your urine by taking sodium bicarbonate.

▶ Drink plenty of fluids—preferably six to eight 8-ounce glasses of water daily—to avoid dehydration.

▶ See your doctor frequently to be sure your kidneys are functioning as they should.

67 Lung Cancer: How to Avoid a Killer

Once upon a time, before cigarettes were invented and air was polluted, lung cancer was unheard of. Today, it's the leading cause of death from cancer in men and women. (About 150,000 Americans die from lung cancer each year, over 85 percent of them can thank cigarettes for the disease.) Since 1987, more women have died each year of lung cancer than breast cancer, which, for over 40 years, was the major cause of cancer death in women.

Lung cancer is especially deadly because the rich network of blood vessels that deliver oxygen from the lungs to the rest of the body can also spread cancer very quickly. By the time it's diagnosed, other organs may be affected.

Symptoms of lung cancer include:

▶ Chronic cough

▶ Blood-streaked sputum

▶ Shortness of breath

▶ Wheezing

▶ Chest discomfort with each breath

► Weight loss

► Fatigue

Depending on the type of lung cancer and how far it's spread, the diseased portions of the lung will be surgically removed; radiation treatment or chemotherapy (or both) will follow.

Lung cancer is difficult to detect in its early, more treatable stages, so the best way to combat the disease is to prevent it. As you might guess, you can do that by eliminating the single greatest cause of lung cancer— smoking cigarettes.

The risk of developing lung cancer is proportional to the number of cigarettes smoked per day. Anyone who smokes two or more packs of cigarettes a day, for instance, runs a risk nearly 25 times greater than that of a nonsmoker (which means that even smoking less than two packs a day still increases your chance of developing lung cancer). The longer a person smokes, and the more deeply the smoke is inhaled, the greater the risk of getting lung cancer.

68 Multiple Sclerosis: You Can Live with It

Normally, delicate nerves are encased in a protective covering called myelin. With multiple sclerosis, the myelin becomes inflamed and eventually dissolves. Over time, scar tissue (sclerosis) accumulates where the myelin used to be. "Multiple" sclerosis occurs in scattered locations in the spinal cord and brain. Nerve impulses, which normally travel at a speed of 225 miles per hour, either slow down considerably or come to a complete halt. This causes the symptoms of MS, which can include:

► Fatigue

► Weakness

► Numbness

► Poor coordination

► Bladder problems (frequent urination, urgency, as well as incontinence)

► Blurred vision, double vision, or transient blindness in one eye

► Muscle spasticity

► Emotional mood swings, irritability, depression, anxiety, euphoria

No one knows what causes MS, but infection and other immunity factors are possibilities. People most susceptible to MS are:

▶ White adults between 20 and 40 years old.

▶ People whose siblings or parents already have the disease.

▶ Women (at a ratio of three women to every two men).

▶ Residents of the northern United States, Canada, and northern Europe.

While no cure exists for multiple sclerosis, you can take several steps to make living with the disease easier. These include:

▶ Treating bacterial infections and fever as soon as they occur.

▶ Getting plenty of rest.

▶ Minimizing stressful situations, especially physically demanding ones, since physical stress seems to aggravate the symptoms.

▶ Avoiding hot showers or baths, since they, too, can aggravate symptoms. (In fact, cool baths or swimming in a pool may improve symptoms by lowering body temperature.)

▶ Maintaining a normal routine at work and at home if activities aren't physically demanding.

▶ Getting regular exercise (physical therapy may be helpful).

▶ Having body massages to help maintain muscle tone.

▶ Getting professional, supportive psychological counseling.

▶ Taking prescribed medication. (This may include antispasmodics, antidepressants, Interferon beta 1-a (Avonex), Interferon beta 1-b (Betaseron), short-term courses of cortisone-like medicines such as intravenous (IV) or oral steroids.

69 Parkinson's Disease: Options to Consider

When Louise first realized that her husband's hands shook while at rest for no reason, she suspected Parkinson's disease. She knew that the disease was also called the shaking palsy, so she asked a doctor about it. Other visible signs revealed that Louise's husband did, in fact, have Parkinson's disease. These symptoms include:

▶ Slow or stiff movement

▶ Stooped posture

▶ Shuffling or dragging the feet

▶ Monotone voice

▶ Blinking less frequently than normal

▶ Lack of spontaneity in facial expression

▶ Difficulty in adjusting positions

▶ Dementia (in advanced stages)

Parkinson's disease results from the degeneration of cells in the part of the brain that produces dopamine, a substance nerves need to function properly. Great strides have been made in treatment, offering new hope for the nearly one million middle-aged and older people who are affected. In most people, the cause is unknown.

Medications such as bromocriptine (brand name Parlodel) and levodopa (brand name Sinemet) increase the dopamine level in the brain For many people, these drugs control symptoms.

Other treatments try to make the person with Parkinson's more comfortable. Warm baths and massages, for example, can help prevent muscle rigidity. Here are some other helpful hints.

▶ Take care to maintain a safe home environment. (Replace razor blades with electric shavers, for example.)

▶ Simplify tasks. (Replace tie shoes with loafers, for instance.)

▶ Include high-fiber foods in the diet (to add bulk) and drink lots of fluids, to prevent constipation.

▶ Get expert physical therapy.

▶ Remain as active as possible.

▶ Get professional help to relieve depression, if necessary.

70 Peptic Ulcers: Tender Treatment for a Sensitive Stomach

Harried, middle-aged business executives aren't the only people who get ulcers. Gastric and duodenal ulcers (grouped under the label peptic ulcers) carve holes into the stomachs and small intestines of all kinds of adults. Men and women alike experience the characteristic symptoms of a peptic ulcer—a gnawing or burning just above the navel within $1\frac{1}{2}$ to 3 hours after eating. The pain feels like indigestion, heartburn, or hunger. It frequently awakens the person at night. Food or antacids generally relieve the pain within minutes.

Persons with a family history of peptic ulcers tend to be at greater risk for getting them. A bacteria called *Heliobacter pylori* may cause about 80% of peptic ulcers. About 20% of peptic ulcers may be caused by the repeated use of aspirin and other nonsteroidal anti-inflammatory drugs (NSAIDs), such as ibuprofen, ketoprofen, and naproxen sodium.

Tests can be done to find out if you have an ulcer and if it is from the *Heliobacter pylori* bacteria. Your doctor can take a blood test, breath test, and get a biopsy of stomach tissue during an endoscopy (looking at your stomach through a tube that's inserted via your mouth). If *Heliobacter pylori* bacteria are present, an antibiotic and acid-blocker should be prescribed.

If you have an ulcer, you can soothe the pain in various ways. Some suggestions are:

► Eat smaller, lighter, more frequent meals for a couple of weeks. Big, heavy lunches and dinners can spell trouble for people with ulcers. Frequent meals tend to take the edge off pain.

► Avoid anything that will stimulate excess stomach acid. That includes coffee (regular and decaffeinated), tea, alcohol, and soft drinks containing caffeine.

► Discontinue use of aspirin and other nonsteroidal anti-inflammatory medicines, which irritate the stomach lining.

► Try antacids (with your physician's okay) on a short-term basis. (Don't try to self-medicate an ulcer. You may soothe the symptoms without treating the problem itself.)

► Don't smoke. Smokers get ulcers more frequently than non-smokers.

► Try to minimize stress in your life. Stress doesn't cause ulcers. But for some people, stress triggers the release of stomach acid—and subsequent ulcer flare-ups.

Consult your physician if you think you have a peptic ulcer or if your stool becomes black and tarry (which can indicate a bleeding ulcer). He or she will prescribe the appropriate tests and treatment.

71 Phlebitis: How to Get Back on Your Feet

When former President Richard Nixon suffered a severe case of phlebitis, it made newspaper headlines. The medical term for his condition is thrombophlebitis: A blood clot forms (thrombosis) and a vein becomes inflamed (phlebitis). Phlebitis is usually caused by infection, injury, or poor blood flow in a vein. It is more common in women over the age of 50.

Superficial phlebitis (SP) occurs just under the skin's surface. The affected area is swollen and feels warm, hard, and tender to the touch. This type seldom showers clots into the bloodstream. It can usually be treated at home.

Deep vein thrombosis (DVT) requires hospitalization and treatment with blood-thinning medication to prevent an embolism from forming. If a blood clot breaks away from the wall of a vein (forming an embolism), it can interfere with the circulation to the limb, or cause death if it reaches the heart or lung. The only symptom may be an aching pain in the limb, but half of persons with DVT have no symptoms. It often develops after prolonged bed rest or major surgery.

Other conditions that can lead to SP and/or DVT include:

- Inactivity (from a sedentary job), a long trip, especially in a cramped space (example: economy class section on a plane)
- Heart failure or heart attack
- Being overweight, in poor physical condition, or older aged
- Trauma to an arm or leg (from a blow or fall)
- Injury to the vein (from injections or intravenous needles)
- Some cancers
- Varicose veins, pregnancy, or estrogen therapy

Only a doctor can tell the difference between SP with or without DVT and DVT alone. If you're diagnosed as having SP without DVT, you'll probably be told to:

- Rest the affected limb and elevate it above the level of your heart until the pain and swelling subside.
- Use aspirin or nonsteroidal anti-inflammatory drugs, such as ibuprofen.
- Avoid bed rest.

To prevent SP and DVT:

- Avoid prolonged periods of uninterrupted sitting or standing.
- Don't sit with your legs crossed.
- Avoid wearing garments that are tight-fitting below the waist, such as garters and knee-high hose. These restrict blood flow.

▶ Wear properly fitting elastic compression stockings for the legs, to help blood flow.

▶ If you're confined to bed, try this: With your feet against a pillow, pretend you're pressing on a gas pedal and then releasing it. Alternate with one foot, then the other.

72 Pneumonia: Tips for a Full Recovery

Pneumonia can develop when the lungs are infected by either bacteria, viruses, fungi, or toxins, causing inflammation. Certain people are at a greater risk for pneumonia than others. They include:

▶ Elderly people, because the body's ability to fight off disease diminishes with age.

▶ People who are hospitalized for other conditions.

▶ Individuals with suppressed cough reflex following a stroke.

▶ Smokers, because tobacco smoke paralyzes the tiny hairs that otherwise help to expel germ-ridden mucus from the lungs.

▶ People who suffer from malnutrition, alcoholism, or viral infections.

▶ People with emphysema or chronic bronchitis.

▶ People with sickle cell anemia.

▶ Cancer patients undergoing radiation treatments or chemo-therapy, both of which wear down the immune system.

Note: These persons should consult their doctor about a vaccine for pneumonia. It is usually given once at age 65. The vaccine may be needed more than once for persons with the above conditions who are under age 65.

To speed recovery from pneumonia:

▶ Get plenty of bed rest.

▶ Use a cool mist humidifier in the room or rooms in which you spend the bulk of your time.

▶ Drink plenty of fluids.

▶ Take any medications your doctor prescribes. Don't suppress coughing, especially if it brings up sputum.

73 Reye's Syndrome: The Single Most Important Safeguard

Parents need to know about Reye's (pronounced "rise") syndrome, a serious and sometimes deadly condition affecting the brain and the liver.

Although no one knows exactly what causes Reye's syndrome, it follows an easily recognized pattern. First, the liver enlarges, due to a buildup of excess fat, and loses its ability to properly metabolize body substances. This in turn causes the brain to swell, and the pressure of the fluid around the brain increases.

Reye's syndrome usually occurs after an upper respiratory tract infection like the flu or chicken pox in children anywhere from infancy to age 19. The child appears to be recovering from the flu or the chicken pox when these new Reye's syndrome symptoms may develop.

- Persistent vomiting
- Confusion or sense of disorientation
- Personality changes (such as irritability or extreme aggressiveness)
- Extreme fatigue or lethargy
- Seizures
- Coma and sometimes death

If you suspect a child has Reye's syndrome, get emergency medical help immediately. Treatment focuses on reducing brain swelling.

One thing doctors do know about Reye's syndrome is that it seems to be associated with the use of aspirin and other medications that contain salicylates in those children with the flu or chicken pox. So doctors strongly recommend against giving aspirin and other medications that contain salicylates to anyone younger than 19 years old during an episode of chicken pox or influenza. Acetaminophen should be substituted, or give no drugs at all.

74 Scoliosis: A Simple Solution to a Common Problem

Coping with the normal physical changes that come with adolescence is trying enough. When out-of-the-ordinary physical changes occur, the problem is doubly discouraging. Such is the case with scoliosis. It generally shows up between the ages of 10 and 15, and affects girls seven to nine times more often than boys. In most cases, no one knows the cause.

At first, scoliosis isn't painful. But it slowly twists the upper portion of the spine. One shoulder may curve one way while the lower back twists another, so that the chest and back are distorted. The spine begins to rotate, and one side of the rib cage becomes more prominent. This is more obvious if the person bends forward at the waist, with the arms hanging freely. In fact, a doctor can detect scoliosis by asking the patient to assume that position during a routine physical or screening for scoliosis.

Adults who have scoliosis should watch for signs of scoliosis in their children.

Scoliosis doesn't always need treatment. In some cases, though, treatment is necessary to prevent heart and lung problems or back pain later in life. There are several treatment options.

▶ Wearing a molded body brace, hidden by clothing, is the most conservative approach. This brace is typically worn most of the day and night for several years. Because the spine grows rapidly during adolescence, wearing a brace at this time can arrest further abnormal curving.

▶ A special form of mild electrical stimulation to the spine is sometimes as effective as brace treatment.

▶ Surgery to straighten the spine is a more radical alternative, used when the spine is severely curved. A thin steel rod is implanted alongside the spine.

In most instances, scoliosis can be sufficiently treated so that the adolescent doesn't suffer any complications as an adult.

75 Sickle Cell Anemia: Information Is the Best Defense

Sickle cell anemia is inherited. It mostly affects blacks. About 1 in 12 African Americans carries the gene for the sickle cell trait (that is, they have the ability to produce children with sickle cell anemia but have no symptoms of the disease). If both parents carry the trait, the chance of having a child with sickle cell anemia is one out of four, or 25 percent.

Sickle cell anemia affects the red blood cells' ability to carry oxygen to the body's tissues. The disease usually doesn't become apparent until the end of the child's first year. The average life expectancy with prompt medical care is now between the ages of 40 and 50.

A blood test can detect sickle cell anemia, but signs and symptoms include the following:

- Pain, ranging from mild to severe, in the chest, joints, back, or abdomen
- Swollen hands and feet
- Jaundice
- Repeated infections, particularly pneumonia or meningitis
- Kidney failure
- Gallstones (at an early age)
- Strokes (at an early age)

For now, no drugs exist to effectively treat sickle cell anemia. At best, treatment is geared toward preventing complications. Painful episodes are treated with painkillers, fluids, and oxygen. The diet is supplemented with folic acid, a B-vitamin. Because people with sickle cell anemia are prone to developing pneumonia, they should be vaccinated against pneumonia.

To prevent sickle cell anemia in offspring, couples, especially African American couples, should have a blood test to determine if they are carriers for the sickle cell trait. Genetic counseling can help them decide what to do.

After conception, sickle cell anemia can be diagnosed by amniocentesis in the second trimester of pregnancy. If the fetus has sickle cell anemia, the parents may elect to terminate the pregnancy.

76 Strokes: You Can Reduce the Risk

Ted was a veteran racquetball player, but suddenly his arms felt weak and numb for no apparent reason, so he decided to check with his doctor. And it's a good thing he did: Tests showed that blood flow to Ted's brain was inadequate. His carotid artery (the artery in the neck that carries blood to the brain) had narrowed from atherosclerosis—something that, if left uncorrected, could lead to a stroke. Thanks to surgery and a change in diet, Ted never had a stroke.

Ted recognized—and heeded—an important warning signal. His follow-up action saved his life.

Strokes (also called cerebrovascular accidents, or apoplexy) are the third leading cause of death in the United States. A stroke can be caused by lack of blood (and therefore lack of oxygen) to the brain, usually due to either atherosclerosis or rupture of a blood vessel in the brain. In either case, the end result is brain damage (and possibly death).

Here's what to do to reduce the risks of a stroke.

- Control your blood pressure. Have it checked regularly and, if necessary, take medication prescribed by your physician.
- Reduce blood levels of cholesterol to below 200 milligrams per deciliter (measured by a blood test).
- Get regular exercise.
- Keep your weight down.
- Don't smoke.
- Keep blood sugar levels under control if you're diabetic.
- Learn to manage stress.

It's important to know the warning signals of a stroke and get immediate medical attention, to minimize the damage. To help you remember what to look out for, the initials of the symptoms spell **DANGER**.

Dizziness
Absent-mindedness, or temporary loss of memory or mental ability
Numbness or weakness in the face, arm, or leg
Garbled speech
Eye problems, including temporary loss of sight in one eye, or double vision
Recent onset of severe headaches

Some people experience a temporary lack of blood supply to the brain or transient ischemic attack (TIA). The symptoms mimic a stroke, but clear within 24 hours. TIAs are a warning that a real stroke may follow, however. So consult your physician immediately if you experience the **DANGER** signs of a stroke, even if they go away.

77 Thyroid Problems: Look for These Signs

The thyroid is a small, butterfly-shaped gland located just in front of the windpipe (trachea) in your throat. Its normal function is to produce L-thyroxine and L-thyronine, hormones that influence thousands of metabolic processes in the body.

Hyperthyroidism occurs when the thyroid produces too much thyroid hormone. Some signs and symptoms are:

▶ Tremors

▶ Mood swings

▶ Weakness

▶ Diarrhea

▶ Heart palpitations

▶ Heat intolerance

▶ Shortened menstrual periods

▶ Unexplained weight loss

▶ Fine hair (or hair loss)

▶ Rapid pulse

▶ Nervousness

▶ Enlarged thyroid gland

Hypothyroidism occurs when the thyroid gland produces too little thyroid hormone to meet the body's requirements. Some signs and symptoms are:

▶ Fatigue and excessive sleeping

▶ Dry, pale skin

▶ Deepening of the voice

▶ Weight gain

▶ Dry hair that tends to fall out

▶ Decrease in appetite

▶ Frequently feeling cold

▶ Puffy face (especially around the eyes)

▶ Heavy menstrual periods

▶ Poor memory

▶ Constipation

▶ Enlarged thyroid gland (in some cases)

Either an oversupply or an undersupply of thyroid hormones could be life threatening, so if you suspect you have a problem, consult your doctor. Treatment for hyperthyroidism includes taking radioactive iodine or having surgery to suppress the thyroid's activity. Treatment for hypo-thyroidism will include supplements of synthetic L-thyroxine to replace what's lacking.

CHAPTER

3

Get Fit, Stay Fit

You can eat the most nutritious food, avail yourself of the best medical care money can buy, and swear off cigarettes and strong drink, but if you don't give your body the activity it needs, you're only partially healthy.

Among its many benefits, getting fit—and staying fit—firms muscles, strengthens the heart and lungs, improves blood circulation, builds strength and endurance, burns off excess calories, strengthens bones, limbers up the joints, reduces stress, enhances self-image, improves digestion, and relieves constipation. And if that weren't enough, evidence shows that exercise triggers the release of beta-endorphin, a hormone that boosts your spirits and makes pain more tolerable.

If fitness could be dispensed in pill form, it would be the single most frequently prescribed medication. But you can't become fit by swallowing a pill, capsule, or liquid. You can, however, take simple, sensible steps to exercise regularly, starting today. This chapter will teach you how to select an activity, set realistic goals, exercise properly, stay motivated, and measure your progress.

Note: Before beginning an exercise program, it's wise to have a medical checkup, especially if you haven't had a physical exam within the past year, you're over 30, you're overweight, or you have a history of high blood pressure, diabetes, or heart trouble. A medical exam can help you avoid orthopedic injuries, cardiovascular complications, or other exercise-related problems.

78 Consider an Exercise Stress Test

An exercise stress test measures the heart's response to physical exertion and can give your doctor an idea of how safe it would be for you to exercise and at what intensity you can exercise with relative safety. If you undergo an exercise test, your doctor will ask you to either pedal a stationary bike or walk on a motorized treadmill that increases in speed or grade. Electrodes placed on your chest will monitor your heart activity. Your blood pressure will be monitored, too.

Should you have an exercise test? It depends. The American College of Sports Medicine recommends an exercise test for those who show signs of heart disease—or run the risk of developing it. They feel an exercise test is a good idea for anyone who:

▶ Is 45 years old or older and healthy.

▶ Is over the age of 35 and has a least one coronary risk factor.

▶ Leads a sedentary life.

▶ Has high blood pressure.

▶ Has high cholesterol. (Most physicians now consider cholesterol readings of more than 240 milligrams per deciliter to be high; levels of 200 to 240 milligrams per deciliter are considered borderline high. Readings below 200 milligrams per deciliter put you at below-average risk for heart disease.)

▶ Smokes cigarettes.

▶ Has an abnormal resting electrocardiogram.

▶ Has diabetes mellitus.

▶ Has a family history of heart disease.

▶ Has experienced chest pains during physical activity.

▶ Has been diagnosed as having a heart ailment, pulmonary (lung) disease, or a metabolic disorder.

79 On Your Mark, Get Set, Exercise

The real battle over starting to exercise takes place in your mind, not in your body. Sure, you know you have to shape up, but you may find it hard to get started.

Here are some excuses to "drop-kick" out of your thoughts.

Exercise takes too much time. Twenty to 30 minutes a day, three to five days a week, is all the exercise you need.

I just don't feel like exercising. Exercise can *relieve* sluggish feelings and a general lack of energy. Something as easy as a brisk walk may do the trick.

I've never been the athletic type. Activities like walking, cycling, or swimming require no special athletic ability, making fitness possible even for outright klutzes.

Exercise is boring. It *can* be, but it doesn't have to be. Vary your exercise routine by bicycling one day, swimming the next, and walking the third day. Make exercise a social event by exercising with friends or your spouse. Exercise to your favorite kind of music to overcome any monotony. You could also explore local parks by foot or bike, or try a new route every so often.

80 Set a Goal, Then Go for It

Goals. They're among the most important aspects of fitness. After all, how can you know when you've arrived if you don't know where you're going?

To make fitness goals more concrete, write them down. To formulate your goals, ask yourself the following questions.

▶ How would I honestly rate my current fitness level? Poor? Fair? Good, but could be better? Am I starting at zero or do I want to improve from one level to the next?

▶ Do I want to increase strength? Endurance? Flexibility? Or all three?

▶ Why do I want to become more fit? To look better? Feel more energetic? Boost my spirits? Prevent health problems?

▶ What will it take to reach this goal? Is it reachable for me?

▶ Will the activities I plan to pursue help me achieve my goal?

▶ What obstacles will I have to overcome, and how will I overcome them? (If exercise interferes with mealtime, for example, schedule dinner for later. Or if you tend to forget your workout clothes, keep a few sets in your car.)

▶ How can I measure my progress? By pounds lost? Change in number of colds I get in a year? Need for less sleep? Lower cholesterol levels?

▶ How will I reward myself along the way? Buy a new sweater? Take a day off to loaf? Call an old friend long-distance?

81 Make an Appointment to Exercise— And Keep It

Like many people, you're probably wondering when you'll find the time to exercise when your days are already jam-packed with job responsibilities, family demands, and other obligations.

It's true that trying to fit something new, like exercise, into a busy schedule takes some doing. But it can be done. Here are some pointers to get you started.

▶ Make an appointment to exercise, just as you would schedule any other important obligation, and write it on your calendar.

▶ Choose an exercise or fitness activity that you'll enjoy, so you'll look forward to your workout and be less tempted to skip it. (More about that in Tips 88 through 93.)

▶ Look for openings in your schedule you may have overlooked—after the kids leave for school in the morning, before dinner, or during lunch hours you normally spend with friends or business colleagues.

And one more thing: Don't give up if you occasionally have to skip your workout because of a cold, bad weather, or emergencies. Perfect attendance isn't important.

82 Exercise Early

What's the best time of day to exercise? A study conducted by the Southwest Health Institute in Phoenix, Arizona, showed that 75 percent of morning exercisers were likely to still be at it one year later, as opposed to 50 percent of those who exercised at midday and 25 percent of those who exercised in the evening. It seems that as the day progresses, would-be exercisers are more likely to think of excuses to avoid working out.

Warm-ups should include the following two activities.

83 Warm Up Properly

No exercise session should begin without a warm-up—a few minutes of light activity to get your muscles primed for real exertion. Warming up increases the benefits of exercise and reduces your risk of injury.

And the body does warm up in the true sense of the word—

increased activity increases blood flow to the muscles, and the body gradually begins to shift gears from relative inactivity to higher performance.

The Stretch

Stretching should take 5 to 10 minutes.

To stretch your arms: Hold one arm straight out from your side, level with the shoulder. Make an arc by raising your arm straight up, then lowering it to your side. Hold your arm out again. Swing it across your chest as far as is comfortable. Swing it toward your back as far as it will comfortably go. Now hold your arm straight out in front of you, bending your elbow in a right angle with the palm toward the floor. Without moving your upper arm, move your forearm straight up and then straight down. Alternate arms.

To stretch your back: Stand with your feet spread apart. Clasp your hands high above your head. Lean your head back and look up. Stretch your shoulder muscles as if you were reaching for the sky. Hold for 5 seconds. Relax. Repeat two to four times.

To stretch your legs: Stand erect and balance yourself with your hand against a wall or chair. Bend one knee, grasp that ankle, and draw the leg up and back. Hold. Pull your foot gently until you feel tension (not pain) in your upper front thigh. Hold for 5 seconds or longer. Repeat with your other leg.

Always stretch slowly, gently, and gradually. (Don't bounce!) Breathe normally—don't hold your breath when you stretch. And don't stretch to the point of pain or discomfort. Rather, stretch to the point where you can feel some tension, but not pain. If you feel any pain or discomfort, stop immediately.

The Quick Warm-Up

Spend 5 minutes performing a less intense rendition of your exercise of choice—like taking a brisk walk before you run. This raises your heart rate slightly and leaves you sweating lightly.

84 Follow Up with a Cool-Down

Cooling down is the reverse of warming up, and it helps your body recover from exercise in three ways. A 5-minute cool-down:

➤ Allows the heart rate to slow down gradually.

▶ Reduces the likelihood that your muscles will feel stiff after exercise because it reduces the buildup of lactic acid.

▶ Prevents blood from pooling in the legs.

As with the warm-up, cool down slowly. Perform the activity at a slower pace, and/or stretch (as described in the previous tip).

85 Get Flexible!

To be truly fit, you need to be limber. The following stretches can help you achieve that goal.

Side Stretch

Stand straight with your legs spread comfortably. Clasp your hands above your head. Lean from the waist as far to the right as is comfortable without moving your hip. Repeat, leaning to the left.

Sitting Stretch

Sit on the floor with your legs extended and at least 6 to 10 inches apart. Keeping your back straight, bend forward with arms outstretched as far as is comfortable and hold the position for 8 to 10 seconds. Don't strain or bounce.

Horizontal Leg Stretch

Lie on your back with both legs outstretched. Be sure to keep the small of your back flat against the floor. Bend your right knee and raise it until your foot is a few inches off the floor. Keeping your leg straight, slide your left leg to the left along the floor. Slide it back and lower the other leg. Repeat, alternating legs.

86 Don't Do These Stretches

The following stretches, although popular, may injure you or aggravate an existing ailment, like a troublesome back or other orthopedic problem. Avoid:

The plow. In this stretch, you lie on your back and raise your legs until your feet are resting on the floor behind your head.

The hurdler's stretch. For this one, sit on the floor with one leg extended forward and the other extended behind you, with the knee bent.

The toe touch. This familiar stretch requires you to bend at the hips to touch your toes, with your legs straight and knees locked.

87 Figure Out Your Target Heart Rate

Exercise physiologists have come up with a formula called the target heart rate to help you determine how fast your heart should beat in order to maximize health benefits without overexerting yourself. The basic idea is to exercise about 70 to 85 percent of your maximum capability for at least 20 or 30 minutes three or four times a week. This safety zone is called the target heart rate zone. (It may be dangerous to run your heart at its maximum attainable rate for a prolonged period.)

Here's a simple way to determine your target heart rate.

1. Before you start to exercise, take your pulse. Place your first two fingers (not your thumb) over the arteries of the opposite wrist, over the area where your skin creases when you flex your wrist and in line with your thumb.

2. Count the number of beats you feel for 10 seconds and multiply by six. (This number represents your resting heart rate.)

3. Take your pulse after warming up, midway through your workout, immediately after stopping exercise, and again after cooling down.

Using the table on page 100, determine whether or not you're within your target heart rate zone, based on your age. If your fastest pulse falls below the range for your age, you might need to exert yourself more while exercising. However, the exercise should never seem more than "somewhat hard." If your pulse exceeds this range, slow down and exercise less intensely.

Note: If your peak pulse rate falls below your target heart rate and your legs feel weak, work on developing endurance—by walking more, perhaps—while you try to increase your heart rate. This can help reduce the risk of musculoskeletal injuries like tendinitis or muscle strain in novice exercisers.

88 Walk Your Way to Fitness

Walking is a great way to keep fit without risking injury or buying lots of special equipment. Since walking is probably the most natural form of exercise, almost anyone can do it with ease.

Figure Out Your Target Heart Rate

Age (years)	Target Heart Rate Zone (beats/minute)*	Maximum Attainable Heart Rate (beats/minute)*
25	140–170	200
30	136–165	194
35	132–160	188
40	128–155	182
45	124–150	175
50	119–145	171
55	115–140	165
60	111–135	159
65	107–130	153

*These values are averages. Your target heart rate range and maximum attainable heart rate may vary depending on your fitness level.

Walking keeps you fit because it:

▶ Improves cardiovascular fitness.

▶ Increases the amount of calories burned.

▶ Enhances muscle tone.

▶ Builds stamina.

▶ Aids digestion and regularity.

▶ Helps to relieve tension.

▶ Enhances feelings of well-being.

Although walking comes naturally, you can maximize comfort and benefits if you:

▶ Warm up by walking slowly for 2 to 3 minutes.

▶ Take a few minutes to stretch before and after walking, especially if you walk briskly.

▶ Wear good walking or running shoes with sufficient arch support.

▶ Walk by stepping down on the back of your heels and rolling onto your toes.

▶ Maintain good posture by keeping your head up, shoulders back, and arms swinging freely at your sides.

▶ Breathe deeply and exhale fully.

▶ Cool down by walking at a slower pace for 3 to 5 minutes before you stop.

89 Pedal for Fitness

Riding a bicycle is good for body and soul. Cycling gets you out in the fresh air, leaves you feeling invigorated, and can do wonders for cardiovascular health. And you don't have to ride fast and furiously to benefit from cycling.

Here's what to do to avoid undue muscle aches when you cycle.

▶ To avoid back and knee problems, take your bike to a bike shop and have the handlebars and seat adjusted to fit you properly. The seat should be adjusted so that when one leg is extended and bent slightly, the ball of your foot contacts the pedal at the lowest point of its revolution. Handlebars should be positioned no lower than your seat.

▶ Stretch your shoulders, back, and legs slowly and gently before and after biking.

For details on how to reduce injuries and accidents when cycling, see Tip 324 in chapter 14, Be Smart, Be Safe.

90 Give Water Exercise a Try

Water exercise (or aquatic exercise, as it's sometimes called) is gaining in popularity among people of all ages. Buoyed up by water, you feel light as a feather, and you can move in ways that are otherwise difficult or impossible yet still tone your muscles and improve your circulation, breathing, and endurance. You weigh 90 percent less in water than you do on land, easing the burden on weight-bearing joints like your hips, knees, and back. That means many people who find it difficult or painful to jog or perform other kinds of weight-bearing activities are able to work out with ease in water. Water exercises take place in the shallow end of a pool, in waist- to chest-deep water, and you can usually hold on to the side of the pool for safety and comfort.

Water exercise is excellent for people who:

▶ Are over 50 years old.

▶ Suffer joint pain.

▶ Have weak leg muscles or back problems.

If any of these descriptions fit you, you might want to consider water exercise.

91 Swim the English Channel (or Its Equivalent)

Imagine the pride you'd feel if you could tell people, "I swam the English Channel." As remarkable as it may sound, you can achieve such a feat, without leaving your hometown. Here's how: Assuming one lap equals 60 feet, keep track of how many laps you swim and convert that figure into miles once a week. The English Channel is 21 miles wide, which is the equivalent of 1,848 laps. Looking at it that way, you'll swim the channel in no time. (The Atlantic Ocean is another matter, however.)

You can apply this motivational tool to walking, bicycling, stair-climbing, or running. Using the table on the opposite page, decide on a goal—climbing a well-known mountain or skyscraper, swimming a famous body of water, walking to a faraway city. Then figure out the distance and get moving.

92 Consider Low-Impact or Nonimpact Aerobics

Fitness activities that involve steady, rhythmic motions of your major muscle groups and burn oxygen for more than a brief spurt are considered aerobic. They force your heart and lungs to work at anywhere from 60 to 85 percent of their capacity. Brisk walking or bicycling, for example, are aerobic. So is aerobic dance—informally choreographed routines that combine calisthenics and dance.

Aerobic dance classes became the rage in the early 1980s, but the shock to bones and tendons caused by repeated jumping and bouncing

Distance Guide for Exercise Goals

Stair Climbing

Peak or Building	Distance	Equivalent*
Mt. Everest	29,028 ft.	49,762 stairs
Mt. Rainier	14,410 ft.	24,703 stairs
Empire State Building	1,250 ft.	2,143 stairs
Eiffel Tower	984 ft.	1,687 stairs

Swimming

Body of Water		
English Channel	21 mi.	1,848 laps
Lake Michigan	118 mi.	10,384 laps
Mississippi River	2,348 mi.	206,624 laps
Atlantic Ocean	4,150 mi.	365,200 laps

Walking/Jogging/Cycling

Route		
New York City to Chicago	831 mi.	
Boston to Seattle	3,123 mi.	
Miami to San Francisco	3,147 mi.	
Great Wall of China	3,950 mi.	

*One stair equals approximately 7 inches. One lap equals 60 feet; 88 laps equal 1 mile. Check the length of your swimming pool.

produced a number of injuries. Now, low-impact and nonimpact aerobics have replaced many higher-intensity aerobic workouts. Both are kinder to your skeleton.

Low-impact aerobics are designed so that:

► Your feet stay close to the floor, and only one foot leaves the floor at a time.

► Only moderate jumping is involved.

► Jerky movements are kept to a minimum.

Nonimpact aerobics are designed so that:

► No jumping is involved.

▶ They rely on large muscles of the thighs (as in knee lifts) rather than muscles in the feet and calves (as in jogging and skipping in place).

▶ They require more arm movement than high-intensity aerobics.

93 Rate Your Aerobics Class

Use this handy ten-point checklist to figure out whether an aerobics class is right for you. (You may have to take a class or two on a trial basis to answer all the questions.)

1. Is the instructor well-qualified? (He or she should be certified by the American College of Sports Medicine or by a national aerobics association.)

2. Is the floor firm yet resilient? (It should be made of either wood, with an airspace or a spring cushion underneath, or polyvinylchloride/urethane. Avoid mats—they can throw you off balance.)

3. Is the room air-conditioned?

4. Is there enough space for each participant to move freely, without crowding?

5. Does the routine include a warm-up and cool-down period?

6. Does the aerobic portion of the class last at least 20 minutes? (Your heart rate should reach but not exceed your target heart rate, as explained in Tip 87.)

7. Are you told how to check your pulse before, during, and after the aerobic portion of the class?

8. Does the routine allow participants to adjust the pace to their individual ability? (You should be able to step up the pace or ease off if you need to.)

9. Does the instructor introduce new routines or music from time to time?

10. Do you feel relaxed or invigorated after class? If you feel sore and exhausted, something's wrong.

"Yes" answers mean you've probably found a class that will suit your needs.

94 Choose an Exercise That Suits Your Body Type

Exercise can do wonders to get rid of unwanted pounds and tone up flabby muscles. But it can't turn a short, stocky person into a tall, willowy reed, or a slightly built person into a brawny bruiser. However, your body type may make you better suited to some activities than to others.

Most people fall into one of three categories: endomorphs, mesomorphs, or ectomorphs, based on their overall build, distribution of body fat, muscle tone, and height. (Some people show characteristics of more than one type.)

Endomorphs may be described as:

▶ Chubby, round, or soft looking.

▶ Broader at the hips than at the shoulders.

▶ Small-boned.

▶ Not very muscular.

▶ Carrying a higher-than-average amount of body fat.

Endomorphs are poor candidates for jogging or any activity that calls for high impact with the ground. They're good candidates for low-impact or nonimpact activities like biking, walking, or swimming, which minimize strain on the body frame.

Mesomorphs are usually described as:

▶ Big-boned, with a strong, muscular physique.

▶ Broad-shouldered, with a narrow waist.

▶ Rugged looking.

Mesomorphs are good candidates for walking, and short-distance running (like 5-kilometer races) but not marathons, martial arts, or sports requiring balance, strength, power, and agility (like power lifting, tennis, or boardsailing).

Ectomorphs are usually described as:

▶ Tall, with a long, slender neck.

▶ Having narrow shoulders, chests, and hips.

▶ Relatively long limbed.

▶ Having small wrists and ankles.

▶ Having little body fat.

▶ Having difficulty developing powerful muscles.

Ectomorphs are poor candidates for swimming (since they have so little body fat for buoyancy) and sprinting. They're good candidates for jogging, skipping rope, basketball, tennis and other racquet sports, and cross-country skiing.

SOURCE: *HealthyLife® on Fitness* (Southfield, Mich.: American Institute for Preventive Medicine, 1987).

95 Find Your Fitness Personality

Body type isn't the only trait that determines which activities are best for you, though. You've probably already given some thought to what you'd like, based on whether you prefer group-participation or solo activities, competitive or noncompetitive pursuits, or outdoor or indoor pastimes.

Finding a fitness activity that suits your personality is also a big factor in how much you'll enjoy exercise and stick with it long enough to reap the benefits. Do any of the following descriptions of fitness personalities sound like you? If so, read the "hint for success" that pertains to each one.

The Weekend Warrior

The weekend warrior is sedentary throughout the work week and binges on exercise or sports over the weekend.

Hint: Adding minimal activity (even as little as 15 minutes twice per week) during the week can help condition your heart and lungs, sustain muscular endurance, and prevent strains or injuries on the weekend.

The Fanatic

The fanatic thinks that if a moderate exercise is good, then a lot is better. He or she always tries to work out a little more, a lot harder, or more intensely than others, and feels anxious and irritable if he or she misses a workout.

Hint: Fitness should be a pleasure, not an addiction or ball and chain.

The Social Butterfly

The social butterfly has difficulty sticking with a solo fitness program, and loves to chat and mingle with other participants in a group.

Hint: Don't always depend on group activities or other people to enable you to meet your fitness goals. Be willing to go it alone if you must.

The Cannonball

The cannonball jumps into a fitness program with a burst of energy and determination but loses enthusiasm a few weeks later.

Hint: Don't try to do too much, too soon, or you'll probably burn out after 2 or 3 weeks. It takes 10 to 12 weeks to start to see the results of your efforts.

The Flipper

The flipper dabbles in one activity, then quickly abandons it for another, and is related to the cannonball. Sometimes he or she may remain inactive for long intervals between flurries of activity.

Hint: Real fitness results from consistent efforts, over the long term.

The Analyst

The analyst loves exercise gadgets and equipment. He or she reads lots of fitness books and magazines and likes to talk about the benefits of exercise.

Hint: This is not a problem if you actually pursue the activities you're learning about. But remember, the important thing is to get out and *move*.

SOURCE: *HealthyLife® on Fitness* (Southfield, Mich.: American Institute for Preventive Medicine, 1987).

96 Take Your Exercise à la Carte

Rodney Dangerfield once quipped, "The trouble with jogging is that by the time you realize you're not in shape for it, it's too far to walk back."

Choosing activities that are right for you is important—otherwise you may lose interest or hurt yourself and drop out.

What's more, no one activity will meet all your needs, so take the "cafeteria approach" to fitness. Try a few things to help you decide what suits you best. And don't rely on one activity—that can get stale. Variety helps you stick with your program, too. For example, if you like to play tennis but your partner is out of the game with a cold one week, you can walk, cycle, or swim as a backup plan.

97 Test Your Fitness Level

How do you measure the success of your fitness program? By how much weight you lose? How many inches you trim off your waistline or hips? How well you sleep at night? How energetic you feel?

These are all worthwhile criteria. Another way to evaluate your fitness level—and assess your progress—is to keep track of your resting heart rate (that is, your pulse rate when you're least active).

The idea is, the lower your resting heart rate, the better shape your heart is in. So as you become more fit, your resting heart rate should drop.

Here's how to measure it.

1. Take your pulse as soon as you wake up in the morning, before you get out of bed.

2. Count the number of beats for 10 seconds and multiply by six. This will give you your pulse in beats per minute.

3. Repeat the following morning. Then calculate the average of the two. (That is, add the two numbers together and divide by two.) This is your resting heart rate.

Calculate your resting heart rate every three months, as conditioning takes some time to have an effect.

98 Take the "Talk Test"

No, this isn't a suggestion that you audition to guest host "The Tonight Show" for Johnny Carson. It's just a simple way for you to tell if you're overdoing it when you exercise. If you're too out of breath to comfortably carry on a conversation with another person as you dance, run, or slam-dunk your way to fitness, you're probably working too hard and should slow down. (On the other hand, you should be working hard enough to break a mild sweat.) And of course, any unusual sign of physical distress (such as chest discomfort, pain of any kind, or dizziness) is a signal to slow down to a stop.

99 Three Ways to Tone Your Stomach

Speaking of ways to gauge fitness, medical experts say that carrying as little as 5 to 10 pounds of excess fat around the torso may be related to health risk factors like elevated cholesterol, blood pressure, and blood sugar levels. So a potbelly may be an obvious sign that you're out of shape, outside and in.

The following exercises, when combined with a weight-control diet and calorie-burning exercise, can help you tone your abdominal muscles. Select the exercise that's right for you. (Anyone with lower back problems shouldn't do the intermediate and advanced exercises.)

Head and shoulder curls (beginning exercise): Lie on your back with your legs bent. Touch your fingertips together behind your head at the base of your skull. Keeping your lower back pressed against the floor and using your abdominal muscles, raise your head and shoulders off the floor at a 30-degree angle. *Important:* Keep your spine, neck, and head in a straight line, and don't jerk up and forward. Breathe in as you raise your torso. Hold this position for a count of five, then exhale as you return to the starting position. Repeat this 10 to 15 times.

Sit-ups with arms crossed (intermediate exercise): Lie on your back with your knees bent and your arms crossed over your chest, each hand grasping the opposite shoulder. Curl up to a sitting position, then down to the starting position. Repeat 10 to 15 times.

Sit-ups with fingers laced behind your neck (advanced exercise): Lie on your back with your knees bent and your feet placed 1 foot apart. Clasp your hands together behind your neck, with your fingers interlaced. Curl up to a sitting position and touch your right elbow to your left knee. (Be careful not to pull your head up with your hands, to avoid strain or injury.) Return to the starting position. Curl up to a sitting position and touch your left elbow to your right knee. Then return to the starting position. Repeat 15 to 25 times.

100 A Shopper's Guide to Exercise Equipment

Treadmills, stationary bikes, trampolines, rowing machines, and cross-country ski simulators have been called dream machines because people sometimes expect belts, cogs, pulleys, and wheels to help make all their fitness dreams come true. And exercise equipment is a universal fixture in many homes as well as health clubs.

This "hardware for soft bodies" can provide a good workout. But you have to understand what the equipment is designed to do for you. A stationary bike, for instance, is good for burning calories, toning the lower body, and conditioning your heart. But it won't tighten your abdominal muscles or strengthen your upper arms.

Once you've decided what type of apparatus you need, you can narrow the selection down to the best choice if you:

► Find out if the company who makes the equipment (and the dealer who sells it) is reputable.

► Talk to other people who own the model you're considering (or one like it).

► Decide if the price fits your budget.

► Test the equipment.

► Determine if it's easy to assemble, install, or move, and what maintenance it requires.

► Look for a reasonable warranty.

► Be sure the equipment will challenge you, so you don't "grow out of it" in a short time.

101 How to Buy Sports Shoes That Fit

A carpenter needs a saw, a painter needs a brush, and an accountant needs a calculator. And anyone who's serious about fitness needs a good pair of shoes (or several, if you're active in more than one activity besides swimming). The right shoes can make the difference between comfort and discomfort, between safety and injury, between performing well and not performing well.

Consider these factors before you buy activewear shoes.

► Are the shoes suitable for the sport or activity for which you intend to wear them? Walking, hiking, racquetball, tennis, aerobics, and so forth require differently designed footwear. But you may want to consider cross-training shoes, suitable for several different activities.

► Can you wiggle your toes in the shoes while sitting and standing? (You should be able to.)

► Does the widest area of your foot correspond to the widest area of the shoe? (To find out, try this: Stand on a piece of paper, bend down, and trace a line around each shoe with a pencil. Then slip off your shoes, stand in the same place, and trace a line around each foot with a different colored pencil. If at any point the outline of your feet is larger than the outline of your shoes, you're squeezing some or all of the bones, ligaments, and muscles in each foot.)

▶ Do the inner seams rub against your foot? (They shouldn't.)

▶ Does the shoe have a firm heel cradle and arch support?

▶ Does the shoe provide adequate shock absorption?

▶ Are the shoes comfortable when you move from side to side or when you walk or jump? Test these movements before you buy.

Good shoes don't need to be "broken in." The shoes you buy should be comfortable from the start.

102 Take These Weather-Wise Steps to Exercise

If you live in a climate with distinctly different seasons, you're lucky: You can vary your fitness program with changing conditions. But weather adds more than interest to your routine; it can affect your body's response to exercise. An exercise done comfortably in one season—like jogging in the spring or fall, for instance—can become unpleasant, or even dangerous, if pursued in summer and winter without allowing for hotter or colder temperatures.

In cold, wintry weather:

▶ Try to cover up all exposed skin on windy, chilly days.

▶ Wear a wool hat. You can lose up to 40 percent of your body heat through your head if it's not covered.

▶ Wear three to five layers of lightweight clothing rather than a single layer or two of heavy clothing. A layer of lightweight polypropylene next to the skin keeps moisture from collecting and chilling you.

▶ Move against the wind on your way out and with the wind on your way home. You'll be cutting down on the windchill factor when you're perspiring the most.

▶ Try to avoid running in open areas. Town houses, office buildings, and homes in subdivisions can help to block chilling winds.

▶ Avoid smoking cigarettes or drinking beverages that contain caffeine or alcohol; such substances increase your susceptibility to the cold.

In warm weather:

▶ Wear lightweight, loose clothing that allows sweat to evaporate easily. Don't wear long-sleeved or full-length sweat suits in hot, humid weather. And don't wear rubberized clothing, which prevents evaporation of sweat, the body's way of keeping you cool.

▶ Use a sunscreen to avoid sunburn.

▶ Exercise at a moderate pace.

▶ Drink at least 8 to 10 ounces of plain water 10 to 15 minutes before you start to exercise. And to compensate for fluids lost through perspiration, drink water during your workout, even if you don't feel thirsty.

▶ Work out in the cooler parts of the day—early morning or after sundown.

103 Eating for Peak Performance

No pill or magic formula can instantly turn you into a superathlete. But eating right can help you perform at your best.

Carbohydrates—from bread, pasta, potatoes, and fruit—provide energy for vigorous activity. So active people need to replenish this fuel frequently. Don't expect to get a quick energy boost from a snack you eat just before starting out, though. Instead, consuming a high-carbohydrate food like skim milk and a banana, whole wheat bread, or a glass of orange juice an hour or two before a workout acts like a time-release capsule of energy.

Because you lose electrolytes (potassium, sodium, magnesium, and calcium) in sweat during vigorous activity, drink plenty of water and eat foods that are rich in these minerals. Almost all fruits and vegetables are rich in potassium, but potatoes, bananas, orange juice, winter squash, cantaloupe, sweet potatoes, and cooked beans are especially high. Sodium is rarely lost in quantities greater than amounts you would normally consume, so you don't need to worry about getting extra. (For food sources of magnesium and calcium, see Tip 110 in chapter 4, Eating for Better Health.)

104 When to Eat If You're Going to Exercise

Is it better to exercise and then eat, or eat and then exercise? Follow these guidelines.

► Don't eat much right before a workout, because your body will divert blood to your muscles and away from your digestive organs, disrupting the process of digestion. Generally, it's best to work out 2 to 3 hours after a meal, or an hour or two after a snack.

► Always eat breakfast. If you exercise before breakfast, you may reduce fatigue if you eat a small amount of food—like a small glass of juice or a piece of toast—15 or 20 minutes before you set out.

► If you exercise before dinner or late in the day, make breakfast and lunch your main meals. To boost energy levels, have a late-afternoon snack.

SOURCE: Adapted from *HealthyLife® on Fitness* (Southfield, Mich.: American Institute for Preventive Medicine, 1987).

105 Treat Sports Injuries with R.I.C.E.

Twisted ankles, painful joints, and stiff, sore muscles are some of the injuries most commonly caused by fitness activities. Continuing to exercise when injured can cause further damage and leave you laid up for weeks or months.

At the first sign of serious discomfort or pain, stop what you're doing and apply R.I.C.E.—rest, ice, compression, and elevation. By following this easy-to-remember formula, you can avoid further injury and speed recovery.

► Rest the injured area for 24 to 48 hours.

► Ice the area for 5 to 20 minutes every hour for the first 48 to 72 hours, or until the area no longer looks or feels hot.

► Compress the area by wrapping it tightly with an elastic bandage for 30 minutes, then unwrap it for 15 minutes. Repeat several times.

► Elevate the area to reduce swelling. Prop it up to keep it elevated while you sleep.

Doctors also recommend taking aspirin to reduce the inflammation and pain, if you can take aspirin safely. Take aspirin with a full glass of water or milk to prevent stomach irritation.

Contact a physician if the following signs or symptoms occur.

▶ Severe pain and swelling

▶ Numbness

▶ Blue discoloration of the skin

▶ Misalignment of the extremity

▶ Inability to move the injured body part

106 If You're Sick, Rest

Some exercise enthusiasts find it difficult to suspend their fitness activities even when they're sick with a cold, flu, sore throat, or fever. Give your body a break. The risks of exercising at this time outweigh the benefits.

A fever is a stress to the body. Some studies have shown that adding to that stress by exercising may prolong the illness. So let your body recover and repair itself before resuming exercise.

If you have a cold but not a temperature, you should still avoid exercise. Exercise increases blood circulation and by doing so, may spread the virus or bacteria responsible for your misery to areas it wouldn't ordinarily reach. Also, your lungs may not be working efficiently when you have a cold, so your exercise capacity drops.

A day or two of rest will do you more good than sticking to your workout schedule.

4

Eating for Better Health

Take this short quiz to test your nutritional savvy.

1. Radicchio is (a) the name of a little boy whose nose grows every time he tells a lie, (b) a teenage slang term for "very, very cool," (c) a kind of lettuce high in iron.

2. Cruciferous vegetables (a) are grown primarily in Crucifera County, California, (b) make wonderful subjects for still life paintings, (c) are rich in vitamins and other substances that seem to prevent cancer.

3. Pectin is (a) the muscle between your trapezius and your collarbone, (b) a spray antiseptic for cuts and scrapes, (c) a type of water-soluble fiber that can lower cholesterol.

4. Omega-3's are (a) high-priced Swiss-made watches, (b) an up-and-coming punk-rock band, (c) substances in fish oils that may help prevent heart disease and other health disorders.

The correct answer in each case is (c). If you're not familiar with these terms, you might need to brush up on your nutritional knowledge. Great strides have been made since the days when all you had to know about good nutrition was the names of the four basic food groups. Consider the following discoveries in the making.

▶ Researchers are studying the cancer-resisting potential of beta-carotene, a plant pigment in apricots, squash, and other yellow-orange fruits and vegetables, which the body converts to vitamin A.

▶ Scientists are discovering that fiber (roughage) does more than keep you regular. Certain kinds of fiber, like pectin, can aid in the elimination of bile acids through the intestinal tract, possibly preventing the development of gallstones and colon cancer.

▶ Tests show that people who eat a lot of mackerel, salmon, and other fish high in omega-3 fatty acids tend to have lower levels of triglycerides and total cholesterol (blood fats implicated in heart disease).

And that's just a taste of the kind of exciting new reports on the link between diet and health. Clearly, there's more to protecting your health than counting food groups or popping a multivitamin pill. You have to eat the right foods. Think of this chapter as a road map to guide you to food choices that lead to tip-top nutritional fitness.

107 Eat Whole Fruit

Have you ever wondered whether drinking a glass of orange juice is much different, nutritionally, than eating an orange? Or whether a glass of apple juice is better than an apple?

Fruit juice is a fine alternative to soda or alcoholic beverages. And in some cases, juice is a rich and convenient source of vitamin C. But whole fruit has some advantages over juice. Ounce for ounce, whole fruit:

▶ Is more filling, and therefore satisfying.

▶ Contains fewer calories.

▶ Has more fiber.

Studies show that fiber (present in fruit but not in juice) helps to regulate metabolism of carbohydrates, so sugar in fruit is absorbed more slowly than the same sugar in fruit juice. And when sugar of any kind moves into the bloodstream more slowly, your body releases less insulin, a hormone that regulates blood sugar levels and keeps them from fluctuating wildly. And you feel better when your blood sugar levels are on an even keel.

Be aware, too, that many "juice drinks" contain only a small percent age of real juice. The rest is water, sweeteners, coloring, and flavoring. Whole fruit, on the other hand, is 100 percent fruit.

108 Keep Produce at Its Peak

Produce—fresh fruits and vegetables—is a gold mine of nutrients, usually with a price to match. To get the most nutrition for the "lettuce" you fork over for fresh produce, follow these suggestions.

▶ Select fruits and vegetables that look crisp or feel firm.

▶ When buying citrus fruits and pineapple, choose fruits that feel heavy for their size.

▶ Don't buy produce that's soft or bruised.

▶ Don't buy more than you can use within a few days or store under refrigeration. Produce kept at room temperature ripens—or spoils—more rapidly. That's fine if you're eager to eat an avocado or bananas, but not so great if you want to be able to use every last orange or lemon in the bag.

▶ Don't soak produce in water—nutrients will leach out.

▶ Pat produce dry after washing, to prolong freshness.

▶ Don't cut vitamin C rich fruits or vegetables like strawberries and peppers until just prior to eating. Exposure to the air destroys vitamin C.

109 A Miniguide to Vitamins

The table on page 118 can help you plan a diet that provides adequate amounts of the essential vitamins indicated. Diet, however, cannot always satisfy the need for all vitamins. Pregnancy, menstruation, illness, crash dieting, food allergies, use of medication, or other circumstances may call for vitamin supplements.

Vitamin	U.S. Reference Daily Intake (RDI)*	Food Sources
A	5,000 International units	Liver, eggs, fortified milk and dairy products. The following contain carotene, which converts to vitamin A after they're eaten: dark green vegetables; deep yellow fruits such as apricots, peaches, cantaloupe, carrots, sweet potatoes, pumpkin, squash.
Thiamine (B$_1$)	1.5 milligrams	Lean meat (especially pork), oysters, organ meats and liver, green peas, legumes, collard greens, oranges, asparagus, whole grains.
Riboflavin (B$_2$)	1.7 milligrams	Organ meats, milk and dairy products, oysters, lean meat, chicken, dark green vegetables, sardines, eggs, tuna, whole grains, legumes.
Niacin (B$_3$)	20 milligrams	Liver, lean meat, fish, poultry, nuts, legumes, dark green vegetables, whole grains. The following are good sources of tryptophan, which can be converted to niacin in your body: milk, eggs, meat.
Pyridoxine (B$_6$)	2 milligrams	Lean meat, liver and other organ meats, fish, nuts, legumes, whole grains, poultry, corn, bananas.
Cyano-cobalamin (B$_{12}$)	6 micrograms	Organ meats, lean meat, egg yolks, dairy products, fish (especially shellfish).

Primary Functions	Deficiency Symptoms
Essential for healthy skin, hair, and mucous membranes. Required for normal vision. Needed for proper tooth and bone development and for resistance to infection.	Night Blindness; dry, rough, scaly skin; susceptibility to infection; dry eyes; stunted bone growth; poor tooth enamel, leading to cavities. (Deficiency disease: hypovitaminosis A.)
Release of energy from the carbohydrates in food, appetite regulation, growth and muscle tone, proper function of heart and nervous system.	Loss of appetite, fatigue, mental confusion, moodiness, irritability, forgetfulness, muscle weakness, leg cramps, enlarged heart. (Deficiency disease: beriberi.)
Helps cells use oxygen. Important in metabolism of protein, fat, and carbohydrates. Helps keep skin and mucous membranes (in mouth and lining of digestive tract) healthy.	Skin disorders, especially cracks at corners of mouth; dermatitis around nose and lips; hypersensitivity to light; reddening of cornea; digestive disturbances.
Participates in metabolism of protein, fat, and carbohydrates. Helps cells use oxygen. Promotes healthy skin, nerves, and digestive tract. Aids digestion and fosters normal appetite.	Skin disorders (especially on parts of body exposed to sun); red, swollen, smooth tongue; digestive tract disturbances, including indigestion and diarrhea; mental disorders, including irritability, depression, anxiety, and mental confusion. (Deficiency disease: pellagra.)
Aids in metabolism of protein, fat, and carbohydrates. Assists in formation of red blood cells and antibodies. Involved in sodium-potassium balance.	Dermatitis, cracks at corners of mouth, smooth tongue, irritability, depression, convulsions, dizziness, anemia.
Aids in formation of red blood cells. Maintains healthy nervous system. Aids metabolism of protein, fat, and carbohydrates. Essential for normal growth and development.	Anemia; numbness and tingling in fingers; degeneration of peripheral nerves, brain, and spinal cord; fatigue; poor growth.

(continued)

Vitamin	U.S. Reference Daily Intake (RDI)*	Food Sources
Folic Acid (Folacin, folate)	400 micrograms	Liver and other organ meats, dark green leafy vegetables, asparagus, lima beans, whole grains, nuts, legumes.
Pantothenic Acid	10 milligrams	In all plant and animal foods, but best sources are organ meats, whole grains, fresh vegetables, egg yolks.
Biotin	300 micrograms	Liver and other organ meats, egg yolks, nuts, legumes, cauliflower, mushrooms, green beans, dark green vegetables.
C (Ascorbic Acid)	60 milligrams	Brussels sprouts, strawberries, oranges, broccoli, green peppers, grapefruit, collard greens, cauliflower, cantaloupe, tangerines, cabbage, tomatoes, asparagus.
D	400 International units	Fortified milk, egg yolks, organ meats, fortified breakfast cereals. Vitamin D is formed in skin exposed to sunlight.

Primary Functions	Deficiency Symptoms
Aids in the formation of hemoglobin in red blood cells. Assists in formation of enzymes and other body cells.	Anemia; red, swollen, smooth tongue; diarrhea; poor growth.
Helps in the metabolism of protein, fat, and carbohydrates. Involved in formation of hormones and nerve-regulating substances.	Fatigue, tingling in hands and feet, severe abdominal cramps, nausea, difficulty sleeping.
Helps release energy from protein. Also involved in metabolism of fats and carbohydrates and formation of fatty acids. Works with other B vitamins.	Deficiencies do not occur under normal circumstances. Raw egg whites can destroy biotin, and metabolic disturbances can interfere with use, causing anemia, nausea, muscular pain, fatigue, depression, poor appetite.
Forms collagen to hold body cells together. Helps maintain walls of blood vessels and capillaries. Helps maintain bones and teeth. Helps heal wounds. Helps absorb iron and aids resistance to infection. Prevents destruction of B vitamins through oxidation.	Weakness; fatigue; loss of appetite; weight loss; irritability; slow growth; increased risk of infection; swollen, inflamed, and bleeding gums; swollen and aching joints; easy bruising; nosebleeds; delayed would healing. (Deficiency disease: scurvy.)
Increases absorption of calcium and phosphorus. Assists in several phases of calcium and phosphorus metabolism, aiding in bone and tooth development. Seems to protect against colon cancer in some way.	During growth years: poor bone and tooth formation, bowed legs, stunted growth, muscle weakness (causing protruding abdomen). Later in life: softening of bones; loss of calcium from bones; pain in pelvis, back, and legs; easily broken bones; muscle twitching and spasms. (Deficiency diseases: rickets in children and osteomalacia in older adults.)

(continued)

Vitamin	U.S. Reference Daily Intake (RDI)*	Food Sources
E	30 International units	Plant oils (used in margarine and salad dressings), wheat germ, green leafy vegetables, nuts, whole grains, liver, egg yolks, legumes, fruits, other vegetables.
K	80 micrograms	Green leafy vegetables, cabbage-family vegetables, liver, egg yolks, milk. (Also, bacteria synthesizes vitamin K in the digestive tract.)

* Reference Daily Intakes (RDIs) have replaced the U.S. Recommended Daily Allowances. RDIs are a compilation of the daily nutrient needs of men and women of all ages. Daily Reference Values (DRVs) on food labels give percentages of RDIs.

110 A Miniguide to Minerals

Nutrients like calcium, iron, and zinc are just as essential as vitamins. The table below shows, in capsule form, how much you need, what foods supply significant amount, and the functions various minerals perform. Use it to plan a mineral-rich menu. (As with vitamins, however, sometimes diet alone can't satisfy the need for certain minerals. Pregnancy, menstruation, illness, crash dieting, food allergies, use of medication, or other circumstances may call for mineral supplements.)

Mineral	U.S. Reference Daily Intake (RDI)*	Food Sources
Calcium	1,000 milligrams	Milk and dairy products, sardines, salmon eaten with bones, oysters, tofu, green leafy vegetables, clams citrus fruit.

Primary Functions	Deficiency Symptoms
Protects essential fatty acids and vitamin A from oxidation. Protects red blood cells. Helps cells use oxygen to yield energy.	Red blood cell breakage and muscle weakness. Deficiency is highly unlikely in humans, as vitamin E is widely distributed in foods and stored in the body.
Aids in formation of blood clotting proteins. Aids in regulation of blood calcium.	Tendency to hemorrhage, delayed blood clotting.

Primary Function	Deficiency Symptoms
Needed for building strong bones and teeth and maintaining strong bones throughout life. Required for normal muscle contraction and relaxation, heart action, nerve function and blood clotting.	Stunted growth in children, weakened bones in adults, bones that break easily. (Deficiency disease: osteoporosis.)

(continued)

Mineral	U.S. Reference Daily Intake (RDI)*	Food Sources
Chromium	120 micrograms	Brewers yeast, meat, clams, whole grains, unrefined foods, cheeses, nuts.
Copper	2 milligrams	Organ meats, shellfish (especially oysters), whole grains, nuts, legumes, lean meat, fish, fruits, vegetables.
Iodine	150 micrograms	Iodized salt, sea salt, seafood, seaweed, foods grown in iodine-rich soil, dairy products from animals fed iodine-rich feed.
Iron	18 milligrams	Organ meats, red meat, fish, shellfish, poultry, enriched breads and cereals, egg yolks, legumes, leafy green vegetables, dried fruits, blackstrap molasses.
Magnesium	400 milligrams	Whole grains (especially wheat germ and bran), nuts, legumes, dark green vegetables, seafood, chocolate, cocoa.
Phosphorus	1,000 milligrams	Milk and dairy products, fish, meat, poultry, egg yolks, nits, legumes, peas, whole grains, processed foods, soft drinks.

Primary Functions	Deficiency Symptoms
Works with insulin to take sugar into cells. Involved in breakdown of sugar to release energy.	Impaired glucose metabolism. (May lead to adult onset diabetes.)
Needed for hemoglobin and to make red blood cells. Forms protective coverings for nerves. Part of several enzymes. May be involved with vitamin C in forming collagen. Needed in respiration and release of energy.	Anemia, bone defects, retarded growth, impaired metabolism.
Part of thyroxide, a hormone secreted by the thyroid gland, which helps to regulate growth, development, reproduction, and metabolic rate (rate at which calories are burned.)	Enlarged thyroid gland (goiter), sluggishness, and weight gain. Can cause sever retardation of developing fetus during pregnancy.
Part of hemoglobin, which carries oxygen to cells. Part of myoglobin, which makes oxygen available for muscle contraction. Needed for use of energy by the cells.	Anemia, fatigue, muscle weakness, headaches, pale skin, inability to concentrate.
Builds protein. Needed to release energy from food. Helps relax muscles after contraction. Helps resist tooth decay. Needed for transmission of nerve impulses.	Confusion, nervousness, disorientation, hallucinations. Muscle weakness can progress to convulsions, and ultimately tetany. (Deficiencies are unlikely unless another medical problem exists.)
Aids in building strong bones and teeth. Activates vitamins for use. Needed to release energy from food. Needed for trans-mission of nerve impulses.	Muscle weakness, loss of appetite, bone pain. (Deficiencies are un-likely unless another medical problem exists.)

(continued)

Mineral	U.S. Reference Daily Intake (RDI)*	Food Sources
Potassium	3,500 milligrams	Lean meat, fresh fruits and vegetables, milk and dairy products, nuts, legumes, most salt substitutes.
Selenium	70 micrograms	Organ meats, seafood, lean meats, eggs, whole grains, wheat germ.
Sodium	2,400 milligrams	Salt, soy sauce, monosodium glutamate (MSG)., most processed foods (especially regular soups, sauces, and cured meats), milk and dairy products.
Zinc	15 milligrams	Liver, egg yolks, oysters, lean meat, fish, poultry, milk and dairy products, whole grains, vegetables.

* Reference Daily Intakes (RDIs) have replaced the U.S. Recommended Daily Allowances. RDIs are a compilation of the daily nutrient needs of men and women of all ages. Daily Reference Values (DRVs) on food labels give percentages of RDIs.

111 Wash That Produce!

As a child, you were probably told to wash your hands before you ate. As an adult, you need to wash your hands and what you eat. Agricultural use of pesticides has doubled over the past two decades, despite research linking certain chemicals to nerve damage, genetic defects, and cancer. Since you don't know which fruits and vegetables have been contaminated

Primary Functions	Deficiency Symptoms
Needed for muscle contraction, heart action, nerve transmission, fluid balance. Involved in making proteins. Needed for maintenance of acid-base balance. Required for formation of glycogen (short-term storage of energy).	Muscle weakness, irregular heartbeat, apathy, confusion and loss of appetite. (Deficiencies are unlikely, unless excessive water loss occurs through vomiting, diarrhea, extreme sweating, or use of diuretics.)
Works with vitamin E to act as antioxidant and protect cell membranes.	Heart muscle abnormalities, anemia (rare).
Needed for normal fluid balance, both inside and outside cells; nerve transmission, acid-base balance, and muscle contraction.	Muscle cramps, weakness, mental apathy, loss of appetite. (Deficiencies are unlikely, unless another medical problem exists.)
Works as part of many enzymes. Present in insulin. Needed for making reproductive hormones, normal sense of taste, and wound healing.	Retarded growth, prolonged wound healing, slow sexual development, loss of taste (and as a result, loss of appetite).

with what poison, the ideal preventive measure is to eat only produce you grow yourself, without use of pesticides. But that's not practical for most people. In lieu of that:

> Whenever possible, buy domestically grown produce instead of imported. Studies have shown that produce grown in the

United States contains lower levels of contaminants than foods grown outside the country.

▶ Be especially careful with peaches, celery, cherries, strawberries, and lettuce. A study conducted by the Natural Resource Defense Council, a San Francisco–based consumer group, found that these items were more likely to be contaminated than others. Corn, cauliflower, bananas, and watermelon were less likely to be affected.

▶ Wash fruits and vegetables in soapy water. Rinse thoroughly, then dry.

SOURCE: "Nutrition Action Health Letter," vol. 16, no. 3. (Washington, D.C.: Center for Science in the Public Interest, April, 1989).

112 Adopt a Bone-Builder Diet

Many people assume their bones stop growing when they become adults. Not so. Bone tissue is continuously dissolving and re-forming. One way to maintain strong bones is to eat foods rich in calcium.

Calcium is the most abundant mineral in the body, but your body can't manufacture it: You have to get all the calcium you need from food. Dairy products such as milk, yogurt, cheese, ice milk, and pudding made with milk are storehouses of calcium. (An 8-ounce serving of milk contains about 300 milligrams of calcium.) Milk and milk products also contain vitamin D and other components that help your body absorb calcium, so dietitians recommend two servings of dairy products a day.

Other sources of calcium include green leafy vegetables, cooked beans, fruit, grain products, canned sardines, and salmon with bones. But you'd have to eat large quantities of these foods to come anywhere close to the amount of calcium present in dairy products.

Use the table, Food Sources of Calcium, on the opposite page to plan a diet that meets your needs for calcium. You can determine how much calcium you need by consulting the table, A Guide to Calcium Needs, on page 130. This table was established by the Food and Nutrition Board of the National Academy of Sciences.

113 Easy Ways to Tolerate Milk

For millions of people, drinking milk isn't so easy. People with lactose intolerance can't digest lactose (the sugar in milk), so they can't drink milk or eat milk products without suffering some or all of the following symptoms.

Food Sources of Calcium

Food	Portion	Calcium (mg)
Swiss cheese	2 oz.	544
Provolone cheese	2 oz.	428
Monterey Jack cheese	2 oz.	424
Yogurt, low-fat	1 cup	415
Cheddar cheese	2 oz.	408
Muenster cheese	2 oz.	406
Colby cheese	2 oz.	388
Brick cheese	2 oz.	382
Sardines, Atlantic, drained	3 oz.	372
American cheese	2 oz.	348
Ricotta cheese, part-skim	½ cup	337
Milk, skim	1 cup	302
Mozzarella cheese	2 oz.	294
Buttermilk	1 cup	285
Limburger cheese	2 oz.	282
Ice milk, soft-serve	1 cup	274
Salmon, sockeye, drained	3 oz.	271
Ice cream	1 cup	176
Ice milk	1 cup	176
Tofu	3 oz.	174
Pizza, cheese	1 med. slice	144
Blackstrap molasses	1 tbsp.	137
Broccoli, raw, cut	1 cup	136
Soy flour, defatted	½ cup	120
Almonds	¼ cup	100
Broccoli, cooked, cut	½ cup	89
Soybeans, cooked	½ cup	88
Parmesan cheese, grated	1 tbsp.	86
Collard greens, cooked	½ cup	74
Dandelion greens, cooked	½ cup	74
Mustard greens, cooked	½ cup	52
Kale, cooked	½ cup	47
Chick-peas, cooked	½ cup	40

SOURCES: Adapted from Agriculture Handbook Nos. 8, 8-1, 456 (Washington, D.C.: U.S. Department of Agriculture).

A Guide to Calcium Needs

Age or Category	Recommended Dietary Allowance* (mg)
Children (1-10 yrs.)	800
Teenagers (11-24 yrs.)	1,200
Adults (25+ yrs.)	800
Pregnant and nursing women	1,200
Pregnant and nursing teenagers	1,600

* RDAs are specific dietary recommendations by age and
   sex categories.

Note: The National Osteoporosis Foundation recommends 1,000 milligrams of calcium a day for adults and 1,500 multigrams of calcium a day for postmenopausal women who are not on estrogen replacement therapy (ERT).

▶ Gas in the lower intestine

▶ Abdominal pain and cramps

▶ Bloating

▶ Diarrhea

▶ Nausea

Intestinal distress may occur within minutes of consuming a food containing lactose and sometimes lasts for hours. The problem is a deficiency of lactase, the enzyme responsible for digesting lactose. The only "cure" for lactose intolerance is a milk-free diet. But because milk and milk products are important sources of calcium, avoiding these foods can deprive you of that essential mineral.

To have your milk and digest it, too, try these maneuvers.

▶ Learn which foods are the most difficult for you to digest and avoid them. Some people with lactose intolerance can tolerate certain dairy products if they eat small portions at a time.

▶ Read food labels carefully. Avoid products containing milk, milk solids, or whey solids.

▶ Pretreat milk with the enzyme lactase, commercially available in powder or capsule form as Lactaid. Added to milk 24 hours before you drink it, lactase predigests most of the lactose so you don't have to. Lactase tablets, taken as a digestive aid, are also available.

▶ Purchase Lactaid brand milk, ice cream, and cheese products, which have been treated with lactase, and are available in many supermarkets.

114 Fiber Up

Fiber is an indigestible carbohydrate. It helps people stay healthy by preventing constipation, and in certain forms seems to lower cholesterol levels and prevent cancer. Yet until recently, fiber was processed out of most grain foods like bread and cereal. In pursuit of good health, we've now welcomed back fiber.

The National Cancer Institute (NCI) recommends that everyone take in 20 to 35 grams of dietary fiber a day. Fruits, vegetables, beans, and grains all contain dietary fiber. Dietary fiber consists of two kinds of fiber: soluble fiber (meaning it dissolves in water) and insoluble fiber (meaning it doesn't dissolve in water).

The following foods are especially good sources of soluble fiber, which may be helpful in lowering cholesterol.

▶ Barley bran

▶ Dried beans, cooked

▶ Legumes

▶ Oat bran

The following foods are especially good sources of insoluble fiber, which may protect against constipation and colon cancer.

▶ Corn bran

▶ Nuts

▶ Vegetables

▶ Wheat bran

Most fruits, vegetables, and grain products contain both soluble and insoluble fiber, though, so eating a wide variety of foods can help you get your fair share of both soluble and insoluble fiber.

Note: Many people rely on breakfast cereals as their main source of fiber. While eating a high-fiber cereal is a good start, it's not the whole answer. Many high-fiber cereals supply 10 to 13 grams of fiber per ¼- to ⅓-cup serving. That's a respectable amount. But to get your fiber quota from high-fiber breakfast cereal alone, you'd need to eat two or three times the manufacturer's suggested serving. It's better to include some fruit, vegetables, and beans in your menu later in the day, to balance out your fiber intake.

115 Be a Smart Meat Eater

With medical science indicting a high-fat diet as a major culprit in various diseases, red meat has fallen into disrepute over the past several years. Many consumers have sworn off steaks, burgers, and chops for poultry and fish. Now the U.S. Department of Agriculture reports that, thanks to changes in breeding and butchering techniques in the meat industry, beef and pork are leaner than they were 25 years ago. Also, certain cuts are considerably less fatty than others.

That's good news, because red meat is a good source of protein, and it's rich in important minerals like iron, zinc, and manganese and B vitamins like thiamine, riboflavin, and niacin.

You can continue to eat beef and pork and minimize your risk of gaining weight or developing high cholesterol levels or heart disease by taking the following steps.

► Check the label or ask your butcher what grade meat you're buying. "Select" (previously known as "good") is the leanest. "Choice" is somewhat higher in fat, and "prime" is the fattiest.

► Limit the amount of lunch meat and frankfurters you eat.

► Be careful buying lunch meat and frankfurters labeled as "lite." Some may technically qualify as low in fat because they contain a high percentage of water, but they're usually a poor buy nutritionally.

► Trim fat from meat before cooking.

► Broil or grill meat rather than frying it.

► Limit servings to 3 to 5 ounces each.

► Eat no more than five to seven servings of meat a week.

116 A Safer Way to Bring Home the Bacon

Meats like bacon, bologna, frankfurters, pepperoni, and salami have been cured to stop the growth of bacteria, delaying spoilage. Curing gives these meats their reddish pink hue and distinctive flavor. Scientists have discovered, however, that nitrites and nitrates, compounds used to cure meats, might be converted into dangerous cancer-causing substances called nitrosamines when cured meats are digested. Luckily, scientists also discovered that vitamin C can help to prevent formation of nitrosamines. So now, meat processors must by law include some form of vitamin C in cured meats.

To further ensure the safe consumption of cured meats:

▶ Don't let bacon or other lunch meats sit unrefrigerated for more than a few minutes. They can still spoil at room temperature.

▶ Cook bacon in a microwave oven. This produces lower levels of nitrosamines than pan frying or oven cooking.

▶ Always drain fat from cooked bacon, since drippings contain twice as many nitrosamines as the meat itself.

Despite these precautions, cured meats are still high in fat and sodium, so you should eat only limited amounts regardless of the threat of nitrosamines.

117 Seven Ways to Make Your Barbecues Healthier

One of the most popular rites of summer is the outdoor cookout. Unfortunately, evidence suggests that foods cooked on a charcoal, gas, or electric grill may be hazardous to your health.

The National Academy of Science has discovered a possible link between the grilling of food and the development of what are believed to be cancer-causing compounds. Some researchers suspect that when high-fat, high-protein foods—like hamburgers—are exposed to the intense, searing heat of barbecue cooking, the fat and protein turn into mutagens—chemicals that can damage the genetic material of cells and possibly cause cancer.

Since the jury is still out on whether or not grilled food definitely causes cancer, it's probably wise to reserve barbecuing for special occasions, rather than grill food regularly. Some other guidelines to reduce the potential risks from eating grilled food include:

▶ Before cooking meat or poultry (or fish, if applicable), trim away fat. And don't baste foods to be grilled with butter or oil.

▶ Keep a spray water bottle handy to douse flare-ups.

▶ Position food well above the heat source.

▶ If noticeable amounts of fat drip and flare up as food cooks, lower the flame or move the food to another part of the grill.

▶ Cook food until it's done, but avoid charring it. The longer food is grilled and the blacker it gets, the higher the risk.

▶ To avoid charring fish and vegetables, wrap them in aluminum foil.

▶ Many foods, like chicken, can be boiled or microwaved before grilling, to reduce fat content and grilling time.

118 Eat Fish More Often

While Eskimos probably eat more fat than any other group of people, very few Eskimos get heart disease. The answer to this medical puzzle seems to lie in their fish-rich diet. Cold-water fish like salmon and mackerel contain abundant amounts of omega-3 fatty acids, special substances that seem to benefit the body by:

▶ Reducing blood levels of harmful cholesterol and other blood fats known as triglycerides.

▶ Preventing blood clots from forming in arteries.

▶ Slowing the growth of breast tumors (according to animal studies).

▶ Relieving the pain of migraine headaches (a vascular problem).

▶ Easing the swelling of rheumatoid arthritis.

Omega-3 fatty acids are best consumed in their natural form, from fish, rather than in supplement form. To get more omega-3 fatty acids into your diet, try to eat seafood rich in omega-3's at least two to four times a week. Some good sources include:

▶ Anchovies

▶ Atlantic mackerel

▶ Chinook or pink salmon

▶ Herring

▶ Lake trout

▶ Norway sardines

▶ Whitefish

119 Drink Water, the Nutrient for Every Cell

Two-thirds of your body is composed of water, making it your body's most vital nutrient. Water:

▶ Provides a valuable source of minerals, like calcium and magnesium.

▶ Helps digest food and absorb nutrients into the body.

▶ Carries nutrients to organs via the bloodstream.

▶ Moistens mucous membranes and lubricates the joints.

▶ Carries away bodily waste products.

▶ Cools the body through perspiration.

Many people underestimate their need for water. The average adult should drink six to eight 8-ounce glasses of water (or its equivalent) a day. You can meet part of that quota by consuming high water content foods. Some examples include:

▶ Iceberg lettuce (95 percent water)

▶ Cantaloupe (91 percent water)

▶ Raw carrots (88 percent water)

120 Make Soup!

People sip, slurp, and spoon soup not only for basic sustenance, but also to stay healthy. Chicken soup really *does* help relieve the nasal stuffiness of a cold. And studies show that soup can help you lose weight. Because soup is mostly liquid, it takes longer to eat than solid food. By the time you've sipped the last spoonful, your brain will have noticed that you've eaten, and shut off your appetite. If you'd quickly gobbled down a sandwich, your brain would still be asking "What's for lunch?"

Here are some tips for making soup that's a bowlful of nutrition.

➤ Use skim milk instead of whole milk for creamed or condensed soups. You'll save calories and add calcium, vitamin D, and protein.

➤ Soups that feature vegetables, beans, or rice add fiber and nutrients to your diet.

➤ Add the liquid left over from cooking vegetables to soup stock.

➤ Season homemade soup with herbs and seasonings like parsley, pepper, garlic powder, and onion powder instead of salt.

➤ If you rely on commercially prepared soup for convenience, try to stick with low-sodium varieties.

121 Shake Salt out of Your Diet

Before refrigeration, salt served as a valuable way to preserve food. Unfortunately, in some people, high-sodium diets are linked to high blood pressure, stroke, and an accumulation of fluid, called edema. (Salt is 40 percent sodium and 60 percent chlorine.)

The taste for salt is acquired, not inborn. So it's possible to wean yourself off salt with no ill effects. We've already suggested you make salt-free soups. Here are some other ideas.

➤ Put away your salt shaker, and forget about using it while cooking or at the table.

➤ Use less seasoned salt, soy sauce, barbecue sauce, or other salty condiments.

➤ Buy only unsalted varieties of snack foods.

➤ Avoid foods prepared with salt brine, like pickles, olives, or sauerkraut.

➤ Limit foods like smoked fish, kippered herring, anchovies, sardines, and caviar.

➤ Prepare meals from fresh ingredients instead of relying heavily on commercial products that contain salt or other sodium compounds.

➤ When dining out, ask that foods be made to order, with no salt.

~~122~~ How to Decode Food Labels

How to Decode Nutrition Facts on Food Labels

Nutrition Facts

Serving Size 1 cup (228g)
Servings Per Container 2

Amount Per Serving

Calories 250   Calories from Fat 110

	%**Daily Value***
Total Fat 12g	**18%**
Saturated Fat 3g	**15%**
Cholesterol 30mg	**10%**
Sodium 470mg	**20%**
Total Carbohydrate 31g 10%	
Dietary Fiber 0g	**0%**
Sugars 5g	
Protein 5g	

Vitamin A 4%	•	Vitamin C 2%
Calcium 20%	•	Iron 4%

*Percent Daily Values are based on a 2,000 calorie diet. Your daily values may be higher or lower depending on your calorie needs:

	Calories:	2,000	2,500
Total Fat	Less than	65g	80g
Sat Fat	Less than	20g	25g
Cholesterol	Less than	300mg	300mg
Sodium	Less than	2,400mg	2,400mg
Total Carbohydrate		300g	375g
Dietary Fiber		25g	30g

Calories per gram:
Fat 9   •   Carbohydrate 4   •   Protein 4

All information on the label is based on the serving size listed. Similar food products have similar serving sizes. This makes it easier to compare foods.

This section lists nutrients important to your health. You can use % Daily Value to see how a food fits into your diet. % Daily Value can also help you compare products.

Only Vit A, Vit C, Calcium and Iron are required to be listed on a label. A food company can list other vitamins and minerals if they want to.

* Daily Values are the label reference numbers. These are set by the government and are based on current recommendations. Some labels list the daily values for a diet of 2,000 and 2,500 calories. Your own nutrient needs may be less than or more than the Daily Values on the label.

Here are some common label terms and what they mean:

Low calorie. Has 40 calories or less per serving

Reduced calorie. Has 25% fewer calories than the regular or reference product.

Sugar-free. Has less than 0.5 grams of sugar per serving.

Sodium-free. Has less than 5 milligrams of sodium per serving.

Very low sodium. Has 35 milligrams or less of sodium per serving.

Low sodium. Has 140 milligrams or less of sodium per serving.

Reduced sodium. Has 25 percent less sodium than the reference product.

Lean. Has less than 10 grams of fat, less than 2 grams of saturated fat, and less than 95 milligrams of cholesterol per serving and per 100 grams.

Low fat. Has 3 grams or less of fat per serving.

Low cholesterol. Has 20 milligrams or less of cholesterol and 2 grams or less of saturated fat per serving.

123 Strategies for Reducing Fats and Cholesterol

Coronary heart disease is the leading cause of premature death among Americans. And it's largely self-inflicted: When vital arteries leading to the heart become clogged by fatty deposits of cholesterol, the blockage can lead to a heart attack. Luckily, a few simple changes in eating habits can reduce your risk of heart disease.

▶ Substitute skim or ¹/₂% milk for 2% or whole milk.

▶ Eat less meat and fewer eggs. A good rule of thumb is no more than 3 to 5 ounces of meat per serving and no more than five to seven servings a week, and no more than three egg yolks per week (unless your physician advises otherwise).

▶ Use one egg yolk and two whites for every two eggs required in a recipe.

▶ Trim all visible fat from meat before cooking. Remove skin from poultry.

▶ Bake, roast, or broil meat, poultry, or fish. Don't fry.

▶ Chill soup made from meat or poultry, then skim off the fat before reheating and serving.

➤ Poach foods like fish or eggs instead of sautéing them in butter.

➤ To cut down on the need for oil in cooking, use a vegetable cooking spray and/or pans with a nonstick surface.

➤ Substitute liquid vegetable oil for solid shortening, and replace butter with oil or soft margarine, and use less.

➤ Limit how much oil-based or creamy salad dressing you use. Substitute oil-free salad dressing, lemon juice, or flavored vinegar.

➤ When you use small amount of fats, use olive oil or canola oil. Some research shows they may protect against heart disease.

➤ Bake, steam, or stir-fry vegetables. Don't deep-fry vegetables or sauté them in lots of butter.

124 Go for the Good Oils

Polyunsaturated or monounsaturated oils are often called the good fats because small amounts may actually help to reduce cholesterol levels. They include:

➤ Canola or rapeseed oil (monounsaturated)

➤ Corn oil (polyunsaturated)

➤ Olive oil (monounsaturated)

➤ Peanut oil (monounsaturated)

➤ Safflower oil (polyunsaturated)

➤ Sesame oil (polyunsaturated)

➤ Soybean oil (polyunsaturated)

Monounsaturated oils are preferred because they lower LDL cholesterol (bad cholesterol) without lowering HDL cholesterol (good cholesterol). Polyunsaturated fats tend to lower both.

125 Plan an Anti-Cancer Diet

The American Cancer Society estimates that one-third of cancer deaths that occur in the U.S. each year is due to dietary factors. It's hard to say exactly how much changing your diet reduces the risk of cancer, but it's fair to say that the following steps can help considerably.

Eat less fat, especially from animal sources. These include foods such as beef, pork, butter, cream, sour cream, and cheese. Choose non-fat and low-fat dairy products and other foods low in fat. Replace fat-rich foods with fruits, vegetables, grains, beans.

Eat more fruits, vegetables, and whole-grain products like cereal and bread. Eat at least 5 servings of fruits and vegetables each day. Fruits and vegetables help protect against some cancers due to the vitamins, minerals, fiber, and plant chemicals they contain. Vary your choices. Foods with whole grains (wheat, rice, oats, and barley) also contain vitamins, minerals, and fiber which have been associated with a lower risk of colon cancer. Have 6 to 11 servings of whole-grain breads, cereals, etc. each day.

Eat fewer cured, grilled, or smoked foods. When eaten in excess, these foods may increase the risk of stomach and esophageal cancer. This increase may be due to one or more of the following: nitrites and nitrates they contain; their high fat content; or changes that occur when they're cooked or processed.

Limit consumption of alcohol, if you drink at all. Combined with cigarette smoking, over-consumption of alcohol has been shown to increase the risk of cancer of the mouth, esophagus, and larynx. Also, alcohol may promote breast cancer regardless of whether you smoke or not. Excessive drinking also contributes to liver cancer. Cancer risk increases with the amount of alcohol consumed. The risk may start to rise having as few as two drinks per day. A drink is defined as 12 ounces of regular beer, 5 ounces of wine, or 1½ ounces of 80-proof distilled spirits, like vodka or whiskey.

Be physically active and maintain a desirable weight. Obesity is associated with an increased risk of cancers of the colon and rectum, prostate, breast (for women past menopause), endometrium, and kidney. Lose weight if you are overweight. Exercise on a regular basis.

126 Get Up and Go with Better Breakfasts

Could you expect to get very far driving a car that is low on gas? Of course not. Yet many people embark on the day's activities without eating breakfast, not even thinking about its effects on their performance. The American Dietetic Association says, "Tests prove that the physical skills, intellectual performance, and attitude toward achievement all suffer in people who don't eat breakfast."

If you could do better with breakfast but don't seem to have the time or the appetite for a morning meal, try these strategies.

▶ Plan your breakfast the night before, so you don't have to deliberate in the morning when you're rushed or half awake.

▶ Pack a quick breakfast "to go" the night before. Bag a couple of cheese cubes, some crackers, and a piece of fruit and eat them on the way to work or school.

▶ Don't limit yourself to traditional breakfast foods like toast and cereal or ham and eggs. Any nutritious food is fine if it appeals to you. If you prefer pita bread stuffed with tuna fish and tomato wedges, for example, help yourself.

▶ If you don't have much of an appetite in the morning, eat small portions. Have half a slice of toast or half a bowl of cereal with a few ounces of milk, for instance. Then eat a piece of fruit or a cup of plain yogurt later, when your appetite wakes up.

▶ Start your day with a good source of vitamin C. Strawberries, grapefruit, and oranges are refreshing wake-up foods, and one serving will meet the recommended allowance for vitamin C.

▶ Include a good source of protein with your breakfast. Research suggests protein foods can help keep you alert. In that respect, milk with cereal or toast is better than just fruit or fruit juice. So is a glass of milk and an English muffin topped with pineapple bits and sprinkled with cinnamon. Avoid ham, sausage, and eggs, though; they're high in saturated fat and, in the case of eggs, cholesterol. Avoid commercial pastries, croissants, and muffins; they tend to be high in sugar, fat, and calories.

127 Getting Your Kids to Eat Right

Persuading your child to develop good eating habits can be a challenge, to say the least. Here are some pointers.

▶ Start your child's day with a good breakfast. Hot cereal is an excellent alternative to oversweetened breakfast foods customarily pitched to kids.

▶ Buy snacks that are low in fat, sugar, and salt. Fresh fruit, unbuttered popcorn, whole-grain muffins, juice, milk, and yogurt are tasty, nutritious foods that appeal to kids. Crackers with small amounts of peanut butter or cheese are also acceptable between-meal treats.

▶ Limit fast-food meals. A steady diet of fast-food menu items tends to be high in fat and generally doesn't provide all the essential nutrients a child needs.

▶ Don't punish or reward behavior with food. Punishing children by withholding food can deprive them of required nutrients. Rewarding them with food can encourage overeating and weight gain.

▶ Set a good example. Children can't be expected to adopt good eating habits if parents don't.

For nutrition-packed school lunches:

▶ Try sandwiches, using turkey, chicken, peanut butter with no added oil or sugar, and low-fat cheese or tuna fish instead of processed lunch meat.

▶ Pack finger foods like grapes, carrot sticks, celery stalks, and other fruit or crunchy vegetables instead of potato chips. Single-serving cans of fruit or applesauce are also handy ways to round out a lunch.

Beware of convenience foods that claim to be nutritious. Here are some of the traps to look out for.

Fruit drinks.   Some contain only a small percentage of fruit juice and considerable amounts of added sugar.

Breakfast bars.   These usually contain lots of sugar and very little in the way of nutrition.

Prepopped popcorn.   Some popcorn products are rife with oil, salt, and artificial coloring.

Teach Teens to Snack Wisely

Once kids reach their teens, they tend to eat what they want, when they want it. But these years of rapid growth and change call for added nutrients—nutrients they might lack if their diets are hit-or-miss. And as their bones grow rapidly, teens need plenty of calcium. Adolescent girls need plenty of iron to offset iron lost due to menstrual flow.

If the right foods are available, between-meal snacking can actually boost a teen's intake of those critical nutrients.

▶ Leftovers, like chicken drumsticks, are high in iron and make good late-night snacks.

▶ Low-fat milk, yogurt, and cheese can provide needed calcium.

▶ Keep the kitchen stocked with whole wheat crackers, sliced watermelon, fruit salad, and other ready-to-eat alternatives to junk food.

▶ Encourage teens to invent their own, easy-to-eat snacks, like "ants on a log"—celery stalks stuffed with peanut butter and dotted with raisins.

128 Nine Tips for Healthier Fast-Food Meals

Fortunately for the 50 million Americans who eat at fast-food restaurants each day, choices are no longer limited to burgers, fries, and shakes. Many chains now offer salads, baked potatoes, soups, and whole wheat products in addition to traditional selections. Here are some suggestions for more nutritious fast-food meals.

▶ Avoid fried foods. Choose baked or broiled instead.

▶ If you order fried food, remove the breading (it sops up most of the grease).

▶ Order pizza with mushrooms, onions, or peppers instead of pepperoni and sausage.

▶ Avoid mayonnaise-laced salads. Instead, opt for fresh, unadorned fruits and vegetables.

▶ Steer clear of bacon bits, croutons, rich salad dressings, and fried noodles.

▶ Use high-sodium condiments like mustard or pickles sparingly. (And don't salt fast food—it doesn't need it.)

▶ Ask for low-fat milk, fruit juice, or plain water instead of milk shakes or soft drinks.

▶ Use low-fat milk instead of cream or nondairy creamer in your coffee or tea.

▶ Avoid high-fat, calorie-rich pastries and desserts—they offer very little nutritionally.

129 What to Know about Irradiated Food

Have you seen the Radura symbol on fruits or vegetables in your supermarket? If so, do you know what it means?

This symbol indicates that the food has been irradiated, a method of food preservation approved for use on produce by the Food and Drug Administration. Irradiation kills microorganisms that spoil food. Irradiated food isn't radioactive, irradiation leaves no residue on food, and it doesn't affect flavor. Proponents of irradiation say it reduces the need for chemicals typically used to keep food fresh longer.

Those who oppose irradiation say essential nutrients in food may be destroyed, that eating food that's been irradiated may cause cancer or other debilitating conditions, and that irradiation may be hazardous to the employees and residents of the area surrounding a food irradiation site. But studies haven't conclusively identified any harmful effects of food irradiation.

CHAPTER

5

Weight Loss: Tipping the Scales in Your Favor

According to a survey conducted by the U.S. Department of Health and Human Services, 37 percent of the people in the United States (27 percent of men, 47 percent of women) are trying to lose weight at any one time.

Put another way, some 60 million Americans are overweight. Why so many? Because overeating is just plain easy—*too* easy. Magazine ads and television commercials for foods tempt us. Food is the focus of many social gatherings. Fast-food restaurants make eating on the run convenient. And quite simply, food tastes good.

Since excess weight contributes to a variety of diseases—including high blood pressure, diabetes, and heart disease—developing strategies to curb overeating is of the utmost importance.

Yet simply making up your mind to eat less may not work. So in this chapter, you will find a smorgasbord of hints that cover a wide range of weight-control strategies. Among other things, you'll learn how to assess your eating habits, find tasty snacks that are less than 100 calories, order less fattening food in a restaurant, and diet during the holidays. In short, you'll learn how to tip the scales in your favor.

130 Determining Your Ideal Body Weight

When assessing your body, it's natural to compare your weight to what others weigh. A better gauge, though, is a weight chart, like the Metropolitan Life Insurance Company's desirable weights table, below.

Desirable Weights for Adults

Men
(wearing shoes with 1″ heels)

Height	Small Frame	Medium Frame	Large Frame
5′ 1″	112–120	118–129	126–141
5′ 2″	115–123	121–133	129–144
5′ 3″	118–126	124–136	133–148
5′ 4″	121–129	127–139	135–152
5′ 5″	124–133	130–143	138–156
5′ 6″	128–137	134–147	142–161
5′ 7″	132–141	138–152	147–166
5′ 8″	136–145	142–156	151–170
5′ 9″	140–150	146–160	155–174
5′ 10″	144–154	150–165	159–179
5′ 11″	148–158	154–170	164–184
6′ 0″	152–162	158–175	168–189
6′ 1″	156–167	162–180	173–194
6′ 2″	160–171	167–185	178–199
6′ 3″	164–175	172–190	182–204

SOURCE: Adapted from *Statistical Bulletin,* Metropolitan Life Insurance Company, vol. 40, no. 3, (November/December, 1959).

NOTE: In indoor clothing, age 25 and over. (For women between 18 and 25, subtract 1 pound for each year under 25.)

Women
(wearing shoes with 2″ heels)

Height	Small Frame	Medium Frame	Large Frame
4′ 8″	92–98	96–107	104–119
4′ 9″	94–101	98–110	106–122
4′ 10″	96–104	101–113	109–125
4′ 11″	99–107	104–116	112–128
5′ 0″	102–110	107–119	115–131
5′ 1″	105–113	110–122	118–134
5′ 2″	108–116	113–126	121–138
5′ 3″	111–119	116–130	125–142
5′ 4″	114–123	120–135	129–146
5′ 5″	118–127	124–139	133–150
5′ 6″	122–131	128–143	137–154
5′ 7″	126–135	132–147	141–158
5′ 8″	130–140	135–151	145–163
5′ 9″	134–144	140–155	149–168
5′ 10″	138–148	144–159	153–173

131 Find Out If You're Overweight or Overfat

Many people fret about how much they weigh. The real issue of concern is what percentage of their body weight is made up of fat. The ideal is about 16 percent for men and about 20 percent for women. Standard height and weight charts ignore this issue.

Here's a simple test to do at home to determine if you are fat, or exceed the average level of body fat.

The Pinch Test

Pinch a fold of skin from these three areas.

- Upper side of upper arm
- Midway up the back of the thighs
- Just to one side of your abdomen

Measure the thickness with a skin caliper or ruler. If you can pinch 1 inch or less of flesh, your body fat level is low or moderate. Every ¼ inch above that represents 10 pounds of excess fat.

Knowing your level of body fat is critical if you've been on a crash diet or if you've lost weight quickly, because unless you've been exercising regularly, the loss may be in muscle tissue, not in actual body fat. In other words, you may *look* slimmer, but still be over*fat*. A scale will not show this, but a measurement of body fat will.

132 Set a Weight-Loss Goal You Can Reach

Do you set out to lose 15, 20, or 30 pounds every year or so, only to find yourself stuck after the first 5 or 10? If so, do you quit out of discouragement?

There may be nothing wrong with your rate of weight loss. Your ability to set realistic goals may be the problem. If you'd like to increase your odds for success, try setting smaller, interim goals you can reach quickly. These are called short-term goals.

First, your goals need to be measurable. For instance, don't tell yourself you have to "lose lots of weight." You can't measure "lots of weight." So decide on a set number of pounds you want to lose. Then, break your overall goal down into realistic minigoals. A realistic minigoal would be to lose 5 pounds in three weeks, for example.

As you achieve your first couple of "minigoals," you'll feel better sooner. After you reach each milestone of 5 or 6 pounds, set the next reachable goal, and so on. Small achievements add up, and keep motivation where dieters need it—high.

133 Figure Out Your Daily Calorie Quota

Calories add up to pounds. So one way to watch your weight is to determine how many calories you should eat each day.

The following formula is designed to produce weight loss of approximately 1 pound per week—a safe amount that's most likely to *stay* off.

1. Determine your goal weight (see the desirable weights table.)

2. Multiply that figure by 10 if you are moderately active. (That is, if you bicycle, walk, swim, or participate in similar activities three or more times a week.) If you are more active than average, (that is, if you participate in aerobic dance, circuit weight training, racquetball, jogging, or other vigorous activities three or more times a week or work at a physically demanding job) multiply by 12. If you are fairly inactive, tend to lose weight slowly, or are over age 45, multiply by 9. (If you rarely, if ever, do anything more strenuous than sewing, reading, or playing cards, you are inactive.)

3. For example: Desirable weight = 130 pounds; activity level = 10 (moderately active); 130 x 10 = 1,300 calories per day.

4. To figure out how many calories a week you should be consuming, multiply the daily total by 7. It's more realistic and practical to try to average a certain number of calories per week than to try to hit an exact number per day, because we all have days when we eat more—or less—than average.

Note: Do not eat less than 1,000 calories per day. It is best not to eat less than 1,200 calories per day. You need this many calories to avoid nutritional deficiencies or serious health consequences.

134 Don't Crash Diet

In their great zeal to be thin, many dieters put their health in jeopardy by trying to lose too much weight too fast. Eating too few calories and rapidly shedding pounds can be unsafe. Your body and your frame of mind can be adversely affected by such drastic changes in eating.

For one thing, dropping 5 to 10 pounds in just a couple of weeks doesn't allow enough time to learn new eating behaviors, so chances are old eating patterns--and the weight--will return. For another, losing weight too rapidly is a strain on your heart and other vital organs, zaps your energy, and increases the risk of nutritional deficiencies. In addition, losing weight rapidly increases muscle loss, which makes it more likely that you will regain the weight.

The following may be signs that you're losing too much weight too fast.

▶ Anemia
▶ Apathy
▶ Depression
▶ Hair loss
▶ Headaches
▶ Irritability
▶ Kidney stones
▶ Lethargy
▶ Listlessness
▶ Liver impairment

If you are uncertain about the calorie content of foods, purchase a calorie guide to make sure your intake does not fall below the levels that physicians say are safe.

135 Trim the Fat and Trim Pounds

The average American consumes about 37 percent of calories from fat. That's about 10 percent too much.

Fat is the most concentrated source of calories. One level tablespoon of oil or shortening, for example, has 120 calories! Yet less than half the fat in most foods is actually visible. So it's a good idea to know which foods harbor hidden fat. Reading labels for fat content is one way to start. Here are some other helpful hints to cut back on fat in the diet.

▶ Reduce the serving size of red meat.
▶ Substitute poultry or fish for red meat.
▶ Trim all visible fat from steaks, chops, and other fatty meats.

▶ Use nonfat or low-fat dairy products like nonfat yogurt or skim milk.

▶ Avoid pastries.

▶ Eat cereal and toast for breakfast instead of eggs and breakfast meats.

▶ Limit consumption of snacks like potato chips and crackers.

▶ Use mustard or nonfat yogurt in place of mayonnaise on sandwiches.

▶ Use less salad dressing or try an oil-free variety.

▶ Use less butter (a teaspoon instead of a tablespoon, for example).

▶ Avoid fried foods.

136 Keep Fat at Bay with Water Each Day

If you're looking for a magic potion to help you lose weight, look no farther than your faucet. Water, often taken for granted, is an important addition to a successful diet. It is recommended that adults drink six to eight 8-ounce glasses of water per day. Reducing diets should include plenty of water because:

▶ Water makes you feel full, thereby suppressing appetite.

▶ Adequate amounts of water will help rid the body of metabolized fat and waste.

▶ Water may help to relieve constipation, which is a common problem when dieting.

Here are some ways to make water more interesting and fun to drink.

▶ Garnish a glass of water with an orange slice or a wedge of lemon or lime.

▶ Drink sparkling water, either plain or mixed with some fruit juice.

▶ Drink flavored bottled water. (Check the labels; many are calorie-free, but many are not!)

▶ Drink water from an attractive goblet or wine glass, or use a special coaster under your water glass.

▶ Take an occasional "water break." Set aside a few minutes at work or home just to relax and drink a refreshing glass of water.

137 Put Your Menu on a Diet

Careful menu planning can make the difference between gaining, maintaining, or losing weight. Look at the caloric differences between the three meal plans shown on the opposite page. Make a point to plan each day's meals in advance and select food items with their caloric value in mind. (Note that you can reduce calories without cutting back drastically on how much you eat simply by selecting low-fat foods.)

138 Develop Supermarket Savvy

A successful weight-control effort begins with smart food purchases.

Here's how to maneuver your way through the supermarket and also stay in control of your weight.

▶ Plan your low-fat meals and snacks in advance, then, using a list, shop only for what you need.

▶ Stay away from the aisles where pastries, potato chips, candies, or other potential problem foods are located.

▶ Shop for food after you've eaten, not when you're hungry. You'll choose food based on clear thinking, not hunger pangs.

▶ Choose fresh foods and vegetables over processed foods, which can deliver unwanted calories in the form of sauces and thickeners.

▶ Don't try to rationalize buying high-calorie snack foods for others in the household. Having them around may very well undermine your weight-control efforts.

▶ Beware of high-calorie foods that, although advertised as "specials," don't do your diet any special favor.

139 Tips for Dining Out without Pigging Out

People who are watching what they eat can stick to their diets anywhere—even in restaurants! Eating establishments don't have to be automatic waistline expanders, if you observe the following recommendations.

▶ Choose a restaurant that offers a wide variety of food, to increase the odds of finding fewer fatty, highly caloric foods.

Calorie Counts for Three Different Menu Plans

4,000 Calories	2,200 Calories	1,200 Calories

Breakfast

2 oz. sausage	1 egg fried in 1 tsp.	1/2 cup oatmeal
2 eggs fried in 2 tsp.	margarine	1 slice dry toast
margarine	1 slice toast with 1 tsp.	1 small orange
2 slices toast with 2 tsp.	margarine	1 cup skim milk
margarine	1/2 cup orange juice	1 cup black coffee
1/2 cup orange juice	1 cup 2% milk	
1 cup whole milk	1 cup coffee with 1 tsp.	
1 cup coffee with 2 tsp.	sugar and 1 tbsp.	
sugar and 2 tbsp.	cream	
cream		

Lunch

Reuben sandwich (2 oz.	Reuben sandwich (same	Chicken sandwich (2 oz.
corned beef, 1 oz.	as on left)	chicken, 1 tsp.
Swiss cheese, 1	12 oz. diet cola	mayonnaise, 2 slices
tbsp. mayonnaise,		whole wheat bread)
sauerkraut, 2 slices		1 medium apple
rye bread)		4 carrot sticks
1 oz. potato chips		12 oz. diet cola
12 oz. cola		

Dinner

2 martinis (3½ oz. each)	1 martini (3½ oz.)	8 oz. sparkling water
T-bone steak (1 lb. raw,	T-bone steak (same as	3 oz. baked fish
6 oz. edible), broiled	on left)	Medium baked potato
Large baked potato,	Medium baked potato,	with 1 tsp. margarine
with 1/4 cup sour	with 1 tsp. margarine	1/2 cup cooked broccoli,
cream	Lettuce salad with 1	with 1/2 tsp.
Lettuce salad with 2	tbsp. Italian dressing	margarine
tbsp. Italian dressing	1/2 cup cooked broccoli,	1/4 cantaloupe
1/2 cup cooked broccoli,	with 1 tsp. margarine	Black coffee
with 1/4 cup		
hollandaise sauce		

Snacks

Cherry pie à la mode	1/6 qt. ice cream	1 cup skim milk
(1/6 of medium pie		2 graham crackers
with 1/6 qt. ice		
cream)		

SOURCE: The Weight No More® program, developed by the American Institute for Preventive Medicine, Southfield, Michigan, 1983, 1989.

► Avoid "all-you-can-eat" restaurants.

► Ask to have the bread basket (or at least the butter dish) removed from the table.

► Refuse french fries, potato chips, and desserts, even if they're included in the price of your meal.

► Ask for food broiled without butter, salad without dressing, and baked or steamed food that's normally fried.

► If servings seem especially large, portion off the excess and put it aside before you begin eating.

► Leave some food on your plate, or take it home for tomorrow's lunch.

► Share one meal with a companion.

► Order à la carte so you won't feel obligated to eat side dishes just because you've paid for them.

Partying Down to a Slimmer You

As with most festive occasions, food plays a prominent role at most parties. It gives people something to look at, something to do, something to talk about, and something to remember. But you don't have to stay home just because you're dieting.

Here are some ways to join the party and not blow your diet.

► At a buffet dinner, first look over all the food presented, then decide what you will and will not eat.

► If possible, inquire ahead of time as to what will be served at a party. If nothing on the menu is allowed on your diet, plan to eat at home first.

► Ask your host or hostess if you can provide a platter of raw vegetables or other low-calorie offering, so you'll be assured of something you can munch on during the party.

► To avoid being tempted to eat hors d'oeuvres and snacks, don't sit near them.

► Politely inform your host and hostess of your diet and ask them not to coax you to overeat.

► Choose mineral water or diet soda instead of alcoholic beverages, or at least alternate them with alcoholic drinks.

► Make a point to socialize with other people or enjoy the entertainment rather than concentrating on eating.

140 Good Cheer for Holiday Dieting

Big holiday coming up? Don't panic. With a good game plan and strategic planning you and your diet can not only survive holidays but you can actually thrive on them. Holidays do not have to be a time of feast or famine—you can strike a happy balance between gorging and self-sacrifice.

▶ Review your eating habits from the previous year's celebration. Does food take center stage at Thanksgiving, Christmas, Fourth of July, and other big holidays? Do you genuinely enjoy foods like fruitcake, for example, or do you just eat them out of custom and tradition?

▶ Decide which customary holiday food habits you could easily change. (If you like to cook out for the Fourth of July, for example, consider barbecued chicken without skin instead of hot dogs.)

▶ Before digging in at a big holiday feast, imagine how you will feel after eating it. Visualize the bloated, uncomfortable, and guilty feelings you've experienced on past occasions.

▶ Forget about being "perfect" on holidays. Stringent dieting may be unrealistic and you could sabotage your efforts by setting standards that are too high. Don't set yourself up for failure by only thinking of what you can't have. Concentrate instead on what is available on your diet plan.

▶ Learn to be festive without depending on alcohol. A drink here, a toast there—the calories of alcohol can add up. Substitute club soda or mineral water for alcohol.

▶ If you're invited to someone's home for dinner, ask if you can contribute a dish, then make it low-calorie. (And be sure to make plenty. Low-calorie foods are usually very popular.)

▶ Remember that the major purpose of the holidays is to enjoy family and friends. Food and alcohol are secondary factors.

141 Selecting Snacks under 100 Calories

Snacking seems to be an integral part of many people's lifestyles, but when you're trying to lose weight, your choices need to be prudent. Whether you crave crunchy, salty, fresh, or sweet foods, there's a variety of food that will satisfy you yet help you lose weight.

The table below lists 25 snacks that are all less than 100 calories each!

Snack Food	Calories
28 gumdrops	97
1/2 cup vanilla ice milk	92
Fudgsicle	91
1 cup tomato soup made with water	90
1/2 cup plain nonfat yogurt with 1/2 cup fresh strawberries	86
5 vanilla wafers	85
2 saltines with 2 tsp. peanut butter	84
6 oz. grapefruit juice	80
1 cup fresh pineapple	77
1 slice raisin bread	70
2 tbsp. raisins	70
10 jelly beans	66
2 graham cracker squares	60
1 sesame breadstick	56
2 cups plain popcorn	50
3 ginger snaps	50
1 oz. slice "reduced-fat" cheese	50
1 cup fresh strawberries	45
1/4 cantaloupe	40
1 medium plum	36
1 medium carrot	30
2 slices melba toast	30
1 cup consommé	29
1 cup diet gelatin	20
2 stalks celery	16

142 How to Turn Your Cookie Jar into an Activities Director

Has your cookie jar always been a source of temptation? Does the urge for a snack send you to the goodie stash on top of the refrigerator or in the kitchen cupboard? Don't get rid of the cookie jar, just get rid of the cookies and use the jar to store reminders of things you can do besides eat. On separate slips of paper, jot down tasks you would like to do or activities you'd enjoy. Be very specific, and stick to tasks which can be completed in 5 to 20 minutes. That rules out things like "Read *War and Peace*," of course. But you could include "Read five pages of *War and Peace*."

Following is a brief list of hypothetical examples to give you ideas.

▶ "Call Aunt Marge from bedroom phone." (Stay out of that kitchen!)

▶ "Get rid of three items of clutter."

▶ "Call Tom to schedule an exercise 'date.' "

▶ "Manicure nails."

Write down as many tasks as you can, one per slip of paper. Then fold each slip and put them in your cookie jar. Next time the urge to snack hits, go raid your cookie jar.

143 Debunking Myths on Exercise and Weight Loss

Exercise is a critical component in any effective weight-control regimen. Unfortunately, some people have misconceptions about weight and exercise. Here are some of the more common popular fallacies.

Myth: Exercise increases your appetite.

Fact: Appetite is actually more manageable after exercise. Furthermore, any slight increase in food intake from physical exercise is more than offset by calories expended by the exercise.

Myth: In order for exercise to be worthwhile, you must work out every day.

Fact: Three times a week for around 20 minutes each time will burn off a significant number of calories. (Of course, if you exercise longer—say, 45 minutes to an hour—you'll burn even more calories.)

Myth: Exercise must be extremely vigorous to achieve weight loss.

Fact: Moderate exercise like walking, if done on a regular basis, can be effective. Daily 30-minute walks can burn up to 15 pounds a year.

Myth: The more you sweat, the faster you lose weight.

Fact: There is no benefit to excessive sweating. It can even be dangerous. So don't overdress for exercise, and don't wear "sauna suits."

Myth: Aerobic exercise is no better than any other form of exercise for weight loss.

Fact: Aerobic exercise (like cycling, walking, or swimming) speeds up your metabolism for 4 to 8 hours after you stop exercising. Therefore, additional calories will be burned off long after you finish working out—an advantage over nonaerobic exercise like weight lifting, which does not speed up your metabolism.

144 Exercise Your Calories Away

Research has shown that dieting alone will not produce permanent weight loss. Any successful weight-loss program should emphasize both what you eat and how you exercise.

Don't just sit around wondering when those extra pounds will come off. Check with your physician first to see if you're ready for exercise, then get moving with the "moderate" and "vigorous" calorie burners in the table below.

Calories Burned by Various Activities

Activities	Energy Costs (cal./hr.)
Sedentary (60–150 cal./hr.)	
Sitting, writing, card playing, etc.	114
Lying down or sleeping	90
Sitting quietly	84
Moderate (150–350 cal./hr.)	
Golf (twosome, carrying clubs)	324
Tennis (recreational, doubles)	312
Swimming (crawl, 20 yds./min.)	288
Volleyball (recreational)	264
Horseback riding (sitting trot)	246
Light housework, cleaning, etc.	246
Dancing (Ballroom)	210
Walking (2 mph)	198
Bicycling (5 mph)	174
Canoeing (2.5 mph)	174

Activities	Energy Costs (cal./hr.)
Vigorous (350 + cal./hr.)	
Circuit weight training	756
Cross-country skiing (5 mph)	690
Jogging (10-min. mi., 6 mph)	654
Bicycling (13 mph)	612
Racquetball	588
Aerobic dancing	546
Swimming (crawl, 45 yds./min.)	522
Football (touch, vigorous)	498
Basketball	450
Tennis (recreational, singles)	450
Scrubbing floors	440
Ice-skating (9 mph)	384
Roller skating (9 mph)	384

SOURCE: Adapted from *Exercise & Weight Control* (Washington, D.C.: President's Council on Physical Fitness and Sports, 1986).

NOTE: Hourly estimates based on values calculated for calories burned per minute for a 150-pound person.

145 Don't Let Appetite Triggers Shoot Down Your Diet

When you eat may be influenced by triggers or cues in the environment. Perhaps you associate eating with events like watching television, talking with friends, or reading. Over time, responding to such frequent cues can lead to weight gain.

The following behavior changes can help to eliminate eating cues that can sabotage your diet.

▶ To make you more aware of your eating cues, keep a diet diary, noting where you were and what you were doing when you ate.

▶ Eat in only one room of the house.

▶ Eat each meal at the same time each day.

▶ Don't do anything else while you're eating.

▶ When you go to parties, focus your attention on the guests, entertainment, surroundings—anything but food and beverages. (See Tip 139.)

▶ Turn down the volume or switch channels during food commercials on television to help you tune out eating cues.

146 Keep a Weight-Loss Diary

Many people enjoy writing in diaries. A written record of your thoughts and experiences allows you to express feelings, look back on good days and bad, and learn from your ups and downs. But a diary can also help you lose weight.

People tend to forget those quick couple of cookies nibbled before lunch or the few bites of food you sampled while preparing supper. It all adds up, though. By keeping a diary of every bite you eat, you'll be more aware of exactly how much you actually consume on a daily basis. (This alerts you to automatic eating you may not be aware of.)

Try it for a week. Write down the following information in a diary.

▶ When you eat.

▶ What you eat and how much.

▶ Where you are at the time.

▶ If you eat alone or with others.

▶ Your mood at the time.

▶ Alternative foods you could have chosen.

▶ After a week, review your diary and ask yourself, "Is there a negative eating pattern here? Can I change it?"

147 Calorie Burners You'd Be Better Off Without

Physical exercise is an excellent way to burn calories. There are some "mental" exercises, however, that we would be better off not engaging in, even though they may burn off a few calories. They are listed in the table on the opposite page.

Exercises in Futility

Activity	Calories Burned
Throwing your weight around (Depending on what you weigh)	25–450
Digging your own grave	222
Beating your head against the wall	221
Chomping at the bit	214
Climbing the walls	193
Running around in circles	187
Making mountains out of molehills	179
Grasping at straws	170
Wrestling with your conscience	150
Swallowing your pride	148
Bending over backward	126
Pushing your luck	103
Beating around the bush	101
Dashing your dreams	98
Jumping to conclusions	87
Putting your foot in your mouth	52
Beating your own drum	42
Spinning your wheels	37
Jumping on the bandwagon	36
Fishing for compliments	29

SOURCE: Adapted from a list developed by Donald McDonald, Northwestern Memorial Hospital, Chicago, Illinois.

148 Knowing When *Not* to Weigh Yourself

If you weigh yourself every day, you'll regret it. Of course, daily weigh-ins are tempting. When you're working so hard to stay on a diet, you're eager to see how you're doing. But weighing yourself more than once a week may undermine your efforts. Here's why:

▶ A moderate, acceptable weekly weight loss is around 1 pound. This comes out to an average of 2.3 ounces per day, which most scales do not register.

▶ You could easily get discouraged if no weight loss is recorded on a particular day. After a week, your weight loss is more likely to register.

▶ As much as 70 percent of your body weight consists of water. Your weight on the scale can go up and down daily due to fluctuations in water, so you can't judge how well you did on your diet yesterday by what you weigh today. Consistent progress over many weeks is a true indication of fat being lost.

▶ Don't become obsessed with the weight registered on your scale. The important issue is whether or not you're learning new eating habits and exercising regularly. As you improve your eating and exercise habits, you will lose weight.

149 How to Help a Heavy Child Lose Weight

A heavy child or teenager carries a psychological burden, especially if he or she is the only family member with a weight problem. What's more, people who are heavy as children have more difficulty in controlling their weight later on, as adults.

Concerned family members can take positive actions that help the child lose weight and promote emotional support at the same time. The basic premise is to make weight control a group effort and not focus on the child. In other words, rather than single out the heavy child for his or her eating habits, the entire family should try to adopt a healthy diet and other weight-control habits.

Focus attention on these activities.

▶ Family participation in fitness or sports activities. Going for a hike or bike ride as a family not only creates an opportunity to exercise, but can bring family members closer together.

▶ Make it a household rule to limit the amount of high-calorie snack foods brought into the home.

▶ Teach all family members how to prepare healthy meals and snacks. Make a commitment to avoid high-fat foods for *everyone's* well-being.

▶ Praise each family member's existing healthy habits. Note who takes the best care of their teeth, hair, or skin, for example.

▶ Set up health goals for each family member so that the heavy child isn't the only one working on improving health.

150 Painless Ways to Eat Less without Starving

It's not always what you eat that determines whether or not you lose weight. Sometimes, small changes in the *way* you eat can help eliminate those extra pounds. Try these suggestions.

▶ Eat smaller amounts of food more often, and eat at least half of your intake earlier in the day (to increase your metabolism). You'll burn off more calories that way. (Eat no more than six times a day—including snacks—however.)

▶ Use small plates, so portions look larger.

▶ Put less food on your fork or spoon, and take smaller bites.

▶ Chew slowly, and pause between mouthfuls.

▶ Wait 10 minutes before snacking. (The urge might pass.)

▶ Don't prepare snacks for other people.

▶ If you feel like bingeing, put on tight clothes—it will discourage you.

▶ Choose more high-fiber and high-water foods like celery, watermelon, and plain popcorn. (You get more to eat without eating very many calories.)

▶ Mentally imagine yourself thinner—it'll keep you going.

▶ Keep low-calorie snacks easily available.

▶ Never skip breakfast.

▶ Don't eat anything after dinner.

▶ Brush your teeth after every meal. (You'll be less inclined to continue nibbling.)

▶ Eat only if you feel relaxed to avoid "nervous munching."

▶ Take the light bulb out of your refrigerator—it will cut down on "search-and-consume" forays.

▶ Drink lots of water every day, to suppress appetite.

▶ Never starve yourself all day in order to eat a special dinner. (You'll be more likely to *over*eat.)

151 Reward Yourself for Weight Loss

When a behavior is followed by a reward, the behavior is more likely to be repeated. So the more you are rewarded for your weight-loss efforts, the more likely you'll continue to succeed.

But you don't have to wait until you lose weight to reward yourself. Rewards should begin the very first day of your diet. (Of course, food should *not* be a reward.)

Here are just a few examples of the kinds of rewards that can help you to adhere to your weight-control plan.

▶ Buy yourself a bouquet of flowers.

▶ Call a friend long-distance.

▶ Give yourself some special "me" time.

▶ Try a new cologne.

▶ Get your car washed.

▶ Have a low-calorie picnic. (The picnic is the reward, not the food.)

▶ Treat yourself to a movie.

▶ Keep a diary of all the improvements you notice while dieting (more stamina, feeling attractive, fitting into smaller-size clothing).

152 How to Survive a Dieting Setback

Everyone experiences occasional setbacks, especially people on diets. The trick is to prevent a minor slip from becoming a major disaster that thwarts your long-term weight-loss goals.

The most determined dieter cheats once in a while—it's only human. Don't chastise yourself or give up because you've had a slip-up in your eating plans. Remember, a temporary setback does not equal a permanent failure!

Here's what to remember when you go astray.

▶ Setbacks are a natural part of learning self-control.

▶ Acknowledge your mistake and plan how you'll respond to a

similar situation the next time. Make it work to your
advantage.

▶ Remember, long-term success is still quite possible.

▶ Give yourself positive feedback. If you eat half of a candy bar,
for instance, praise yourself for not eating the whole thing.

153 Practice Positive Imagery
to Avoid Bingeing

Research has shown that we can strongly influence our behavior by
what we think, whether it's positive or negative. Use this four-step approach to avoid the urge to binge or overeat.

1. Write down a reason to control a binge (for example, "I'll die of a
heart attack," "I look fat," "My stamina will be reduced," "I'm out
of control").

2. Then formulate a clear image of this negative consequence in
your mind. Concentrate on it for a full 20 seconds.

3. Now write a brief description of a positive mental picture. This
should be a pleasant image that is soothing to you (for example,
watching a sunset or taking a peaceful stroll in a park).

4. Imagine this scene and concentrate on it for a full 20 seconds.

The chances are that this image will short-circuit the desire to binge.

154 Lose Weight by Cleaning Up
Your Psychological Pollution

Smile when you push away those french fries, because maintaining
a positive attitude is important for anyone watching their weight. And it
requires some extra effort because—let's face it—trying to lose weight is
probably not your idea of fun.

Basically there are two kinds of attitudes you can adopt: negative or
positive.

▶ People with a negative attitude undermine their own efforts.
They see weight loss as a form of self-denial only, an ordeal to
be suffered through. People with a negative attitude perceive

that something of great value has been denied. They pollute their minds with this negative thinking in much the same way that we pollute our air and water. As a result, they soon begin to feel sorry for themselves and end up eating to relieve those feelings of loss and denial.

▶ People with a positive attitude approach weight control as an opportunity for improvement, self-enhancement, and self-control. A positive attitude enables a dieter to focus on what can be gained in terms of satisfaction, self-esteem, and better health rather than what is lost.

To clean up your "psychological pollution," stick to your goals, memorize or write down this credo, called the Dieter's Dictum, and repeat it to yourself often.

I do not think of weight control as "giving up my problem foods." To give something up denotes that it has some value. Overeating has no value to me. I view eating management as "getting rid of my problem foods" much like I get rid of the week's garbage.

SOURCE: Many of the hints in this chapter were adapted from the Weight No More® program, developed by the American Institute for Preventive Medicine, Southfield, Michigan, 1983, 1989.

CHAPTER

6

Success over Stress

Stress kills. Witness the downing of an Iranian civilian airliner by a U.S. Navy ship in July 1988.

Two hundred ninety people died because radar operators on the American ship, the *Vincennes*, mistakenly convinced themselves that the aircraft was hostile and about to attack their ship. (It wasn't.) The fiasco was blamed on crew error arising from the psychological stress of facing combat for the first time.

A dramatic example, perhaps, but telling. Threats—real or perceived—create stress. As for what triggers stress, suffice it to say that any change in the status quo—good or bad, real or imagined—causes stress. Marriage or divorce, job loss or the threat of being fired, even the disappointment of not getting a coveted promotion, all create stress. So do countless other situations.

Inside, your body reacts to stress by preparing to *do* something—fight, kick, scream, cry, run away. But in most situations, none of these options is acceptable. The adrenaline flows, blood pressure increases, breathing speeds up—for what? You can't usually fight or flee, so you just stew in your own juices. And then you get sick. In fact, the American Academy of Family Physicians states that approximately two-thirds of all visits to family doctors are for stress-related disorders. And obvious discomforts—like insomnia or headaches—aren't the only health problems that have been linked to stress. Heart disease, low back pain, and alcoholism—along with just about every disease affected by the immune system—are at least partly affected by the inability to handle what life dishes out. So even if you don't end up firing on civilian aircraft, you might end up seriously hurting yourself.

The good news, though, is that you don't have to stew under stress. You can learn to view changes as challenges, opportunities, or blessings—anything but threats. In this chapter, you'll learn a variety of skills that can enable you to cope more effectively with stress. Some tips will help you prevent stress, while others can short-circuit a stress response once you feel it coming on. As a result, you'll live a happier and healthier life.

155 How to Cope with Emotional Fender Benders

Death, divorce, or disease may top the list of major stressors, but a pileup of minor hassles can be just as stressful. Those petty annoyances and irritations—like waiting in line, getting overcharged by the dry cleaner, or tripping over your kid's skateboard for the hundredth time—can leave you tense or frustrated. But like death and taxes, minor hassles are equally impossible to avoid.

What you need are ways to buffer their impact. One survey found that people most frequently shield themselves against these kinds of stresses by:

▶ Sharing their feelings with a spouse or romantic partner.

▶ Sharing their feelings with friends.

▶ Completing a task that gives them satisfaction.

▶ Getting enough sleep.

▶ Maintaining good health.

To further offset the emotional damage wrought by minor hassles, think of things that are going *right*. Ask yourself:

▶ Did you hear any good news today?

▶ Did you arrive anywhere on time—or *earlier* than expected?

▶ Did anything you were expecting to receive arrive on time?

▶ Did anyone pay you a compliment?

Focusing on the positive in this way is good psychological protection against the effects of chronic stress.

156 Five Simple Ways to Reduce Stress

Sometimes stress is subtle. But very often, stress practically hits you in the face. When that happens, practice these easy techniques.

▶ Get some physical exercise. A quick walk around the block frees your mind from what's bugging you, gets your blood circulating, and boosts flagging energy levels. *Regular* exercise—with a green light from your doctor—is even better.

▶ Take a warm bath or shower, which tends to relax tense muscles and calm nerves.

▶ Talk over your troubles with a friend, relative, or professional counselor. A "sympathetic other" can sometimes help you to see a problem more clearly—or help you think of practical solutions.

▶ Count to ten when you're so upset you want to scream. It buys you time, so you can reflect on what's bothering you and calm down.

▶ Pour yourself a cup of warm herbal tea. Sip it slowly and savor its soothing warmth and aroma.

157 "Rehearse" for Stressful Events

If you've ever mentally rehearsed a speech before you gave it, you may already have some idea of how advance playacting can help you prepare for stressful situations. (Athletes, musicians, salespeople, and actors do it all the time.) The idea is to *imagine* yourself feeling calm and confident in an otherwise stressful situation, so you can relax more easily when the situation arises. Here's how it's done.

▶ Close your eyes and unwind, releasing every bit of muscular tension your body has accumulated.

▶ For a minute or two, concentrate on simply feeling relaxed.

▶ For the next minute or so, think of yourself actually doing whatever you're practicing for, rather than observing yourself doing it.

▶ Concentrate again on feelings of calmness.

▶ Visualize the event once again, and re-create as many details as possible. (What is the setting? What are you wearing? Who else is present?)

▶ Imagine yourself continuing to feel calm as you successfully handle the anticipated situation.

▶ Imagine a positive outcome—your boss congratulating you on a job well done, your spouse volunteering to pitch in around the house, and so forth.

Use this technique to prepare for any stressful situation—your performance review, a confrontation with your spouse, or other tense occasion. Practice twice a day for 5 minutes each time (preferably when you first wake up in the morning and when you're ready to go to sleep at night). Imagining that you're confident and successful increases the likelihood that you *will* be confident and successful in real life, because you're creating new mental pictures of yourself. After practicing regularly for a few weeks to prepare for various events, you'll be able to relax when the real situations occur.

SOURCE: Smokeless® program, developed by the American Institute for Preventive Medicine, Southfield, Michigan, 1983, 1989.

158 How to Relax, Muscle by Muscle

Contradictory as it may sound, you can learn a lot about relaxation from tension. By alternately tensing and relaxing your muscles, group by group, you can induce a wonderful sense of head-to-toe relaxation.

Dubbed Progressive Deep Muscle Relaxation by Edmund Jacobson, M.D., who invented the technique, this exercise requires only a few minutes to master and is an efficient way to release accumulated tension. (It's often called Progressive Relaxation, for short.)

Here's how to perform Progressive Relaxation.

1. Sit in a chair and close your eyes. Rest your forearms on the sides of the chair, palms downward.

2. Take a few slow, deep breaths.

3. Concentrate on whatever muscle tension you may be feeling, but do nothing about it.

4. Command yourself to "tense" and tighten a muscle group for 5 seconds, then tell yourself to "relax" and let the tension dissolve for 30 seconds. Follow this sequence for each body part listed below.

— Bend both arms at the elbows and wrists. Make a fist with each hand. Relax.

— Press your back against the chair. Relax.

— Tighten your abdomen. Relax.

— Lift and extend your lower legs. Relax.

— Tighten your jaw. Relax.

— Squinch your eyes. Relax.

— Tuck your chin against your chest. Relax.

5. Continue to breathe slowly and deeply.

6. Concentrate on the overall sensation of relaxation and allow your body to go limp like a rag doll. Let your head and shoulders drop forward.

7. Imagine you feel energizing warmth flowing through your body.

8. Slowly open your eyes and note how refreshed you feel.

Note: Don't hold your breath during the tensing phase, and don't tighten any region of the body that's weak or injured.

159 Use Your Imagination to Unwind

Imagination can make a cloudy day sunny—and overpower stress. Here are three ways to create mental pictures that offset daily stressors.

Music. Choose a recording you find soothing. Find a quiet, calming environment in which to listen to it. Feel yourself become part of this calming environment of sound, a physical extension of every note. If your thoughts stray, simply release them and refocus on the music. When the music ends, compare the way you feel to how you felt before listening to it. (You should feel more relaxed.)

Colors. Imagine two colors, one (like bright red) representing tension, and the other (like pale blue) representing relaxation. Close your eyes and imagine that your muscles are the "tense" color. Then imagine each muscle changing to the "relaxation" color. End the exercise by imagining that your entire body is now a vivid hue of the relaxation color (like vivid blue), symbolizing complete relaxation.

Paint a picture. If you have trouble visualizing abstract concepts like tension and relaxation, substitute concrete images that connote these feelings. Use symbols that can interact, like jagged rocks to symbolize tension and rolling waves to symbolize relaxation. Then imagine the waves slowly smoothing out the surface of the rocks. An alternative: Imagine warm sunlight (relaxation) gradually melting icicles (tension) until they disappear.

160 "Remember" to Relax with Biofeedback

Whenever you're tense, your pulse speeds up, your muscles tighten, your skin perspires, and your hand temperature increases. These changes can be easily monitored by a biofeedback machine, a device that provides "feedback" in the form of sounds or lights that go off in response to the tension and relaxation. Then by doing specific relaxation exercises like autogenic training (see the following tip), Progressive Relaxation (see Tip 158), or imagery (see the previous tip), you can alter the physical stress responses. In short, the machine tells you when you're tense so you can know how it feels—and then learn to relax.

You've probably already used some forms of biofeedback without even realizing it. When you weigh yourself, the numbers on the scale showing how many pounds you weigh—and how much you have to lose—are biofeedback. When you take your temperature with a thermometer, that's biofeedback, too. Biofeedback machines are much more sophisticated than a thermometer or scale, and it takes a professionally trained biofeedback therapist to coach you on how to use them.

Yet, while most biofeedback techniques require coaching, you can practice the following methods on your own.

Take your pulse. A rapid pulse is a sign of tension. So taking your pulse before and after practicing a relaxation technique can tell you whether you're relaxing or not.

Measure your hand temperature. A simple hand-held thermometer can show you whether or not you're relaxing effectively. (The warmer your hand, the greater the degree of relaxation.)

Take a good look at yourself. Stand in front of a full-length mirror and look for signs of tension in your face, shoulders, or neck. Are your eyes red, puffy, or tired? Are your lips pursed? Is your jaw tight? What is your appearance telling you about your frame of mind? If stress is written all over your face, take steps to relax.

161 Command Yourself to Relax

Imagine scraping your nails across a blackboard or biting into a raw lemon. Either thought probably made you cringe—the power of suggestion is that strong. Used correctly, suggestion is yet another effective stress-management tool.

A technique called autogenic training is based on the power of suggestion and was developed many years ago to reduce muscle tension in chronic headache sufferers. Basically, you give yourself a series of verbal commands geared to induce feelings of either heaviness or warmth. "Heaviness" commands promote muscle relaxation; "warmth" commands relax the blood vessels, so blood flows more freely, triggering sensations of warmth. Together, the two sensations promote relaxation.

Here's how it's done.

1. Choose a quiet environment with no distractions. Dim the lights and wear comfortable clothing. Sit in a comfortable chair and close your eyes.

2. Start with your right arm (if you're right-handed) or your left arm (if you're left-handed), and slowly give yourself these verbal clues:

— My arm is heavy. (Repeat three times for each arm.)

— My leg is heavy. (Repeat three times for each leg.)

— Both my arms and legs feel heavy. (Repeat three times.) It might help to visualize small weights attached to your arms and legs.

3. Follow the same sequence for the "warmth" commands:

— My arm is warm. (Repeat three times for each arm.)

— My leg is warm. (Repeat three times for each leg.)

— Both my arms and legs feel warm. (Repeat three times. It might help to imagine your arms and legs submerged in warm bath water or basking in sunlight.)

4. To complete the exercise, take a deep breath and say, "I am calm."

Note: People with certain medical or psychiatric conditions (like severe depression) shouldn't practice relaxation without first checking with their physicians.

162 Float Away Stress

Imagine yourself effortlessly floating in water that's about 93.5°F—not too hot, not too cold. You're in total darkness. All is silent except for the comforting sounds of your own breathing. In this pleasurable and totally stress-free environment, every muscle feels deeply relaxed. Your thoughts wander, but you don't really think about much of anything.

What you're experiencing is R.E.S.T. (Restricted Environmental Stimulation Therapy)—more commonly known as flotation therapy. In this stimulus-free setting, your heart and breathing slow down, muscle tension dissolves, and stressful feelings disappear. To achieve this state of bliss, all you have to do is sign up for a session in a float tank at a flotation center. The tank is slightly longer than a bathtub and contains very salty water that allows you to effortlessly float on your back. Some tanks have no lighting or sound; others are in a room that is dimly lit and has recorded music of your choice piped in. Float sessions last for an hour or so.

Flotation has benefits other than reducing stress.

▶ Listening to instructional tapes while floating can sharpen learning skills.

▶ Flotation can help to control blood pressure.

▶ Regular flotation sessions can help to alleviate arthritic pain, other types of chronic pain, and nausea resulting from chemotherapy.

Note: Flotation may not be appropriate for everyone. Anyone who is being treated for a mental health problem should check with his or her therapist before considering flotation therapy.

163 Don't Be Afraid to Cry

Most people say they feel better after a good cry, and tears of joy, sadness, or relief may be a very healthy outlet for stress. Tears of joy, for example, relieve the intense emotions generated by happy occasions. But shedding emotional tears also seems to alleviate stress in a more subtle manner.

University of Minnesota researchers who are studying the chemical composition of tears have isolated two important chemicals, leucine-enkephalin and prolactin, in emotionally shed tears. The researchers say that leucine-enkephalin may be an endorphin, one of the natural pain relievers released by the brain in response to stress. William Frey, Ph.D., a biochemist and the leader of the research team, suspects that tears cleanse the body of substances that accumulate under stress. In other words, crying seems to be an appropriate way to respond to stress. (Tears released in response to an unemotional activity, like cutting an onion, didn't contain such chemicals.)

Conversely, to resist crying may be harmful to your health. It's possible that men develop more stress-related illness because they don't cry as freely as women do.

So if you feel like crying, let the tears flow.

164 Laugh Your Cares Away

Laughter's medicinal powers have been recognized for centuries. The ancient Greeks believed laughter was an essential part of the healing process. And studies now show that laughter can promote better blood circulation, stimulate digestion, lower blood pressure, and prompt the brain to release endorphins and other compounds that reduce pain. So don't be surprised if some day you hear your doctor say, "Take two aspirins and call me with a joke in the morning."

To get your healthful daily ration of giggles and guffaws:

➤ Pretend you're viewing your surroundings through the lens of "Candid Camera." Focus on silly and offbeat things people do. This helps you lighten up and brightens your outlook.

➤ Take some time each day to read or listen to something funny—the comics or a taped comedian, for example.

➤ Don't just smile—laugh out loud.

➤ When confronted by a rude salesperson or an overbearing co-worker, imagine them wearing nothing but a diaper—they'll seem less intimidating.

➤ Try to incorporate good-natured humor in meetings, memos, and conversations. Humor helps to develop trust, sell ideas, and strengthen relationships.

➤ Always keep humor upbeat and positive. Laughter generated at someone else's expense is counterproductive.

➤ Don't be afraid to laugh at yourself.

➤ And remember, he (or she) who laughs, lasts.

165 Learn to Accept Criticism

Are you thin-skinned? If critical remarks (or perceived criticism) are unduly painful for you, learning to put them in perspective can reduce their impact.

But why does criticism hurt in the first place? Part of the reason is fear that the criticism may be warranted—that you are indeed too fat, too slow, too loud, or whatever barb has been lobbed in your direction. The other factor may be low self-esteem. If you don't feel so good about yourself, you're more apt to take criticism to heart. On the other hand, if you feel fairly self-assured, the negative remarks of others are more likely to bounce off.

Still, a fair amount of criticism may be valid—and just what you need to correct a fault. In order to decide just how much attention a critical remark warrants—or what you should make of it—ask yourself:

► Does the criticism seem reasonable? Is there some truth to what was said? (Perhaps you should pay attention to the remark.)

► Have I been criticized by other people on the same issue? (If so, maybe it warrants attention.)

► Does the person making the critical remark know what he or she is talking about? (If he or she is a self-appointed critic-at-large, ignore the remark.)

► Was the remark really directed at me, or was the critic venting general frustration, anger, or bitterness at something over which I have no control? (If criticism stems from general dissatisfaction, let it slide.)

► Is the criticism based on a difference of opinion? (If so, don't overreact.)

If you decide that the criticism is valid, you can consider taking positive steps to improve. If it's unwarranted, forget it.

166 Just Say No to Stressful Thoughts

When nagging thoughts or worries stand in the way of feeling good, a technique called thought stopping is an effective way to eradicate them. The trick is to recognize negative thoughts, then reduce their impact.

Here's an example: You're so distressed by a petty remark a co-worker makes, you can't concentrate on anything else, and you dwell on it for hours. Here's what to do.

1. Isolate the stressful thought.
2. Close your eyes and focus on it briefly.
3. Count to three.
4. Shout "Stop!" (Or, if others are in earshot, imagine a stop sign, a flashing red light, or the word "stop" in bold letters.)
5. If the thought's still present, repeat steps 3 to 5.

6. Resume normal activity, feeling better.

You can use this technique anytime you find yourself obsessed with negative thoughts. (If work problems dominate your thoughts, substitute an "off duty" sign for the stop sign in the exercise described above.)

167 Ward Off Worry in Five Easy Steps

We're a nation of worrywarts. The National Institute of Mental Health reports that anxiety is the most frequently reported mental health problem. Nearly 13 million Americans spend the better part of their day feeling anxious. That's a lot of worry.

What *is* worry, anyway? It is a stream of thoughts focused on the fear of what *might* happen.

Here's a five-step plan to minimize needless worry, developed by psychologist Thomas Borkovec, Ph.D., at Pennsylvania State University. The idea is to acknowledge that you have something worth worrying about, but limit the time you spend worrying to a reasonable level.

1. Identify your own symptoms of worry, like inability to concentrate, sweaty palms, or feeling as though you've got butterflies in your stomach.

2. Set aside a period of ½ hour every day for the sole purpose of worrying.

3. Write down a list of things that you plan to worry about during the assigned period.

4. Use your worry time as a problem-solving session, to work on solutions and remedies.

5. If you find yourself worrying at other times of the day, distract yourself by actively pursuing a chore or deliberately thinking about something else, or use thought stopping (see the previous tip).

168 Slow Down!

Most people expect too much of themselves. Attempts to accomplish too much in a short period of time causes lots of unnecessary stress. The result is something doctors call hurry sickness, a constant state of rushing around trying to meet an endless line-up of self-imposed deadlines. Stress is the inevitable by-product of this frenetic level of activity.

Here's how to turn your activity meter to "slow" instead of "go."

► Leave your wristwatch at home on days you don't absolutely have to be somewhere on time.

► Practice doing one thing at a time instead of two or three things at once (like talking on the phone and reading your mail).

► Make a deliberate effort to speak more slowly. Don't cut other people off in midsentence.

► Walk at a slow, steady pace, not a racewalker's clip.

► Smile and greet people instead of occupying your thoughts with where you're headed or what you're going to do next.

► Drive no faster than the posted speed limit.

► Get used to waiting in line without getting agitated.

► Allow a buffer zone of 15 minutes between appointments, to give your brain and body some stress-free "breathing space."

► Schedule some free time into every day. It's not a waste of time to rest and do nothing.

► Take time to "smell the roses"—that is, to notice beauty and appreciate the little things in life.

169 Budget Your Time

Time: We can't make it, borrow it, sell it, or stop it. All we can do is spend it. Time is egalitarian, too. We each receive exactly the same amount: 24 hours a day, seven days a week. Yet some people use their time far more effectively than others. How do they accomplish this miracle?

Make a "to do" list.   Write down what you have to do, what you ought to do, and what you'd like to do. Then systematically check off items that you get done. This is gratifying, and gives you some idea of your progress.

Prioritize.   Categorize every activity as either A (top priority; must be done soon), B (less priority; should be done fairly soon), and C (least priorty; can wait indefinitely). Forced to decide among various tasks, you'll know what to spend your time on.

Avoid overcommitment.   Know your personal limitations, how much time you have available, and what you can realistically expect to accomplish.

Know the difference between activity and productivity.
Activity—making a lot of phone calls, reorganizing your paperwork—
may or may not lead to accomplishment. Productivity—taking steps toward a solution or goal—leads to results. Whenever possible, choose to
be productive rather than active.

Analyze the time wasters in your day. Make a list of activities
that steal time away from productive work: people who drop in to chat
and hang around too long, unsolicited phone calls or meetings you don't
really need to attend. Then devise ways to eliminate intrusions.

Create quiet time. Let people know when you're available and
when you can't be interrupted. Close your door and turn on your answer-
ing machine (or have someone take your calls), if necessary.

Plan for your personal prime time. If you're like most people,
you probably feel more energetic and productive at some times than at
others. Take advantage of your peak performance time, and plan to tackle
your most demanding tasks then. Leave routine tasks for off-peak times.

Don't be a perfectionist. Do your best, but realize that not everything has to be perfect. Too much attention to detail may be a waste of
time. Again, prioritize.

Avoid indecision. When you're unsure of what to do, ask yourself, "What is the best use of my time right now?"

170 Seven Ways to Cure Workaholism

Time off is good behavior, especially for people who work, work,
work all the time. When work overpowers all other activity, stress develops. Long hours, with little relief, generally leads to:

▶ Less productivity or inefficiency.

▶ Neglected family and social life.

▶ Distorted concepts of what's important and what's not.

So often, though, a workaholic is the last to realize a problem exists.
People who have trouble separating themselves from their jobs may feel
that their personal worth is measured by how much they produce at work
and little else.

Ask your spouse or a close friend if they think you're a workaholic.
If the answer is yes, here are some ways to create a healthier balance between work and play.

**Gradually cut down the number of hours you work each day or
week.** Avoid radical changes, but take measurable steps, like making it

a rule not to work on weekends. (If that means you have to cut your work-load proportionally by skipping unimportant tasks or delegating some work, so be it.)

Plan time for recreation in your schedule as though it were an important commitment. (It is.) Set aside some time for fun, however brief, every day.

Get some physical exercise every day. Take a walk, do some stretching, or participate in some other nonstressful, noncompetitive activity.

Avoid talking shop over lunch. Go on a picnic or meet an old friend and talk about something unrelated to work.

Choose a hobby that contrasts with the kind of work you do. If you work on highly technical mental problems all day, take up a handcraft hobby like woodworking or needlework. If you stay indoors all day, take up an outdoor activity like gardening or bicycling.

Select leisure activities carefully. You need at least one activity you can share with family or friends.

Refuse to feel guilty when you're not working. This is probably the most important step of all.

171 If You Can't Alter Traffic, Alter Your Mood

Cars are inching along bumper to bumper. The weather is foul. You've already been late to work twice this week. Every muscle in your body is beginning to feel tense.

What a way to start the morning. Boy, are you in for a bad day!

Auto commutes don't have to be "stress on wheels," though. Here are some ways to avoid commuter stress.

▶ Before you set out, listen to radio traffic reports to find out if and where traffic is tied up.

▶ Take less heavily traveled routes.

▶ Leave 10 to 15 minutes earlier, to allow for unexpected delays.

▶ Look at a map and plan alternate routes should you encounter unexpected slow-downs along the way.

If, despite such avoidance tactics, you end up caught in traffic anyway, don't let stress get the best of you. Some hints:

▶ Loosen your grip on the steering wheel.

▶ Take a few deep breaths.

▶ Don't dwell on negative factors over which you have no control, like rude drivers or the odds of arriving late.

▶ Listen to a radio talk show or all-news station.

▶ Play some audio cassettes of pleasant music, narrated books, or self-improvement courses. (Learn French on your way to work, for example.)

▶ Keep a notebook and pencil or a cassette recorder handy to make notes for planning your day, make shopping lists, and so forth.

Not only do these strategies help you make good use of otherwise wasted time, you might actually enjoy the drive!

172 Keep Cool in a Crisis

If you're going through a crisis, your view of the world probably isn't too rosy. Sudden, sometimes unexplainable events like loss of a job, death of a loved one, or illness or injury throw people into an emotional abyss. It's a crowded abyss, too: The National Institute of Mental Health estimates that in any six-month period, nearly 30 million Americans face some kind of crisis.

Much of the stress triggered by a crisis arises from our perception of the event—whether we view a crisis as a challenge or a threat, an opportunity or a ticket to doom. Here are some skills that are useful for putting crises into perspective and surviving with minimal damage to emotional health.

▶ Visualize the future in positive, healing ways. Imagine yourself feeling good again and being happy. When people imagine themselves behaving in a particular way, the likelihood that things will turn out as expected increases.

▶ Learn to physically relax, using any of the techniques described at the beginning of this chapter. It's hard to feel tense when your body is completely relaxed.

▶ Be realistic when you describe your situation to yourself and others. Avoid exaggerating or using emotionally charged words like "never," "always," or "hate."

▶ Take one day at a time. Set goals you can measure and achieve, and don't demand too much of yourself.

▶ Don't allow yourself to get bogged down in self-pity, but be

willing to accept help from others. Love, friendship, and social
support are powerful coping tools for managing stress.

▶ Remember, you're not alone. Whatever you're going through,
others have experienced and survived. You will, too.

173 Burned Out? Try This

You may think that only corporate go-getters suffer burnout. Not
so. Burnout can and does strike workers of all sorts—construction workers, office workers, homemakers, artists—anyone who's under continu-
ous pressure to perform or achieve. Also, anyone who's just plain tired of
what they're doing can burn out.

Burnout isn't something that hits out of the blue. Rather, burnout
is a long, slow process arising from repeated frustration and unmet expectations. Some symptoms of burnout include:

▶ Loss of energy

▶ Weariness

▶ Self-doubt

▶ Reduced efficiency

▶ Apathy

Different people respond to burnout in different ways: by feeling
guilty or irritable, denying anything's wrong, blaming others, or working
even harder. These responses are futile, though, and only fan the flames.

Here's what you can do to prevent burnout or nip it in the bud.

▶ Pay attention to any signals your body is sending. Insomnia,
overeating, and other minor complaints may be signs of
burnout.

▶ Ask yourself what you really expect to accomplish in your
career or personal life. Are your expectations realistic? If not,
reevaluate your goals and make sure they're reachable. This is
especially useful if you often find yourself describing your
workload as "impossible," "ridiculous," or "overwhelming."

▶ Mentally distance yourself from your work.

▶ Treat yourself to something special from time to time. A
pleasant break, a change of scenery, or a slight indulgence can

reduce some of the resentment that often leads to burnout.

▶ Reduce work hours if possible. Take breaks. Learn to delegate some tasks—anything to prevent yourself from feeling like a galley slave.

▶ Learn meditation or practice other relaxation techniques (see Tips 158 through 161) to help you through stressful periods. Most can be mastered quickly and easily.

▶ Pursue some kind of physical activity. But be careful not to choose exercise that reinforces the feeling of hopelessness. If your job is highly competitive, you may have to avoid playing highly competitive sports, for example. Something simple, like walking, may be better.

174 Make Stress Work for You

Slay your dragons and eat them for lunch! (Figuratively speaking, that is.) Lots of people have learned to tame stress by refusing to accept defeat in the face of negative forces. Instead, they meet stress head on, with a positive outcome. In other words, if you can use a negative event (like losing your job) to motivate you to take positive action (like getting a *better* job), you can beat stress at its own game.

Here's how you can make stress work for you, not against you.

▶ Try not to think of setbacks as defeats.

▶ View stress as an energizer. Consider each new demand as a challenge, no matter how forbidding it may seem.

▶ Always ask yourself, "What's the best that can happen?" rather than "What's the worst possible outcome?"

▶ Pause between skirmishes. Allow for rest and recuperation before facing each challenge.

▶ Take charge. Although you can't control other people's actions, you can control your response to what comes your way. When it comes to managing your emotions, you're the boss.

▶ Don't try to please everyone—you can't. (Do aim to please yourself occasionally, though.)

▶ Get the big picture. Think in terms of long-range goals, not just day-to-day problems.

175 Stop Family Friction Before It Starts

Stress resistance begins at home. What better way to help your family withstand the rapid change, constant disruptions, and various surprises life dishes out than to estabish a stable "base of operations" at home. Psychologists and other mental health professionals have found that families who work and play together as a cohesive unit can survive a crisis like unemployment or illness better than those with poor coping skills.

Here are some guidelines for insulating your family against stress.

▶ Take time to talk things over and be good companions to one another.

▶ Hold regular family conferences or meetings. Use this time to set mutual goals, present grievances, or discuss future plans. Take turns heading these meetings. Plan an agenda, so everyone gets an opportunity to speak and so that important issues aren't overlooked.

▶ Teach the value of being a good listener. Pay attention to what others say. Learn to "hear between the lines." And ask questions if you don't understand what your spouse or children are trying to tell you.

▶ Establish family traditions tied to significant occasions, like birthdays or holidays, that can be celebrated together.

▶ Learn the value of compromise.

▶ Be flexible, and shift gears if the situation calls for it. Flexibility is especially important if one parent goes back to work after managing the household full time, or if one wage earner loses his or her job or gets sick.

▶ Allow for individual strengths and interests. Don't compare brothers and sisters to one another, and allow family members to have "their own space."

▶ Discourage competition between family members.

▶ Don't overemphasize academic and financial status.

176 Remember: Kids Are People, Too

Don't think for one minute that kids lead stress-free lives. Carefree as childhood may seem to adults, children experience stresses that are as real to them as car payments and broken water heaters are to you.

Coach your children in stress management so they can learn to handle setbacks and disappointments. Here's how:

▶ Find a calm, quiet time to discuss with your children what it feels like to be stressed. Choose simple examples that are appropriate to their age levels.

▶ Ask your children about any physical signs of stress they may be experiencing, like upset stomach or sweaty palms.

▶ Teach your children that they can calm down, and show them how to make themselves feel better.

— Tell your children to take a slow, deep breath and imagine that they are sucking in air through their feet. Then tell them to exhale all the "stressed" air out of their bodies and let go of tense feelings.

— Tell your children to imagine a comforting mental image. Suggest they picture themselves somewhere associated with relaxation—safe in bed, at a favorite playground, on the sofa with the family pet, sitting in Dad's lap, or something similar. Encourage them to include as many details as possible in this image, to make it clear and memorable.

▶ Encourage your children to practice deep breathing or conjure up a comforting mental image whenever they feel stressed.

SOURCE: Many of the hints in this chapter were adapted from the Systematic Stress Management™ program, developed by the American Institute for Preventive Medicine, Southfield, Michigan, 1989.

CHAPTER

7

Your Emotions and Your Health

If the average person comes down with a cold, sprains a knee, or suffers a heart attack, there's no hesitation about seeking treatment. And the person lets friends and co-workers know about the problem. Most people are allowed time off for physical illness or surgery.

Mental health is another matter, however. Many people deny troublesome feelings, hesitate to tell others what's bothering them, and believe only crazy people need professional help. And the idea of giving workers time off for a "mental health day" (in place of a sick day) is not widely accepted.

Yet mental health problems deserve as much attention as physical disease or injury. Research has discovered a link between good mental health and a strong immune system. A long-term study conducted at Western Electric Corporation showed that depressed middle-aged men were twice as likely to die of cancer than happier co-workers. Another study showed that 60 percent of widows surveyed experienced a major health problem within one year of their husbands' deaths. Also, University of Michigan researchers found that lonely, socially isolated adults run the same risk of dying before their time as do cigarette smokers.

Evidently, a healthy mental outlook is essential to a healthy body. And the tips in this chapter can help heal mental hurts like anger, jealousy, guilt, depression, and phobias, among others. You'll discover how elements of your environment—like music, weather, and pets—can help you feel better. You'll also find out how to locate a trustworthy therapist, should you need professional counseling.

177 How to Manage Anger

Yelling, throwing things, and generally blowing your top aren't the only signs of anger. Sulking, nagging, and crying are also common expressions of anger.

Besides alienating others, chronic anger can contribute to a variety of unpleasant ills, including headaches, skin rashes, stomach upsets— even high blood pressure.

If you tend to get angry easily and often, take these steps to help you control this negative reaction.

▶ Count to ten at the first twinge of anger, and take three or four slow, deep breaths. The angry impulse may pass.

▶ If it's convenient and you feel a major outburst coming on, take a short walk until you calm down.

▶ Don't resort to nagging or door slamming. If someone says or does something that bothers you, discuss it calmly.

▶ Distract yourself. If you're stuck in traffic, for example, try to accept the delay and recognize that it's beyond your control. Pounding the horn and cursing at other drivers only prolongs your agitation. Instead of sounding off, play pleasant music on the radio or listen to an interesting program. (See Tip 171 in chapter 6, Success over Stress.)

178 Overcoming Jealousy

It's normal to feel a little jealous if a co-worker is promoted to a position you covet or if someone flirts with your spouse. But if you're so jealous that you're miserable and preoccupied with resentful thoughts, jealousy can be debilitating.

Jealousy arises from the belief that others are better off, from fear of losing someone (or something), or from distrust of others. To control or overcome jealousy:

▶ Admit to yourself that you feel jealous. Only then can you begin to deal with your feelings constructively.

▶ Be happy for others' gains and accomplishments, and use your jealousy in a positive way by motivating yourself to achieve what you admire in others.

▶ Remind yourself of your own unique qualities.

Unfounded jealousy can ruin a marital or romantic relationship. If you find yourself thinking suspicious thoughts about your spouse or lover, distract yourself by doing something constructive like a home repair project. Also, don't make it a habit to check up on the other person or question his or her activities or companions.

179 Get Rid of Guilt

Guilt is a by-product of all the "shoulds" people accumulate on their mental lists of "things to do." To help you distinguish between what's right for you to do and what you do because you're guilt ridden:

▶ Don't let others' values dictate the way you live your life. Decide for yourself what's important to you, what you value, or the way you wish to be.

▶ Don't expect to be pleasant, wise, and even-tempered at all times. It's normal to feel irritable or angry occasionally. Feeling guilty about negative emotions is futile.

▶ Forgive yourself for mistakes in judgment. Learn something from your mistakes. Make them work for you in the future.

▶ Take satisfaction in your accomplishments, rather than dwelling on your shortcomings.

180 Put an End to Depression

Life changes, such as the birth of a baby, divorce, death of a loved one, or loss of a job can and do leave people depressed. So can worrying about financial problems or illness. But sometimes you may feel empty and depressed for no apparent reason. Symptoms of depression include:

▶ Persistent feelings of sadness or emptiness

▶ Feelings of helplessness, hopelessness, guilt, and worthlessness

▶ Loss of interest in pleasurable activities, including sex

▶ Sleep disturbances

▶ Loss of energy or enthusiasm

▶ Difficulty in concentrating or making decisions

▶ Ongoing physical symptoms, such as headaches or digestive disorders, that don't respond to treatment

To overcome mild, hard-to-explain depression, try these approaches.

▶ Substitute a positive thought for every negative thought that pops into your head.

▶ Associate with congenial people, not negative people. They'll lift your morale.

▶ To focus your attention away from yourself, do something to help someone else.

▶ Get some physical exercise every day, even if it's just taking the dog for a walk. If you can do something more exhilarating, like biking, playing tennis, or chopping firewood, that's even better.

▶ Do something different. Walk or drive to someplace new, or try a new restaurant.

▶ Challenge yourself with a new project. It doesn't have to be difficult, but it should be enjoyable.

If you feel depressed for three weeks or longer, see a doctor. There may be a physical cause for the way you feel. Also, check with your doctor or pharmacist about any medication you may be taking. Depression is sometimes a side effect of a drug.

181 Defeat the Holiday Blues

The Christmas season (and other holidays, to a lesser degree) leave millions of people blue, not joyful. Contributing factors include:

▶ Family members who live far away

▶ Memories of a loved one who has passed away

▶ Financial problems

▶ Fatigue and feelings of being overwhelmed by tasks and obligations associated with the holidays

▶ Idealistic expectations

Some ways to prevent the holiday blues include the following.

▶ Begin holiday preparations well in advance, to avoid becoming overwhelmed.

▶ Delegate chores like writing greeting cards or baking cookies to other members of the household.

▶ Don't drink alcohol if it makes you moody and depressed.

▶ Don't expect everything—food, decorations, family
get-togethers—to be perfect for the holidays.

▶ Don't spend beyond your budget.

▶ If keeping old holiday traditions is painful, start new ones.

▶ If you expect to be alone for the holidays, don't wait to be
invited somewhere; invite people over.

182 A Cure for the Winter Doldrums

Many people start to feel depressed in November and continue to
feel as dark and dreary as the weather until the spring thaw. Scientists call
severe depression that sets in during winter Seasonal Affective Disorder
(SAD). Light and temperature play a significant role in SAD. Daylight
prompts the brain to release chemicals that spark feelings of energy. For
about 5 percent of the population, their mood grows darker when days
grow shorter. Daily exposure to full-spectrum fluorescent light, which re-
sembles sunlight, can help cure SAD.

Other tips for overcoming SAD include:

▶ Get outside as much as possible. SAD sufferers report they
benefit more by exposure to early morning light than to light
later in the day.

▶ Keep the drapes in your house open and the window shades
raised during daylight hours.

▶ Sit near windows, and gaze outside periodically.

▶ On cloudy days, turn on bright lights.

▶ Don't isolate yourself during winter. Visit friends, go to
museums, see shows—anything to get out and about.

▶ Try to take your vacation in the winter instead of in the summer.

183 Managing Grief

Many people associate grief with the death of a loved one. But grief
can also follow in the wake of job loss, a debilitating illness or injury, or
divorce. And grief is a normal and natural emotion characterized by feelings that ebb and flow. One day you may feel that grief is behind you,
only to find that the pain returns the next.

Grief usually consists of five stages: shock, denial, and anger, then depression, and finally acceptance. It takes some people longer than others to accept a loss and recover, so grief shouldn't be ignored or rushed. The following can help overcome grief.

▶ Don't hide your emotions or feel embarrassed about grief.

▶ Turn to supportive friends and family members for help and understanding.

▶ Cope with anger over your loss by writing in a journal, pursuing a physical activity, or otherwise venting your feelings in a constructive way.

▶ Don't overeat or use alcohol and drugs in response to grief.

▶ Be sure to eat a well-planned, nutritious diet and get enough rest and exercise, to boost your resistance to disease during your period of despair.

▶ Avoid spending birthdays, holidays, or other momentous occasions alone.

▶ Put off major decisions or changes until your grief has passed, since your judgment will be cloudy at this time.

▶ Expect temporary setbacks. The path for working through loss is neither straight nor smooth.

▶ If you feel overwhelmed and unable to function, seek professional counseling.

184 Take the Fear out of Phobias

We can all recall experiences when we were afraid of something—going to the dentist, perhaps, or driving in a thunderstorm, or being home alone as a child. These fears are usually short-lived and don't disrupt our lives. A phobia, in contrast, is a severe, recurring, irrational fear that triggers dramatic physical and psychological changes, such as heart palpitations, sweating, vomiting, a feeling of suffocation, and sometimes even a sense of impending death. People with phobias go to extremes to avoid the object or situation they fear. A person who's afraid of driving on the expressway, for example, may travel on side roads only, no matter how inconvenient.

Some of the more common phobias include:

▶ Claustrophobia (fear of enclosed spaces)

▶ Agoraphobia (fear of open spaces)

▶ Ailurophobia (fear of cats)

▶ Hematophobia (fear of blood)

▶ Nyctophobia (fear of the night)

A behavior modification technique known as desensitization combines mental imagery and relaxation training. Taught by psychologists or other mental health professionals, desensitization cures phobias in about 80 percent of those affected by the problem. Contact your community mental health agency for where to go for help if you think you could benefit from desensitization treatment.

185 Feel Better with Music

You might call music solace on the air waves. Dentists play music to reduce their patients' anxiety. Hospitals pipe tunes into delivery rooms. And supermarkets broadcast music to keep shoppers rolling along. And the right kind of music can soothe your nerves. Soft, slow, low-pitched music lowers heart rate and blood pressure and relaxes muscles, while loud, fast, high-pitched music creates tension.

Consequently, soothing music is now used to reduce anxiety and pain associated with medical procedures and other unpleasantries.

Here's how to put soothing music to work for you.

▶ To relax, select music that has a regular rhythm with no extremes in pitch. Bach's "Air on the G String," Pachelbel's "Canon in D," Haydn's "Cello Concerto in C," and Debussy's "Claire de Lune" are good examples.

▶ To pull yourself out of a glum mood, listen to music that's snappy and upbeat.

▶ To quiet a crying baby, play soft music with a tempo that's the same as the human heart rate (70 to 80 beats per minute).

▶ To increase work productivity, turn on an easy listening radio station. The music format is usually geared to the changes in mood people routinely experience in the course of the day: Bright and cheery music to get going in the morning, stimulating tunes during the prelunch slump, and relaxing music to wind down at day's end.

186 Feeling Low? Get a Pet!

Who doesn't feel warm and happy watching a puppy or a kitten at play? Americans dote over their house pets, and for good reason: Pets offer companionship, and they improve our mental and physical well-being.

Pets brighten the lives of those who are anxious, lonely, or depressed because they:

▶ Give a person something to nurture and care for.

▶ Offer a sense of being wanted and needed.

▶ Offer nonjudgmental acceptance.

▶ Decrease feelings of isolation.

▶ Provide a feeling of safety for those living alone.

A study of elderly people who were depressed, disabled, or uncommunicative found that pets transformed their lives. Individuals became more communicative and less depressed, and they overcame some of their physical disabilities. Other research has found that cuddling a furry pet or watching fish swim in an aquarium lowers high blood pressure and reduces feelings of anxiety.

People-oriented pets like cats and dogs bring families closer together and help to reduce household tension. Studies show that families with pets spend more time playing with the pet and have fewer family arguments.

187 Develop a Cancer-Resistant Attitude

Of all the diseases known to man, cancer is the most feared. And even though cancer in its various forms strikes about one-third of the people in the United States, doctors are still at a loss to explain exactly what causes it. Factors like smoking, exposure to toxic substances like asbestos or radiation, and high-fat diets have been associated with causing cancer. But something else is afoot. Why, for example, does one cigarette smoker get lung cancer and another does not?

Researchers are looking into the existence of a cancer-prone personality—attitudes and behavior that, all else being equal, make certain people more likely than others to develop cancer. Numerous studies indicate that these traits may point to a cancer-prone disposition:

▶ A passive, unemotional outlook on life

▶ Suppression of feelings

▶ Allowing anger to build up

▶ Withdrawal or feelings of hopelessness and helplessness when something bad happens

▶ An emotionally troubled childhood

People with these characteristics are more likely to get cancer, and when they do, they accept the condition passively and are likely to die in a shorter period of time.

Doctors explain the apparent relationship between cancer and personality by theorizing that a lifetime of built-up emotions causes a release of hormones that interferes with the body's natural defenses against disease. To resist cancer, then, people should actively try to solve conflicts within their control and should suppress or let go of feelings about conflicts that they can't change. In fact, researchers have found that people who survive cancer tend to be feisty, demanding, and express their feelings easily.

188 How to Spot a Possible Suicide

If someone you know talks about suicide, take them seriously. Comments like "They're better off without me," "I won't have to worry about my life much longer," or "I wish I were dead" are warning signs of desperation. Also, watch for these suicidal signs.

▶ Feelings of worthlessness, hopelessness, and helplessness

▶ Sleep disturbances

▶ Difficulty thinking, concentrating, or making decisions

▶ Spending time alone or not associating with others

▶ Giving away personal possessions

Suicide prevention "don'ts" include:

▶ Don't ignore a threat of suicide.

▶ Don't keep someone's threat of suicide a secret.

▶ Don't dare or challenge someone who has threatened to commit suicide.

▶ Don't leave a person alone if they talk about suicide.

What to do instead.

▶ Ask how the person plans to carry out the suicide. Has he or she acquired a gun or pills?

▶ Waste no time in finding help. Contact friends, family members, family doctor, clergy, a crisis intervention center, and/or a suicide prevention hotline.

▶ Let the person know you care. Reassure the person that treatments are available to help him or her work through problems, no matter how hopeless they seem.

▶ Encourage the individual to continue to work or participate in hobbies, sports, or other activities.

189 When to Seek Professional Help

There may be times when sympathy and reassurance from a concerned friend aren't enough to help you handle a personal problem. A crisis may arise that's more than you can handle. Or lots of everyday problems pile up—and wear you down. If that happens, you may need a skilled professional to help you cope with your distress or solve your problems.

Therapists offer more than sympathy: They monitor their clients' conditions carefully and guide them through planned treatment. The goal of therapy is to help people develop skills to effectively deal with their problems on their own.

The following are signs that you may need the help of a therapist.

▶ Prolonged depression

▶ Extreme shifts in mood

▶ Panic attacks or other episodes of overwhelming fear and anxiety

▶ Recurrent displays of anger

▶ Abuse of alcohol or drugs

▶ Abusing others or experiencing abuse from others

▶ Eating disorders, including bulimia (bingeing followed by self-induced vomiting after eating)

▶ Obsessive-compulsive behavior (preoccupation with recurrent thoughts and senseless repetitive behavior that interferes with daily living)

▶ Learning that you have a debilitating or terminal disease

Therapy is also helpful for people who have lost their jobs, experienced divorces, lost loved ones through death, or face similar crises.

People who experience hallucinations, hear voices, or think about suicide, or who feel out of control and fear they'll commit a violent act, need help immediately.

190 How to Find a Therapist You Trust

Say you're having trouble overcoming guilt, grief, depression, anger, resentment, or other emotional problems and you decide you need counseling. Two factors are critical to successful counseling. One is the therapist's qualifications and credentials. The second is your relationship with the therapist.

Research shows that whether or not you like and trust your therapist is more critical to success than the method of counseling or treatment the therapist uses.

Use the following checklist to decide if the therapist you're considering is right for you.

▶ Summarize your problem and ask if the therapist has treated people with a problem similar to yours.

▶ Tell the therapist what you expect to get out of therapy, and find out what approach the therapist uses. Will the therapist's method of treatment help you reach your goal?

▶ Do you feel confident with the therapist's experience?

▶ Ask the therapist how long you are likely to need therapy. (Don't expect a quick and easy fix, though. Therapy is usually a slow process, and some problems take months to resolve.)

▶ Find out if your medical insurance will cover all or part of the cost of the proposed treatment.

If you need marriage counseling or sex therapy, your spouse should accompany you for treatment to be effective.

CHAPTER

8

Freedom from Substance Abuse

People smoke, drink alcohol, or abuse drugs for various reasons. Many find that nicotine, alcohol, and other psychoactive substances take the edge off tension, add excitement to otherwise boring routines, or make them more sociable. Whether you're addicted to cigarettes or cigars, wine coolers or whiskey sours, prescription tranquilizers or cocaine, the net effect on your health is the same: Take away the euphoria and temporary lift or thrill, and you're left with a body that's aching to break free but can't live without its physical and/or psychological crutches.

Problem is, you can't live with them, either. The use of tobacco products is responsible for over 400,000 premature deaths each year, because of its role in heart disease, strokes, emphysema, and cancer—yet more than 25% of adult Americans continue to smoke. It's ironic: "To your health"—in various languages—is a customary toast. Yet in excess, alcohol is unhealthy. Alcohol causes problems for about 10 percent of the population—it can destroy families, careers, and the drinker's health.

Other drug abuse produces many of the same sad results. Yet never before have so many people of all ages used illicit drugs like marijuana, cocaine, and heroin. Even prescription drugs like sleeping pills and sedatives, are used—and abused—extensively.

This chapter will present sound strategies to help you (or someone you care about) break free of a number of common dependencies.

191 Take the Nicotine Dependency Test

One of the ingredients that makes cigarettes addictive is nicotine. One researcher says, "If cigarettes didn't contain nicotine, people would be no more inclined to smoke them than they would be to blow bubbles."

Some smokers are more dependent on nicotine than others. The test below can help you determine just how hooked you may be. (If you're seriously hooked, you may want to consider nicotine reduction therapy, discussed in Tip 196.)

Nicotine Dependency Test

	0 Points	1 Point	2 Points	Score
1. How soon after you wake up do you smoke your first cigarette?	After 30 min.	Within 30 min.		————
2. Do you find it difficult to refrain from smoking in places where it is forbidden, such as libraries, theaters, or doctors' offices?	No	Yes		————
3. Which of all the cigarettes you smoke in a day is the most satisfying?	Any other than the first one in the morning.	The first one in the morning.		————
4. How many cigarettes a day do you smoke?	1–15	16–25	More than 26	————
5. Do you smoke more during the morning than during the rest of the day?	No	Yes		————
6. Do you continue to smoke even on days you are so ill that you remain in bed?	No	Yes		————

	0 Points	1 Point	2 Points	Score
7. Does the brand you smoke have a low (up to 0.4 mg.), medium (0.5 to 0.9 mg.), or high (1.0 mg. or more) nicotine content?	Low	Medium	High	_____
8. How often do you inhale the smoke from your cigarette?	Never	Sometimes	Always	_____
			TOTAL	_____

SOURCE: Test developed by Karl-Olov Fagerstrom, Ph.D., Smoking Withdrawal Clinic, Ulleraker Hospital, Uppsala, Sweden.

How to score: Scores of 7 or higher indicate that you are highly dependent on nicotine. Scores of 6 or less indicate that you have a low to moderate nicotine dependence.

192 Blow Out Your Birthday Candles— If You Can

Do you have trouble blowing out the candles on your birthday cake? Do you get winded dashing up a short flight of stairs? If you're a smoker, diminished lung power may be to blame for these failed feats.

Take this simple test to determine your lung capacity (that is, the amount of air your lungs hold in reserve).

1. Strike a match. When the flame is burning steadily, hold it about 6 inches from your mouth.

2. Inhale deeply, then try to blow out the match by exhaling quickly through your mouth, *without* pursing your lips. Try more than once, if you must.

3. If you can't blow out the match, your lung capacity may be impaired. See your doctor.

193 Seven Answers to Smokers' Excuses

Despite reams of evidence that says smoking is harmful, many smokers continue to smoke. Below are seven common rationales smokers use to justify why they smoke—with rebuttals that explain why they're incorrect.

I'll gain weight if I quit. People don't gain weight because they quit smoking; they gain weight because they eat more. Ex-smokers gain an average of 5 to 10 pounds. But you can lose it—or keep from gaining—if you get more exercise and stay away from fatty foods and nervous snacking. (See chapter 5, Weight Loss: Tipping the Scales in Your Favor.)

I need cigarettes to relax. Nicotine is actually a stimulant; it prompts the nervous system and the adrenal glands to trigger the release of adrenaline, the "fight or flight" hormone. Adrenaline leaves you feeling wired, not relaxed.

I know lots of people who smoke—they're still healthy. We all know people like this, but they're the exception rather than the rule. The odds are stacked against you.

Cigarettes won't hurt me—I'm in good shape. Don't bet on it. Even if you don't die from smoking, you'll almost certainly experience some degree of disability—like difficulty breathing, a hacking cough, high blood pressure, or heart disease—and eventually be forced to quit. Why not quit now, before the damage is done?

I've tried to quit—dozens of times. It's no use. If you've tried to quit smoking 17 times—and failed 17 times—each attempt increases the likelihood that you'll succeed on a subsequent attempt. Most ex-smokers made many attempts before they finally succeeded.

Quitting is too difficult. If you once quit for a short time but were in total agony each and every day, remember that no one ever died from quitting. You'll get through it.

I can't imagine life without cigarettes. You weren't born smoking; you acquired the habit. You survived before you smoked, and you'll survive after you quit.

SOURCE: Adapted from "Tobacco Tattler," by Don R. Powell, Ph.D., *Your Patient and Cancer* (May 1984).

194 The Hidden Costs of Cigarettes

Do you realize how much it costs for the privilege of being a cigarette smoker? A pack here, a carton there—in a year, it adds up. And it's not getting any cheaper!

The table below shows the *minimum* amount you can save if you or a family member quits smoking now. The figures are based on an average cost of $2.25 per pack of cigarettes. (Some brands cost more.) And the totals don't include the interest the amount spent would earn if you put it in the bank.

The Cumulative Cost of Cigarettes ($)

| | Number of Packs a Day | | | | |
	1	1½	2	2½	3
Day	2.25	3.38	4.50	5.63	6.75
Week	15.75	23.66	31.50	39.41	47.25
Month	67.50	101.40	135.00	168.90	202.50
Year	821.25	1,233.70	1,642.50	2,054.95	2,463.75
10 Years	8,212.50	12,337.00	16,425.00	20,549.50	24,637.50
20 Years	16,425.00	24,674.00	32,850.00	41,099.00	49,275.00
30 Years	24,637.50	37,011.00	49,275.00	61,648.50	73,912.50
40 Years	32,850.00	49,348.00	65,700.00	82,198.00	98,550.00

SOURCE: The Smokeless® program, developed by the American Institute for Preventive Medicine, Farmington Hills, Michigan, 1983, 1989, 1993.

What's more, these totals don't reflect other, hidden expenses of smoking, which include the cost of:

- Lighters and other smoking paraphernalia
- Cigarette burns on clothing, carpeting, and furniture
- Extra dry cleaning
- Mouthwashes, colognes, and special toothpastes
- Missed work days
- Extra medical and dental care

▶ Increased life and health insurance rates

These hidden costs can add up to another $700 or more per year for the average smoker. Most smokers can't afford *not* to quit. (See the following tip for hints on how to quit smoking for good.)

195 The "Warm Pheasant" Plan to Quit Smoking

You've heard of quitting cigarettes cold turkey—all at once, in an unflinching moment of resolution. Well, that works for some, but not all, smokers. In fact, there are as many ways to quit smoking as there are brands of cigarettes for sale. If you're like Mark Twain (who said, "Quitting smoking is easy. I've done it over a hundred times"), you might want to try the "warm pheasant" method. Unlike the cold turkey approach, this three-phase plan allows you to continue to smoke, while you prepare to quit, psychologically and physically.

Phase I: Preparing to Quit

This phase takes approximately one week.

1. Mark a "quit" date on your calendar one week in advance.
2. Keep track of each cigarette you smoke by making a slash mark on a piece of paper tucked in the wrapper of your cigarette pack.
3. Every time you have an urge to light up, wait 10 minutes.
4. Collect your cigarette butts in a "butt bottle." (The mere sight of so many spent cigarettes will graphically demonstrate just how much you really smoke in a week.)

Phase II: Quitting

This phase takes approximately one to two weeks.

1. Throw away all your cigarettes and hide all smoking paraphernalia, like matches, lighters, ashtrays, and so forth.
2. Whenever you have an urge to smoke, take a deep breath through your mouth and slowly exhale through pursed lips. Repeat five to ten times.
3. Change your routine, to eliminate familiar smoking cues. If you always light up when driving to work, take a different route. Or substitute a walk for your usual coffee—and cigarette—break. Or

sit in a chair you don't customarily use when relaxing or watching television at home.

4. Take up activities you don't normally associate with smoking. Enroll in a cooking class, visit a nonsmoking friend, or go swimming at your local Y, for example.

5. Keep your hands busy by holding something—a pen, a Nerf Ball, or a binder clip, for example.

6. In place of cigarettes, substitute other things that will provide oral gratification, like sugarless gum or mints, toothpicks, or coffee stirrers.

7. Avoid drinking coffee and alcohol or eating foods high in sugar, like candy and pastries. They cause biochemical changes in the body that increases your desire for a cigarette.

8. Create a "ciggy bank" and put the money you used to spend on cigarettes in a jar. Watch it add up.

9. Place a rubber band on your wrist and snap it every time you get an urge to smoke.

Phase III: Staying off Cigarettes

Allow three months for this final phase.

1. Always remember that the craving to smoke will pass, whether you smoke or not.

2. Renew your commitment to stay off cigarettes each day.

3. Beware of saboteurs—usually other smokers—who may try to encourage you to light up. Assert your right *not* to smoke.

4. Talk to a nonsmoking buddy for support.

5. Make a list of good things you've noticed since you quit—food tastes better, you cough less, your clothes don't smell bad, and so forth.

6. Continue to practice the behavior modification techniques listed in the quitting phase.

SOURCE: The Smokeless® program, developed by the American Institute for Preventive Medicine, Southfield, Michigan, 1983, 1989.

196 Nicotine Gum Can Help Smokers Quit

Until lately, many people assumed cigarette smoking was just a bad habit (albeit an unhealthy one). In 1988, the *Surgeon General's Report on*

Smoking and Health changed that view. After reviewing over 2,000 scientific studies, the report confirmed what many scientists suspected: Smoking cigarettes is addictive, because they contain nicotine. So in order for you to quit smoking, you need to break the physical addiction as well as the psychological habit.

A technique called nicotine replacement therapy can help break that stranglehold. By either wearing a nicotine transdermal patch or by chewing a nicotine gum called Nicorette, smokers absorb small amounts of nicotine. These little doses enable them to reduce their nicotine cravings and wean themselves off cigarettes with little anxiety, irritability, sleepiness, headaches, or other symptoms that make nicotine withdrawal such torture. (Some say nicotine withdrawal is worse than heroin withdrawal—or close to it.)

If you think nicotine replacement therapy might help you to quit smoking:

▶ Take the Nicotine Dependency Test in Tip 191. If you score 7 or higher, consider using nicotine replacement therapy.

▶ Discuss this option with your physician. People who are pregnant or have high blood pressure or heart disease need to weigh the hazards of smoking with the possible danger of absorbing nicotine from a patch or the gum.

▶ Follow all package insert instructions if you use a patch or Nicorette.

In order for nicotine replacement therapy to work, a smoker should also follow the kind of behavior modification techniques outlined in the previous tip. Or you can attend a reputable stop-smoking program. Studies have shown that combining a nicotine patch or Nicorette with a stop-smoking program can triple your chances for success.

197 Wean Yourself off Pipes or Cigars

A generation ago, smoking a cigar after dinner or puffing on a pipe was a popular habit among men. Fortunately, using these two forms of tobacco has steadily declined over the past 25 years. Unfortunately, those who still enjoy smoking pipes or cigars run higher risks of cancer of the larynx, pharynx, and esophagus. If you happen to inhale pipe or cigar smoke, you also run the same risk of diseases associated with cigarette smoking— namely, lung cancer, emphysema, stroke, and heart disease.

As with cigarettes, smoking a pipe or cigars is ingrained with other routine activities. To disassociate smoking from other habits—and gradually break away from a pipe or cigars—follow these seven steps.

1. Pay attention to your smoking behavior for a few days. Note when and where you like to smoke (key rooms in the house, car, office, after meals, and so forth).

2. Instead of lighting up at your customary time, wait an hour. Do this for several days.

3. Smoke in one area only, like the back porch. Don't smoke anywhere else.

4. Extend your 1-hour delay to 2 hours. Do this for another week.

5. Don't read, watch television, or perform other "automatic" activities while you smoke.

6. Finish only half the cigar or bowl of pipe tobacco. Discard the rest.

7. Finally, don't smoke your pipe or cigar at all.

198 Snuff Out Smokeless Tobacco

Regardless of whether you smoke it, chew it, or just place it between your cheek and gums, all forms of tobacco are hazardous to your health. "Snuff" and chewing tobacco were once considered safe alternatives to cigarettes. They're not. People who use smokeless tobacco absorb nicotine through the mucous membrane of the mouth. Nicotine absorbed in this way is no less addictive than nicotine inhaled from cigarettes. People who pack tobacco in their mouths or chew it run a high risk of cancer of the mouth and a precancerous condition called leukoplakia (a whitish, wrinkling of the mouth lining, with thickening of the area that comes in contact with the tobacco).

The best way to avoid these risks, of course, is to never use smokeless tobacco. But if you already use it, here are some suggestions to help you give it up.

▶ Ignore the appeals of sports figures who promote smokeless tobacco in advertisements.

▶ Use substitutes like gum, mints, or toothpicks.

▶ Distract yourself with other activities.

▶ Reward yourself each day you don't chew tobacco.

199 Help Someone Quit Smoking

Nagging does no good. Sarcasm has no beneficial effect. Threats, harassment, yelling, and pleading leave the object of your attention feeling demeaned and resentful. So, how can you truly help someone kick the cigarette habit?

If someone close to you has decided to quit, here's how you can help.

▶ Let the smoker know you support his or her efforts and that you care about the person whether or not he or she is successful in quitting.

▶ Offer to babysit, prepare meals, or do other favors to help reduce stress for the other person for the first few days after he or she has decided to quit.

▶ Don't tell the other person what to do. You can suggest ways to make quitting easier, but don't nag or dictate.

▶ Sincerely praise the quitter's efforts. Comment on how much more in control he or she is.

200 Alcohol: Know Your Limit—And Stick to It

The tables, The Effects of Alcohol, on the opposite page, and Know Your Limit, on page 208, show approximately how much you have to drink to reach various levels of blood alcohol content (BAC), and what effect alcohol has at those levels.

These are only rough guides, however. How much you drink isn't the only factor that determines how intoxicated you become. Other factors explain why one person seems to be able to "hold their liquor" (or beer or wine) while another can't. How tipsy you get when you drink depends on:

How much you've eaten. You get drunk faster on an empty stomach; food slows down the body's absorption of alcohol.

How long it takes you to finish a drink. The body metabolizes alcohol at ⅓ ounce per hour—a little less than the amount in a 12-ounce beer, a 5-ounce glass of wine, or a mixed drink with 1½ ounces of 80-proof liquor. So downing two or three drinks in an hour is more intoxicating than sipping those same drinks over the course of an evening.

What you drink. Generally, the higher the concentration of alcohol, the more quickly alcohol is absorbed. Vodka, for example. is 40 or 50 percent alcohol, so it's absorbed faster than beer, which averages 3.2 to 5 percent alcohol.

Carbonation. Carbonated drinks like champagne are absorbed faster than noncarbonated drinks, like wine.

Your weight. Given equal amounts of alcohol consumed in 1 hour, a lighter person will reach a higher blood alcohol level than a heavier person.

Your age. Given equal amounts of alcohol, older people generally achieve higher blood alcohol levels than younger people.

The Effects of Alcohol

As the amount of alcohol in your blood increases, your mental and physical reactions to it change. Here's a rough guide to the physical and psychological effects of alcohol consumption.

Alcohol in Blood (%)	Typical Effects
0.05	Loosening of judgment, thought, and restraint. Release of tension, carefree sensation.
0.08	Tension and inhibitions of everyday life lessened.
0.10*	Voluntary motor action affected; hand and arm movements, walk, and speech clumsy.
0.20	Severe impairment. Staggering; loud, incoherent speech. Emotionally unstable. One hundred times greater risk of traffic accident.
0.30	Deeper areas of brain affected, causing confusion and stupor.
0.40	When asleep, difficult to arouse. Incapable of voluntary action. Equivalent to surgical anesthesia.
0.50	Coma. Anesthesia of center controlling breathing and heartbeat. Death.

*For most states, a blood alcohol content (BAC) of 0.10 is the indicator for driving while intoxicated.

Know Your Limit

Body Weight (lbs.)	Number of Drinks Consumed in a 2-Hour Period*									
100	1	2	3	4	5	6	7	8	9	10
120	1	2	3	4	5	6	7	8	9	10
140	1	2	3	4	5	6	7	8	9	10
160	1	2	3	4	5	6	7	8	9	10
180	1	2	3	4	5	6	7	8	9	10
200	1	2	3	4	5	6	7	8	9	10
220	1	2	3	4	5	6	7	8	9	10
240	1	2	3	4	5	6	7	8	9	10

Be Careful Driving (BAC† to 0.05%)	Driving May Be Impaired (BAC† 0.05–0.09%)	Do Not Drive— Intoxication (BAC† 0.10% & up)‡

NOTE: This chart provides averages only. Individuals may vary, and factors such as food in the stomach, medication, and fatigue can affect your tolerance.

*One drink equals 1½ oz. of 80-proof liquor, 12 oz. of beer, or 5 oz. of wine.

†Blood alcohol content.

‡The BAC percentages for impairment and intoxication vary from state to state.

201 Smart Tips for Business Drinking

Sloshing down three martinis at a business lunch went out with wide ties and bell-bottom pants. As one investment banker quipped, "No one's going to trust you to handle their money, services, or products if you get smashed over lunch."

Keep in mind that business is business. Others' impressions of you can make or break a deal—or a career. Alcohol is served at many business functions, yet more and more people are choosing not to drink.

If you choose to drink, here's what you can do to manage your alcohol intake and its effects.

▶ Don't feel you have to "keep up" with associates who drink.

▶ Remember that drinking isn't the main purpose of the get-together. Keep your underlying mission in mind, and stay clear headed.

▶ If you're nervous about the meeting, it might be better to avoid alcohol altogether, since you may drink too fast or too much and end up fuzzier than usual because of your anxiety.

If you attend a business dinner:

▶ Have only one predinner drink, if any.

▶ If champagne is served, sip it very slowly.

▶ Drink water with the meal.

▶ Avoid finishing each drink.

202 How to Head Off a Hangover

Oh, the throbbing head . . . the queasy stomach . . . the thundering vibrations from the smallest movement. It's the morning after a night of too much to drink, and now you're miserable with a full-blown hangover. You'd be willing to try almost anything to get rid of it.

Unfortunately, the only real cure for a hangover is to wait it out. But meanwhile, you suffer. To ease the discomfort:

▶ Get as much rest as you can.

▶ Avoid bright lights.

▶ Take aspirin (or an aspirin substitute) to help ease the overall ache.

You don't have to suffer a hangover every time you drink, though. These tips can save you a lot of self-induced misery.

▶ Eat a high-fat source of protein, like cheese or meat, to help prevent the nausea or heartburn associated with drinking.

▶ Avoid drinks that are more likely than others to cause a hangover. Bourbon, scotch, red wine, and peach schnapps contain congeners, substances that give flavor to liquor and produce longer-lasting hangovers. In contrast, vodka and gin are low in congeners.

▶ Most important, don't overdo it.

203 Face Up to Your Drinking Habits

Are you a social drinker or a problem drinker? If you have any doubts, you probably have a problem or are developing one. Alcoholics Anonymous has developed the following quiz to help you determine if you have a drinking problem.

1. Have you ever decided to stop drinking for a week or so, but lasted only a few days?   Yes _____   No _____

2. Do you wish people would mind their own business about your drinking and stop telling you what to do?   Yes _____   No _____

3. Have you ever switched from one kind of drink to another in the hope that this would keep you from getting drunk? Yes _____   No _____

4. Have you had a drink in the morning during the past year? Yes _____   No _____

5. Do you envy people who can drink without getting into trouble? Yes _____   No _____

6. Have you had problems connected with drinking during the past year?   Yes _____   No _____

7. Has your drinking caused trouble at home? Yes _____   No _____

8. Do you ever try to get extra drinks at a party because you're not served enough?   Yes _____   No _____

9. Do you tell yourself you can stop drinking any time you want, even though you keep getting drunk when you don't mean to? Yes _____   No _____

10. Have you missed days of work because of drinking? Yes _____   No _____

11. Do you have blackouts?   Yes _____   No _____

12. Have you ever felt your life would be better if you did not drink? Yes _____   No _____

How to score: If you answer yes to four questions or more, chances are you have a problem and should seek professional help.

SOURCE: *Is AA for You?* reprinted with permission of Alcoholics Anonymous World Services, Inc., New York.

204 Where to Get Help for a Drinking Problem

Problem drinkers can go about conquering their problem in a variety of ways, depending on their needs.

Psychotherapy. Counseling, one-on-one with a therapist or in group sessions, focuses on feelings and situations related to drinking. The goal is to help an individual cope with emotional problems and other stresses so that he or she no longer relies on alcohol.

Support groups. Organized groups like Alcoholics Anonymous provide assistance, encouragement, and guidance (including a 12-step recovery plan) for members who share an alcohol problem.

Medication. One called Naltrexone, blocks the craving for alcohol and the pleasure of getting high. Another one, called Antabuse, causes physical reactions, such as vomiting, when drinking alcohol. Antabuse is rarely used.

Alcohol treatment centers. Affiliated with hospitals, medical clinics, or community health centers, alcohol treatment centers generally combine more than one approach. People who need help are either treated as an outpatient or admitted as an inpatient, depending on how serious the problem is.

For help determining the best approach, you can consult the following resources.

Your family physician. A doctor who knows the drinker (and the drinker's family) can determine what type of treatment would be appropriate. Also, anyone with a history of heavy drinking should have a thorough medical exam to uncover any medical conditions that may have been caused or aggravated by alcohol abuse.

Family service agencies. Most communities have agencies that run outpatient alcoholic treatment programs or can refer you to one. Look in your telephone directory or contact your local social services department.

Your religious adviser. Talk with your priest, minister, or rabbi.

205 Teach Your Kids Not to Drink

Underage drinking is a growing problem. All too often, teenage drinking leads to:

▶ Traffic accidents (many of them fatal)

▶ Destruction of property

▶ Violent or antisocial behavior

▶ Poor academic performance

▶ Disciplinary problems

▶ Withdrawal from social activities

▶ Problems coping with stress

If you suspect (or know) your teenager drinks, don't ignore it. To discourage or prevent underage drinking:

▶ Be a good role model. The best example you can set is to not drink. But if you choose to drink, drink responsibly. Children of alcoholics are four times as likely to develop a drinking problem as children of nonalcoholic parents.

▶ Show your children that you love them. Be affectionate, and show them you care and are interested in them.

▶ Make an effort to organize family activities. It may be hard to compete with your son's or daughter's peers for their attention at times, but make the effort anyway. Shared hobbies and sports can create bonds and strengthen a teen's resistance to outside influences.

▶ Discuss the potential risks and consequences of alcohol use before it becomes a problem. Answer questions honestly and let your children know how you feel about them drinking before the situation arises.

▶ Tell your children to never get into a car with a drunk driver. Promise you'll pick them up anytime, anywhere, no questions asked, if they call you instead of putting themselves at risk.

206 If You Suspect Narcotics Overdose, Act Fast

Horse. Harry. Scag. Junk. Lords. Schoolboy. Morpho. Hocus. Unkie. Powder. Joy. Snow. Miss Emma. Dollies. These are just a few of the street names for narcotic drugs.

Heroin, morphine, and cocaine are the three most common illegally used drugs. Each is powerfully addictive. Obvious symptoms of ongoing drug use include:

▶ Euphoria

▶ Drowsiness

▶ Apathy

▶ Mood swings

▶ Constricted pupils

▶ Flushed skin

▶ Red, raw nostrils (in cocaine users)

▶ Scars, "tracks," or abscesses at injection sites on the arms or legs

Signs of overdose include:

▶ Constricted, pinpoint pupils

▶ Clammy skin, with a bluish tint

▶ Slow pulse

▶ Shallow breathing (which can lead to respiratory arrest)

▶ Convulsions

▶ Coma

If you suspect someone has overdosed on drugs, call an ambulance or drive the victim to the nearest hospital emergency room *immediately.*

207 Stay Tuned to Hidden Signs of Substance Abuse in Teens

Some parents feel like they have to sleep with both eyes open when their chidren are growing up. Adolescence is a natural period of experimentation. Coupled with the profound physical and emotional changes kids undergo at this time, using drugs (including alcohol) is a potential problem—and a serious one.

Aside from the obvious clues—like the smell of marijuana drifting from your son or daughter's bedroom—other, more subtle signs of substance abuse include:

▶ Borrowing money frequently, or stealing

▶ A short fuse; becoming easily irritated or frustrated

▶ Sleeping or eating more or less than usual

▶ Sudden, noticeable weight loss

► Unusual moodiness or withdrawal
► Lack of interest in appearance, or poor personal hygiene habits
► Secretiveness about new friends or personal belongings
► Decline in academic performance

If you notice any of these symptoms, don't preach, lecture, or lash out. Instead, discuss the substance use calmly and frankly. Let your children know you're concerned, and let them know why: Their use of alcohol and other drugs is not only illegal, it's also not too smart.

Be firm; tell your children what you intend to do if they continue to abuse alcohol or other drugs, and follow through.

Why Smoking Marijuana Is a Mistake

Marijuana is the most commonly used illicit drug around. It's a mild hallucinogen that may also produce euphoria, apathy, poor coordination, reddened eyes, increased appetite, increased heart rate, panic attacks, and short-term memory loss.

Doesn't sound like too much fun. So why do kids smoke pot? For the same reason they drink alcohol or smoke cigarettes: It's wrong, it's risky, and their friends coax them into it. The only way to persuade your kids not to try pot is to give them the facts. Tell them that:

► Driving when you're high on pot is as dangerous as driving when you've been drinking.

► Smoking one joint is the equivalent of smoking 16 cigarettes in terms of reduced vital capacity.

► In males, marijuana decreases sperm count and lowers blood levels of testosterone (the primary male hormone)—in effect, reducing virility.

► In females, marijuana may increase the risk of miscarriage.

► In everyone, marijuana slows learning, impairs memory, and muddles your thinking and understanding, making you tired and fuzzy brained.

Hopefully, marijuana won't appeal to your youngsters once they realize how it affects their brains, lungs, hearts, and the rest of their bodies.

Warn Your Kids Not to Sniff Inhalants

As unappealing as it may sound to adults, some children deliberately inhale the vapors from household products to produce a cheap and dangerous—yet legal—high. The sniffer's repertoire includes glue, nail polish remover, paint, lacquer thinner, cleaning fluid, or plastic cement—precisely the types of products that usually carry a warning on the label saying, "Use in a well-ventilated area. Do not inhale fumes."

Alarmingly, the kids who are most likely to try this are usually about 12 years old. As parents, here's what you can do.

➤ Look for signs of abuse—nausea, sneezing, coughing, disorientation, or evidence of hallucinations.

➤ Warn your child that deliberately sniffing toxic fumes can lead to leukemia, a fatal blood disease, or sudden death.

208 Don't Be Seduced by Cocaine

As recently as the late 1970s, cocaine was considered almost perfect, as illegal drugs go: It apparently offered no threat of addiction, only the promise of pleasure and euphoria. How wrong that belief turned out to be. Cocaine lures users toward a titillating but short-lived high, followed by a gripping physical and psychological dependency. Coke users quickly reach a point where they don't know how to exist without it. Inhaled, snorted, or injected, cocaine traps you into thinking you *need* it—to have fun, to be productive, to get through life.

Toxic levels can cause psychotic reactions that can last from two to four days. (In short, it makes you crazy.) Added to that are the real and present dangers of seizures or a fatal stroke or heart attack, even among first-time coke users.

If you've experimented with cocaine—or know someone who uses it—look for these danger signs.

➤ Preoccupation with thoughts of doing cocaine.

➤ Feeling the need to use cocaine before any social or business event.

➤ Setting limits to cocaine use, then breaking them again and again.

➤ Using the drug nonstop for periods of an entire day or longer.

➤ Lying to family and friends about your cocaine use.

➤ Finding that cocaine is hurting your work, your health, and your relationships with others.

If you think that you or someone you care about has a cocaine problem, get help fast. (See appendix B for the addresses and phone numbers to call for professional—and confidential—help with drug problems.)

209 If You Take Valium, Beware

Diazepam (better known as Valium) was developed as an anti-anxiety drug for people under stress. And it's still an effective drug if used properly. Chronic use, however, can carry serious risks, including addiction. People who stop taking Valium after more than three to four weeks can experience the following withdrawal symptoms.

▶ Increased, uncontrollable anxiety

▶ Jitteriness, nervousness, and tremors

▶ Distorted senses of taste and smell

▶ Difficulty sleeping

In short, the drug could leave you worse off than you were before you started taking it. At that point, the best way to withdraw from the drug is to wean yourself away gradually, under a doctor's supervision. He or she will reduce your dosage over a period of several weeks.

For people who suffer disabling anxiety, Valium can be a useful short-term aid. To avoid dependence, though, keep in mind that:

▶ Only the smallest dose necessary should be taken.

▶ Valium shouldn't be used for more than three or four weeks.

▶ Once the anxiety-producing circumstances are under control, Valium should be discontinued.

▶ If you're taking Valium for ongoing anxiety, take "drug holidays" away from the drug for two-day intervals every three or four weeks.

Note: Don't mix Valium—or other similar anti-anxiety drugs—and alcohol. And don't take Valium if you're pregnant or think you might be pregnant; it can damage a growing fetus.

210 Use Caution with Sleeping Pills

Used improperly, prescription sleeping pills (called sedative-hypnotics) can be as addictive as alcohol and can produce unpleasant withdrawal symptoms if stopped abruptly.

You can develop a tolerance to sleeping pills in as little as two weeks of frequent use. In other words, you need higher and higher amounts to fall asleep. Older people should be especially cautious about taking sleeping pills, since their tolerance for medication is usually lower than middle-aged or younger adults.

If you or someone you're close to takes prescription sleeping pills, possible signs of misuse include:

▶ Taking sleeping pills nightly for more than two weeks.

▶ Needing to take higher doses to fall asleep.

▶ Increasing the dosage without consulting the doctor.

If you've become dependent on sleeping pills, don't quit cold turkey—you're apt to suffer confusion, slurred speech, drowsiness, difficulty concentrating, relentless insomnia, and possibly death. So contact your doctor for instructions on how to wean yourself off the drug. (If you've been tortured with insomnia, see Tip 4 in chapter 1, Fast Relief for Everyday Health Problems.)

9

Women's Health Problems

On the average, women outlive men by about seven years. Doctors credit female biology for 40 percent of that lead and healthier lifestyle for the remaining 60 percent. Fewer women smoke, drink, or meet with fatal accidents than do men. But researchers worry that women will lose their edge on health and longevity if the number of women who smoke continues to increase, and if the stress created by trying to raise a family and work outside the home also continues to mount.

Women can take steps to preserve their health, though. This chapter is packed with tips that address the specific health needs of women. You'll find out how to protect against breast and cervical cancers. You'll learn what questions to ask and what alternatives to consider if you're told you need a hysterectomy. And you'll discover how to manage premenstrual syndrome (PMS), avoid toxic shock syndrome, and relieve breast pain and swelling. And, if you've decided to postpone having a family, you'll learn how to have a safe pregnancy after age 35. So you'll discover how to keep that healthy edge no matter what your age.

211 Examine Your Breasts, Save Your Life

When detected and treated early, breast cancer is curable. And most breast lumps are discovered by women themselves, not by a doctor or mammography (low-dosage x-rays of the breast). Although most lumps are benign, it's wise to examine your breasts once a month for changes that could indicate cancer. (Examine your breasts at the same time each month, preferably within a week following your menstrual period. The breasts will be less tender or swollen and easier to examine at that time.)

Here's how to examine your breasts.

1. Stand in front of a mirror and visually examine both breasts for dimpling; changes in color, texture, or shape; nipple discharge or bleeding; scaliness around the nipple; or veins that weren't visible before.

2. Lie down. Raise your left arm and place your left hand under your head. With the fingers of your right hand, press against the top portion of the left breast. Using a circular motion, feel for lumps or thickened tissue. Moving in a clockwise direction, examine the entire breast, including the portion of breast tissue that extends into your armpit.

3. Gently squeeze the nipple and the darkened area surrounding the nipple. Note any discharge.

4. Examine the right breast, repeating steps 1 through 3.

You can also perform this exam while you're standing in the shower. If you detect any abnormalities, contact your physician.

212 Relief for Breast Pain and Swelling

If you should discover a lump in your breast, don't panic: Chances are it's benign (noncancerous). Many benign breast lumps turn out to be cysts filled with fluid, and they sometimes cause pain. They can occur as a single lump or in clusters that give a "lumpy" feel and appearance to the breast.

The presence of multiple benign breast cysts is known as fibrocystic breast disease. Symptoms include tenderness and pain in one or both breasts about one week before a menstrual period. A nonbloody nipple discharge may also be present.

No one knows what causes fibrocystic disease, but doctors suspect it's due to an increase in estrogen or prolactin levels. For some women, breast pain can be severe and disabling.

To reduce breast pain:

▶ Limit salt and sodium intake, to prevent fluid buildup in the breasts.

▶ Wear a bra that provides good support. (You may want to wear a bra while you sleep, too.)

▶ For severe discomfort, apply ice packs to your breasts two to three times a day.

▶ If an area of the breast feels warm, with swelling and redness, contact your doctor. These could be signs of infection, which can be treated with antibiotics.

▶ Cut down on caffeine. Some studies indicate that women who are heavy coffee drinkers and suffer from fibrocystic disease find relief when they cut their caffeine intake.

▶ Oral contraceptives eliminate breast pain for some women. Or your doctor may prescribe Danazol, a prescription medication, to reduce pain.

▶ Vitamin E (400 international units per day) or diuretics (water pills) may reduce breast pain.

In any case, it's important to report any breast lumps or discomfort to your doctor even if you've had only benign problems so far.

213 A Low-Fat Diet to Protect against Breast Cancer

Several factors determine who will and will not get breast cancer. Women who menstruated earlier than average, who had no children or a late first pregnancy, or who entered menopause late are at higher-than-average risk. So are women whose mother or sister had breast cancer.

Another risk factor is diet—an element you can control in two ways.

▶ Control your weight and cut back on the amount of fat in your diet. Many studies suggest that a high-fat diet and being overweight increase the risk of breast cancer.

▶ Limit your alcohol intake. Some research has shown that women who have three or more drinks a week increase their risk of breast cancer.

214 Real Solutions to PMS

Four out of ten menstruating women suffer premenstrual syndrome (PMS)—bloating, irritability, headache, insomnia, diarrhea, food cravings, and sometimes personality change or severe mood swings. Here's what helps to ease the troublesome symptoms.

▶ Exercise, such as swimming, walking, or bicycling, performed three times a week for 20 minutes at a time, alleviates fluid retention and relaxes muscles.

▶ A diet low in salt, fat, and sugar and high in protein and fiber (from whole grains, fruits, and vegetables) reduces breast tenderness and helps eliminate excess estrogen (a hormone that may contribute to PMS).

▶ Avoid caffeine, alcohol, and nicotine for two weeks before your period is due.

▶ Vitamins E and B$_6$, calcium, magnesium, and the amino acid L-tyrosine seem to help some women. (Before trying vitamin therapy, however, you should consult your physician for guidance.)

▶ If PMS disrupts your sleep, take naps.

▶ Practice relaxation techniques like deep breathing, meditation, yoga, or soaking in a hot tub.

215 Relief for Menstrual Cramps

Menstrual cramps may be accompanied by backache, fatigue, vomiting, diarrhea, and headaches. Sometimes, distress is severe enough to leave women debilitated for the first one to three days of their periods.
To relieve menstrual cramps:

▶ Drink chamomile or mint tea.

▶ Whenever possible, lie on your back, supporting your knees with a pillow.

▶ Hold a heating pad or hot-water bottle on your abdomen.

▶ Gently massage your abdomen.

▶ Do mild exercises like stretching, walking, or biking.

▶ Take aspirin, ibuprofen, or other over-the-counter medication formulated for relief of menstrual discomfort.

If these measures don't alleviate pain—or a heavy schedule prevents you from crawling into bed with a hot-water bottle for three days a month—see your doctor. He or she may prescribe nonsteroidal anti-inflammatory medicines or other medication to help menstrual pain.

216 When to See a Gynecologist

If you experience any of these symptoms, see a gynecologist.

▶ Heavy, painful, irregular, or missed menstrual periods

▶ Bleeding between menstrual periods

▶ Lower abdominal pain or cramping

▶ Vaginal irritation, discharge, or painful intercourse

▶ Bleeding after intercourse

▶ Lumps, thickening, or tenderness in the breasts

Also see a gynecologist for a yearly checkup even if you have no symptoms. Have a checkup more often if you are at high risk for cervical cancer (see Tip 221).

217 Protect Yourself against Toxic Shock Syndrome

Toxic shock syndrome (TSS) is a potentially fatal illness caused by bacteria. Symptoms are:

▶ High fever

▶ Muscle aches

▶ Vomiting

▶ Diarrhea

▶ Sunburnlike rash

▶ Rapid pulse

► Dizziness

► Fainting

If you experience these symptoms during your menstrual period (or any other time), act fast: Contact your doctor or go to a hospital emergency room immediately.

Women should take the following precautions to prevent TSS.

► Never use tampons if you've experienced TSS in the past. Use sanitary napkins instead of tampons whenever possible, or alternate tampons with sanitary pads during a menstrual period. Don't use superabsorbent tampons.

► Lubricate the tampon applicator with a water-soluble (non-greasy) lubricant like K-Y jelly before insertion.

► Change tampons and sanitary pads every 4 to 6 hours, or more frequently.

218 Get Rid of Yeast Infections

Sooner or later, every woman suffers a yeast infection, which occurs when the normal environment of the vagina is disrupted and small amounts of yeast begin to multiply. Symptoms include: itching, irritation, and redness around the vulva and labia; a thick, white discharge; and burning when you urinate or have sex.

To get rid of a yeast infection, douche with a mild solution of 1 to 3 tablespoons of vinegar diluted in a quart of warm water. Repeat once a day (but not longer than a week) until the symptoms subside. If symptoms persist, consult your physician.

You can prevent yeast infections by taking these personal hygiene measures.

► Wear underpants and panty hose with cotton crotches.

► Change underwear and workout clothes immediately after exercising.

► Use unscented tampons or sanitary pads.

► Change tampons and sanitary pads frequently.

► Don't use bath oils, bubble baths, or feminine hygiene sprays.

► Dry the vaginal area thoroughly after you shower, bathe, or swim.

219 Be Alert for Pelvic Inflammatory Disease

If you experience pain and discomfort in your lower abdomen, accompanied by a mild fever, call your doctor. The pain may mimic appendicitis or an ectopic pregnancy, but you may have a pelvic inflammatory disease (PID) in your fallopian tubes or other reproductive organs. If neglected, PID can cause permanent damage and leave you infertile. Follow your physician's instructions; treatment will probably include bed rest and antibiotics.

PID is transmitted sexually, and using an intrauterine device (IUD) increases the chances for infection. If you have been diagnosed as having PID, your sexual partner should be treated also, and your physician should remove the IUD.

220 What You Should Know about Pap Tests

A Pap test examines cells scraped from the cervix for abnormal changes that could indicate cancer. The American College of Obstetricians and Gynecologists recommends that women have a yearly Pap test. An annual test is especially important if you are at higher than average risk for cervical cancer. You are at higher risk if you became sexually active before the age of 18, have multiple sex partners, have a history of pelvic infections, have ever had an abnormal Pap smear, have a history of precancerous changes of the cervix, or if your mother took diethylstilbestrol (DES) when she was pregnant with you.

To help ensure accurate results, avoid douching, using vaginal medications, or having sexual intercourse for 24 hours before the test.

221 Cut Your Risk of Cervical Cancer

To reduce your risk of developing cervical cancer:

➤ Have a Pap smear at least once a year and more often if you are at increased risk (that is, if you have multiple sex partners, if you became sexually active at an early age, if you have a human papilloma virus, if your partner is uncircumcised, if you had frequent and early pregnancies, or if your mother took the drug diethylstilbestrol, or DES, when she was pregnant with you).

➤ Don't smoke.

➤ Limit your sexual activity to monagamous relationships.

▶ If you have more than one sexual relationship, use barrier protective methods, such as a condom, diaphragm, or cervical cap with a spermicide.

▶ Contact your gynecologist if you have pain during intercourse or bleeding or spotting between periods.

222 The Facts about Fibroids

Sometimes lower abdominal pain, heavy menstrual periods, or midcycle bleeding signals the presence of fibroid tumors—round, hard balls of smooth muscle that develop inside the uterine walls. Some women also experience frequent urination, constipation, or abdominal swelling. And for some women, fibroids cause no discomfort at all and are discovered during a routine pelvic exam.

Fibroids are benign—that is, they aren't cancerous—but they can interfere with conception and pregnancy. Since fibroids are most common during the childbearing years, they can be a problem even if they don't cause any discomfort.

If your doctor says that you need a hysterectomy for fibroids, get a second opinion, especially if you still want to have children. Depending on the number, size, and location of fibroids, your uterus may or may not have to be removed.

One option is myomectomy, a limited procedure that cuts out the fibroids but leaves the uterus intact. Or your doctor may prescribe progesterone or a tumor-shrinking drug called gonadotropin-releasing hormone (GnRH). Yet another option, if you take birth control pills, is to switch to a progesterone-only pill or other nonhormonal method of birth control, since estrogen seems to stimulate the growth of fibroids. (For similar reasons, fibroids almost always shrink after menopause.)

Even if your condition warrants removing your uterus, you may be able to keep your ovaries, thus avoiding a surgically induced menopause. To find out what's best for you, discuss the pros and cons of all the possible options with your doctor.

223 The Right and Wrong Reasons for a Hysterectomy

Over the past few years, some women, doctors, and medical insurance providers have questioned the need for hysterectomy (surgical removal of the uterus). Alternative therapies have evolved to treat some of the conditions that hysterectomy has routinely been used for. Consequently, the number of unnecessary hysterectomies performed is on the decline.

Hysterectomies are still warranted for:

▶ Large fibroids

▶ Severe hemorrhaging not controlled with medication

▶ Irreversible damage from an untreated infection

▶ Cancer of the cervix or uterus

▶ Endometriosis

Alternative treatments exist for heavy, painful periods, fibroid tumors, endometriosis, and prolapsed uterus. If these conditions don't respond to more conservative treatment, then a hysterectomy may be warranted. So if you're told you need a hysterectomy:

▶ Ask about alternatives to surgery.

▶ Ask for specific details about the condition you're being treated for and the expected outcome of surgery.

▶ Ask if your ovaries can be spared, to prevent shutting off the release of estrogen and, subsequently, premature menopause.

▶ Don't hesitate to get a second opinion if you question the need for a hysterectomy.

224 If You Take the Pill, Don't Smoke

Studies published by the U.S. Department of Health and Human Services indicate that women who smoke and take birth control pills may increase their risk for a heart attack, especially if they're over 35. So if you smoke, don't take the Pill. And if you must take the Pill, don't smoke.

225 Want to Have a Baby? Try This

Many couples don't conceive as quickly as they'd like to. You can improve your chances of getting pregnant if you follow these measures.

► Avoid alcohol, tobacco, and marijuana.

► Avoid foods and beverages that contain caffeine.

► Avoid extreme overweight or underweight.

► Lie on your back with your hips elevated by a pillow for approximately 30 minutes after intercourse.

► Know when your ovaries release eggs, and time intercourse for your fertile period. Ovulation normally occurs 14 to 16 days after the start of your period. Signs of ovulation include a dull ache in either the lower right or left side of the abdomen; clear, elastic vaginal mucus; and a slightly elevated temperature.

You can buy an ovulation predictor kit at most drugstores. The kit contains sticks which, when dipped in urine, turn blue if you're ovulating. Or you can keep track of your fertile days with a special basal thermometer, also available at drugstores. Having intercourse when your temperature drops approximately 0.4 F increases your chances of conception.

If you fail to conceive after one year of trying, consult your gynecologist or a fertility specialist. A number of factors can prevent conception. (See also Tip 243 in chapter 10, Men's Health Problems, for information on how men can enhance fertility.)

226 Tips for a Healthier, Easier Pregnancy

Healthy moms tend to have healthy babies. If you plan to become pregnant, take the following steps to help your baby get off to a good start.

► Have a complete medical exam, including a gynecological exam. A number of medical conditions, including obesity, high blood pressure, diabetes, smoking, alcohol use, nutritional deficiencies, and Rh negative blood factor (after the first pregnancy) can jeopardize the health of mother and child.

► Check with your doctor about the effects of any prescription or over-the-counter medication you take.

► If you have a chronic medical condition, ask your doctor how it may affect your pregnancy and whether or not you should change or adjust your medication.

► If you use and IUD or take birth control pills, use an alternative form of birth control for 1-2 months before trying to become pregnant.

▶ If you're markedly overweight, plan to lose excess pounds before becoming pregnant.

▶ Exercise regularly.

▶ Consider genetic tests or counseling if you or your husband has a family history of genetic disorders, if you are 35 or older, or if your husband is 60 or older.

You and your baby will do best if you follow these guidelines.

▶ Ask your doctor or a dietitian to outline a meal plan that meet the special nutritional needs created by pregnancy,

▶ Avoid caffeine, alcohol, nicotine, and illicit drugs, as they can harm you and your unborn baby.

▶ Consult your doctor before taking any medication.

▶ Ask your doctor what prenatal vitamin/mineral supplement you should take.

▶ Follow your health care provider's advice about weight gain. The recommended weight gain for the woman of average weight is between 25 to 35 pounds. A small boned, petite woman will probably be at the lower end of the scale and a larger, big boned woman will be on the higher end.

▶ Continue to exercise in moderation (see Tip 229).

▶ Practice relaxation and other stress control techniques. (Doctors think emotional stress may constrict the blood supply to the uterus and placenta, the baby's sole source of oxygen and nutrients.)

▶ Enroll in childbirth preparation classes.

▶ If you own a cat, arrange for someone else to empty the litter box. Cat excrement can transmit a disease called toxoplasmosis If you're infected while pregnant, your baby may be stillborn, born prematurely, or suffer serious damage to the brain, eyes, or other parts of the body.

227 Safe Pregnancy after Thirty-Five

Age is not the biggest factor in a healthy pregnancy. The biggest factor is the good health of the mother.

Becoming pregnant after the age of 35, however, poses a number of potential problems. Chances for conception decrease with age. The incidence of miscarriage and premature birth is slightly higher in later-life pregnancies. So is the likelihood that the mother will develop diabetes or high blood pressure. The chances that a baby will be born with a genetic defect increases, too. So along with other health considerations, a pregnant woman in her mid-thirties or older should:

▶ Discuss with her doctor, in detail, her pregnancy plans, risk factors, and measures she needs to take for a healthy pregnancy.

▶ Talk to her doctor about prenatal genetic tests.

About Amniocentesis

Usually performed between week 15 and 18 of the pregnancy, amniocentesis can detect Down's syndrome, Tay-Sachs disease, sickle cell anemia, Rh incompatibility, or spina bifida. (Amniocentesis will also reveal the sex of the child, but it's never done for that purpose alone.) The doctor uses a long needle to draw out a sample of amniotic fluid, which is tested for genetic abnormalities. The test itself presents some risk—there is about 1 chance in 100 to 1 chance in 200 that a miscarriage may occur within three weeks after the procedure is performed.

Amniocentesis is justified under the following conditions.

▶ The pregnant woman is 35 years old or older.

▶ Someone in the mother's or father's immediate family (a parent, sibling, or child) has a genetic or metabolic disorder.

▶ There is a family history of hemophilia (a bleeding disorder) or spina bifida (a neural tube defect).

▶ An earlier pregnancy produced a baby with chromosome abnormalities.

Amniocentesis can't detect abnormalities such as a club foot or cleft palate, so normal results don't necessarily guarantee a normal baby. Another technique called chorionic villous sampling (CVS) analyzes a small sample of the placenta and can be performed much earlier than amniocentesis, (in weeks 8 to 12). The earlier testing is done, the more time the prospective parents and their doctor have to decide on the best course of action.

228 How Long Expectant Mothers Can Stay on the Job

With more than half the women in the United States working full time, many want to know how long they can continue to work if they become pregnant. What's safe? What's wise? What's right for you?

It depends. The Council on Scientific Affairs of the American Medical Association studied the effects of pregnancy on work performance and came up with the guidelines presented in the table below. (As you can see, some women can work until the day they're wheeled into the delivery room with no ill effects.) Of course, you and your physician are the best judges of how work affects your pregnancy and vice versa.

How Long Expectant Women Continue to Work

Job Demands	Week of Pregnancy
Secretarial and light clerical	40
Professional and managerial	40
Sitting, with light tasks	40
Standing	
Prolonged (more than 4 hrs.)	24
Intermittent	
(more than 30 min. per hr.)	32
(less than 30 min. per hr.)	40
Stooping and bending below knee level	
Repetitive (more than 10 times per hr.)	20
Intermittent	
(less than 10 but more than 2 times per hr.)	28
(Less than 2 times per hr.)	40

Job Demands	Week of Pregnancy
Climbing vertical ladders and poles	
Repetitive (more than 4 times per 8-hr. shift)	20
Intermittent (less than 4 times per 8-hr. shift)	28
Climbing up and down stairs	
Repetitive (more than 4 times per 8-hr. shift)	28
Intermittent (less than 4 times per 8-hr. shift)	40
Lifting	
Repetitive	
(50 lbs. or more)	20
(less than 50 but more than 25 lbs.)	24
(less than 25 lbs.)	40
Intermittent	
(50 lbs. or more)	30
(less than 50 lbs.)	40

SOURCE: Council on Scientific Affairs, "Effects of Pregnancy on Work Performance," *Journal of the American Medical Association*, vol. 251, no. 15 (April 20, 1984). Copyright 1984, American Medical Association.

229 Smart Ways to Exercise during Pregnancy

Exercise can help ease muscular aches and pains and other discomforts women sometimes experience during their pregnancies. Yoga, walking, swimming, and other forms of low-impact or stretching exercises are best.

Check with your doctor if you've never exercised, and follow these safety guidelines for exercising during pregnancy.

► Wait 1 to 2 hours after eating to exercise.

► Drink one or two 8-ounce glasses of water before you start to exercise.

► Don't do exercises that involve jumping, twisting, or strenuous activity.

► Keep your heart rate below 140 beats a minute.

► Don't become overheated.

► After the fourth month of pregnancy, avoid exercises in which you lie flat on your back.

► If you always or nearly always feel tired for more than 2 hours after exercise, see your doctor.

230 Breast Care for Nursing Mothers

Breastfeeding your baby is one of the most fulfilling experiences in life. But if nursing leaves your breasts tender and sore, satisfaction gives way to discomfort. Proper breast care can minimize this problem, though.

► Wear good support bras throughout your pregnancy.

► Wear a nursing bra day and night as long as your baby is breastfeeding.

► Avoid wearing bras that have a plastic liner.

► Change your bra or breast pads when they become damp or wet.

► Alternate breasts when nursing.

► Avoid nursing your baby more than 20 minutes on each breast.

► Don't pull the baby away from your breast. Instead, break the suction by gently inserting your finger between the baby's mouth and your breast.

► Expect some temporary swelling for the first few days you breastfeed. Warm showers and ice packs can relieve discomfort.

► Wash your breasts daily, using warm water and a soft cloth. Don't use soap; it can dry your skin and irritate your breasts.

► Apply a cream or ointment to your breasts after your baby

nurses. Doctors recommend lanolin, cocoa butter, wet tea bags, or special breast creams.

If your breasts are red, inflamed, and painful despite precautions, consult your doctor.

231 Riding Out Postpartum Blues

If you're like most mothers, you've eagerly awaited the birth of your child. So why do you burst into tears for no good reason now that your baby is home? Why can't you seem to get organized?

It's simple: You've got postpartum blues, or the "baby blues." And approximately six out of ten new mothers experience this peculiar mood change to some degree, typically on the third day following childbirth. Postpartum blues are blamed on hormonal changes, fatigue, and the adjustments required by a new baby.

Take these steps to help alleviate the baby blues.

▶ Arrange for household help when you and the baby come home.

▶ Nap when your baby naps.

▶ Plan to spend some time away from home with your husband or friends (or both), even in the first week that you're home and even if it's just for an hour or two.

Postpartum blues should last no longer than a week. If you feel blue, overwhelmed, and unable to cope for more than a week, contact your doctor. You may have postpartum depression, which affects about 15 percent of new mothers. It can last for months and interfere with normal functioning. Your doctor may prescribe medication or recommend professional counseling.

232 Plan for a Healthier, Happier Menopause

Some women dread menopause, associating the change of life with hot flashes, painful intercourse, mood swings, and the spectre of old age. As with menstruation and childbearing, menopause is a rite of passage that has some discomforts. But you can help to prevent or alleviate many of them.

▶ To maintain a positive outlook, share your feelings with friends, stay active, and take an interest in others in your community.

▶ To alleviate mood swings, cut down on caffeine, alcohol, and sweets.

▶ To combat insomnia, drink a cup of herbal tea, such as chamomile, before bedtime.

Kegel exercises (named for the individual who invented them) can help to keep your pelvic and vaginal muscles toned, preventing a prolapsed uterus or poor bladder control, both of which sometimes accompany menopause. To feel these muscles at work, stop and start your urine flow in midstream the next time you use the toilet. Then practice the two simple exercises that follow.

▶ Squeeze the pelvic/vaginal muscles for 3 seconds, then relax them for 3 seconds. Do this ten times, three times a day.

▶ Squeeze and relax the same muscles as quickly as possible. Repeat ten times, three times a day.

233 How to Take the Heat out of Hot Flashes

Women typically describe a hot flash as a wave of suffocating warmth that starts in the chest, works its way to the neck and face, and hits as often as every 90 minutes. Hot flashes aren't usually obvious to others, but women who have hot flashes find them uncomfortable and embarrassing.

To reduce the discomfort of hot flashes, try these tactics.

▶ Wear lightweight clothes made of natural fibers.

▶ Limit or avoid beverages that contain caffeine or alcohol.

▶ Avoid rich food or heavy meals.

▶ Take 400 international units of vitamin E daily. (Consult your doctor first, though.)

If you suffer from night sweats (hot flashes that occur as you sleep):

▶ Wear loose-fitting cotton nightwear.

▶ Keep the room cool.

234 Simple Solutions for Vaginal Dryness

At menopause, estrogen levels drop. The decline in estrogen production is responsible for atrophic vaginitis, or vaginal dryness. Intercourse may be painful or difficult. Here are some ways to deal with this problem.

➤ Don't use deodorant soaps or scented products in the vaginal area.

➤ Use a water-soluble lubricant, such as K-Y jelly, to facilitate penetration during intercourse. Avoid oils or petroleum-based products—they encourage infection.

➤ Ask your physician about intravaginal estrogen cream.

➤ If you still experience pain during intercourse, or if you notice a pink-tinged discharge, or experience burning when you urinate, contact your doctor. You may have an infection.

235 Tactics to Prevent Osteoporosis

Everyone's bones lose density after age 40. In women, menopause accelerates the loss, especially if they're thin or small-boned, have red or blond hair or freckles, are of Oriental or northern European descent, or have never had any children. Smoking, a sedentary life, taking corticosteroids, and eating too few calcium-containing foods also increase the risk. And the earlier you reach menopause, the higher the risk. (Women who have a family history of osteoporosis, hyperthyroidism, hyperparathyroidism, and certain forms of bone cancer are also at risk.)

To prevent or slow osteoporosis, take these steps now.

➤ Be sure your diet includes a minimum of 1,000 milligrams of calcium a day (if you're premenopausal) or 1,500 milligrams a day (if you're postmenopausal and not on estrogen replacement therapy). As mentioned in Tip 112 in chapter 4, Eating for Better Health, high-calcium foods include low-fat dairy products and soft-boned fish like salmon and sardines. Beans and bean sprouts, soybean curd, broccoli, kale, and sunflower seeds contain small amounts of calcium, too. Avoid supplements derived from dolomite or bone meal, however.

➤ Cut back on sodium and salt.

➤ Begin a program of regular, weight-bearing exercise like walking, jogging, biking, or low-impact or non-impact aerobics.

➤ Ask your doctor about estrogen replacement therapy (ERT), alendronate sodium (Fosamax), and Calcitonin.

236 Look into Estrogen Replacement Therapy

Many of the symptoms typical of menopause can be attributed to one factor: a drop in circulating levels of estrogen, the principal female hormone. Consequently, replacing estrogen by means of pills, injections, vaginal creams, or skin patches can relieve vaginal dryness, insomnia, and hot flashes and can protect against osteoporosis and other common consequences of menopause. Today, lower doses of estrogen are given than previously used, and are given in conjunction with progesterone.

Estrogen replacement therapy (ERT) is not risk-free, however. Some women experience an increased risk of uterine cancer, gallstones, high blood pressure, thrombophlebitis, and, less seriously, nausea, breast tenderness, or fluid retention. Consequently, ERT should never be used in women who have a history of blood clots or breast or uterine cancer. And ERT should be used with caution in women who have or have had high blood pressure, diabetes, gallbladder disease, liver disease, fibroid tumors of the uterus, or cancer of the ovaries.

ERT is worth considering if you experience menopause (either naturally or because of removal of the ovaries) before the age of 40 or if you are at high risk for osteoporosis, as discussed in the previous tip. It may also be appropriate if you suffer recurrent vaginal and urinary tract infections or are bothered by hot flashes, insomnia, or vaginal dryness. (Incidentally, ERT may bestow one major benefit on women: A study conducted at the University of Southern California School of Medicine showed that women who took estrogen were less likely to die from a heart attack than women who didn't take estrogen.)

If you're taking estrogen and experience any of the following symptoms, contact your doctor.

► Hair loss
► Facial pigmentation
► Skin rash
► Abnormal vaginal bleeding
► Warm, red, tender calves

237 Protect Yourself against Rape

No rape prevention strategy is foolproof. But you can avoid making yourself an easy victim by taking the following precautions.

In your home:

- Change all the locks after moving into a new home or apartment.
- Use deadbolt locks on your doors and secure your windows so that they can't be opened more than 5 inches from the outside.
- Keep the shades or drapes drawn after dark and turn on any outside lights.
- Don't open your door to anyone you don't know.
- Don't list your first name in the phone book or on your mailbox.

Use these tactics when you're away from home.

- In an elevator, stand near the control buttons, and avoid riding an elevator alone with a stranger.
- On the street, walk purposefully. Don't stroll along aimlessly; stay alert to possible danger. Avoid walking along dark alleys, close to doorways, and past untrustworthy-looking people.
- Carry a whistle or a stickpin.
- When walking to your car, have your keys in your hand, get into your car quickly, and lock the doors immediately. (You can also use your keys as a weapon, if you have to defend yourself.)
- To avoid getting stranded, keep your car well maintained, and don't let it get low on fuel.
- If you have car trouble, stay in your car with the doors locked and the windows closed. Turn on your emergency flashers and wait for police or other help to arrive.
- If someone approaches your car, crack the window and ask them to send help. Don't let the person into your car.
- Don't hitchhike, and don't pick up hitchhikers.
- Don't go out on single dates unless you know the person well.

If you suspect trouble, here's what to do.

- Don't enter your house or car if you suspect someone has broken in. Call the police from the nearest telephone.
- If you're walking and suspect someone is following you, go into a public building and get help or call the police.
- If you're driving and suspect someone is following you, don't go home. Instead, drive to a police station or a friend's house.

CHAPTER

10

Men's Health Problems

The average life expectancy of a boy born today is 72 years. That's about a 3-year gain over the life expectancy of boys born 10 years ago. But before men sprain their wrists patting themelves on the back, keep in mind that their average life expectancy still lags behind that of women, who can expect to live about 79 years. Why the difference?

Attitude may be part of the explanation. Traditionally, men have been taught to ignore pain and show little concern for their health. Or they believe that "real men" don't admit to physical weakness of any sort—or that some kind of innate strength wards off illness.

Fortunately, that attitude is beginning to change. Many men now realize that being born male doesn't automatically make them too tough to get sick—and that it's not unmanly to ask for medical help when they need it.

Certain health problems—some minor, some major—are unique to men. Others affect men more often, or affect men in a different way than they affect women. This chapter will help you recognize the symptoms of exclusively male problems like prostate trouble, testicular cancer, and impotence. It will also provide tips on protecting yourself against nuisances like jock itch and baldness. Hopefully, the information here—combined with the tips throughout this book—will give men the edge they need to live longer, healthier lives.

238 Alternatives to Baldness

Almost all men worry about going bald, especially if their fathers and grandfathers went bald. Worry builds when men hit their thirties and they notice their hair is thinning.

Don't be taken in by fraudulent claims for vitamin formulas, massage oils, lotions, or ointments that promise to cure baldness. No existing potion or ointment will produce a full head of hair. The only remedy that comes close is the drug Minoxidil (Rogaine), originally developed as a blood pressure medication. Minoxidil has shown promising results for some (but not all) cases of baldness.

Another option is a hair transplant, or "punch grafts." A surgeon cuts out plugs of the bald portion of the scalp and replaces them with plugs from the hair-bearing portion of the scalp (usually the back). The transplanted hair falls out and new hair grows in a month or so. It takes about 250 plugs—at a cost of several thousand dollars—to fill in a receding hairline. In the meantime, the tufts of hair give your scalp a pegboard appearance.

If you choose to wear a hairpiece, be sure it matches your natural hair and fits properly. And remember to keep your hairpiece as clean and well-groomed as your own hair.

See your doctor if you suffer sudden hair loss—you may have a medical problem.

239 Loosen Your Tie and See Better

Dressing for success may propel you toward the top, but not toward top-notch vision. Research at Cornell University suggests a necktie that is knotted too tightly can interfere with blood flow to the brain and sensory organs—namely, your eyes. Computer operators, pilots, draftsmen, and other professionals who need to pay close attention to visual details may be hampered by the "tie that binds."

One sure way to prevent this problem is to avoid wearing a tie altogether. But in some occupations, wearing a tie is standard attire. If you must wear a tie:

▶ Buy shirts with plenty of neck room.

▶ Leave your shirt collar unbuttoned beneath your tie.

▶ Don't knot your tie so tightly that you can't slip a finger between the shirt collar and your neck.

▶ If feasible, loosen or remove your necktie from time to time throughout the day.

240 Stop Snoring for Good

You've probably heard funny stories about snorers. On camping trips they are forced to sleep in their own tents. At home, neighbors make them close their windows. Spouses sleep in separate bedrooms.

Well, snoring isn't so funny if you're the one who's ostracized—or if you have to put up with someone who snores. (Nine out of ten snorers are men, and most of them are age 40 or over.)

Here are some tips to help you stop snoring.

▶ Sleep on your side. Prop an extra pillow behind your back so you won't roll over. Try sleeping on a narrow sofa for a few nights to get accustomed to staying on your side.

▶ Sew a marble or tennis ball into a pocket on the back of your pajamas. The discomfort it causes will remind you to sleep on your side.

▶ If you must sleep on your back, raise the head of the bed with bricks or blocks. Elevating the head in this way can prevent the tongue from falling against the back of the throat, which can cause snoring.

▶ If you are heavy, lose weight. Excess fatty tissue in the throat can cause snoring.

▶ Don't drink alcohol or eat a heavy meal within 3 hours before bedtime. For some reason, both seem to foster snoring.

▶ Take an antihistamine or decongestant before retiring to relieve nasal congestion (which can also contribute to snoring).

▶ Try over-the-counter "nasal strips". These help keep nasal passages unobstructed.

If the problem persists—or if your bed partner notices that you stop breathing for several seconds in the midst of snoring—see an ear, nose, and throat specialist or a physician who specializes in sleep disorders. You may have a medical problem that needs attention.

241 Prevent Jock Itch

"Jock itch" may have an athletic ring to it, but men who suffer the problem aren't sports about it. Jock itch is typified by redness, itching and scaliness in the groin and thigh area, and it's caused by a fungus infection.

Jock itch gets its name because an athletic supporter worn during a workout, then stored in a dark, poorly ventilated locker, and then worn again without being laundered provides the ideal environment in which the fungi thrive. (Under similar conditions, women's clothing can develop this problem, too.)

To relieve jock itch and prevent future attacks:

▶ Don't wear tight, close-fitting clothing. Boxer shorts are recommended for men.

▶ Change underwear frequently—especially after work, if you have a job that leaves you hot and sweaty.

▶ Bathe or shower immediately after a workout.

▶ Apply talc or other powder to the groin area.

▶ Don't store damp clothing in a locker or gym bag between wearings. Wash workout clothes after each wearing.

▶ Sleep in the buff.

An antifungal cream, powder, or lotion like tolnaftate (brand name Tinactin) may also help relieve jock itch. It takes up to two weeks to work. If your problem persists despite these measures, consult your doctor for help.

242 Overcoming Impotence

Just about every man will experience an episode of impotence—failure to achieve or maintain an adequate erection for sexual intercourse—at least once in his life. The cause may be psychological, physical, or a combination of both. Inhibitions, guilt, performance anxiety, and stress can trigger the problem. So can atherosclerosis, hormonal disorders, high blood pressure, diabetes, neurological problems, and certain types of surgery on the genitourinary system. Alcohol and some medications can also produce impotence.

If you have a frequent or ongoing problem with impotence, consult a physician. Physician referral services and hospitals with support groups for impotent men can help you locate a qualified doctor. Your medical history and the results of certain tests can provide important clues to help diagnose the problem and dictate what kind of treatment may help.

▶ If the cause is psychological, your doctor may suggest you consult a therapist who specializes in sexual dysfunction.

▶ If you have a hormonal disorder, your doctor may prescribe hormone injections or pills.

▶ Some men require surgery to restore sexual function. A device known as a penile implant, for instance, can help produce erections.

Avoid over-the-counter products like vitamins, creams, exercises, and various gadgets marketed as cures for impotence. They don't work.

243 Reversing Male Infertility

If a man has been unsuccessful at fathering a child, he'll probably be checked for two kinds of problems: low sperm count (too few sperm per given volume of semen) and poor sperm motility (sperm that are poor swimmers and have trouble fertilizing an egg).

Factors that can reduce fertility in men include:

▶ Extreme overweight.

▶ Heavy smoking. (Smoking has been associated with low sperm count and poor sperm motility.)

▶ Drug and alcohol use. (Marijuana and alcohol lower production of testosterone, a hormone produced by the testicles.)

▶ Wearing tight, restrictive underwear. (Clothing that holds the testicles too close to the body heats them up and thus interferes with sperm production, which is temperature sensitive.)

▶ Work that requires you to sit for long periods of time (for reasons similar to those above).

▶ Frequent use of saunas or hot tubs.

▶ Prolonged occupational exposure to lead, zinc, copper, or radiation. (Pollutants can disrupt the production, quality, and transportation of sperm.)

▶ Prolonged abstinence from sex.

▶ Use of lubricants like petroleum jelly and K-Y Jelly, which can kill or immobilize sperm.

▶ Infection or other illness. (These hamper the testicles' ability to do their job.)

▶ A varicocele (a congenital defect in the blood vessels to the testes).

For many men, restoring fertility is simply a matter of switching to boxer shorts, quitting smoking, losing weight, or making other adjustments. Be patient, though. It may take two or three months to restore fertility. If your partner still doesn't conceive, see a doctor who specializes in treating infertility.

~~244~~ Facts and Fallacies about Vasectomies

Sterilization is the ultimate method of birth control. Vasectornies are safe and can be performed in about 30 minutes under local anesthesia. (The procedure involves surgical removal of part of the vas deferens or sperm duct.) You don't even have to go to the hospital.

Some common misconceptions make many men reluctant to consider a vasectomy. Vasectomy does not lower your sex drive, leave you impotent, or cause hardening of the arteries. And a vasectomy won't reduce pleasurable sensations during sex.

If you're considering a vasectomy:

▶ Consult a urologist who specializes in genitourinary surgery.

▶ Make sure all your questions are answered satisfactorily.

▶ Think the matter over carefully before you take action.

~~245~~ Help for an Enlarged Prostate

If they live long enough, most men will eventually suffer from an enlarged prostate gland—what doctors call a benign prostatic hypertrophy. An enlarged prostate is troublesome but not usually life threatening. The symptoms are:

▶ Frequent urination, especially during the night

▶ Delay in onset of urine flow

▶ Diminished urine flow

These symptoms indicate that your prostate gland has enlarged enough to partially obstruct the flow of urine. Serious complications, such as kidney damage or kidney infection, could arise. So report these symptoms to your doctor. Most likely, surgery will be required.: Because an enlarged prostate can lead to kidney problems, contact your doctor immediately if you experience:

▶ A burning sensation when you urinate
▶ Pain in the lower back, groin, or testicles
▶ Fever and chills

An enlarged prostate does not necessarily indicate the presence of prostate cancer. A digital rectal exam can be done in your doctor's office to screen for prostate cancer. A blood test called a PSA may also be done.

246 How to Perform a Testicular Exam

Early detection of testicular cancer—by a monthly self-exam—can lead to a complete cure 90 to 95 percent of the time. It's best performed when the scrotum is relaxed, after a warm bath or shower. Here's how it's done.

▶ Use a lotion or soapy lather to reduce friction and make it easier to detect abnormalities.
▶ Check both testicles, one at a time, by rolling the testes between the fingers. If you feel any lumps, enlargement, or change in consistency, see your doctor. Also, report any sense of heaviness or pain.

247 Men Need Calcium, Too

Much has been written about the importance of calcium for women's health, but men need calcium, too. Although osteoporosis is more prevalent in women, it can strike men. And recent studies have suggested that calcium may play some role in controlling blood pressure for some people—something that's worth asking your physician about.

In addition to eating foods high in calcium—like fat-free or low-fat milk, cheese, and yogurt—you can protect your bones by performing a weight-bearing exercise like walking regularly, by avoiding over-consumption of alcohol, and by getting your fair share of vitamin D (from either fortified milk or sunshine).

Medications like cortisone or Dilantin can interfere with calcium absorption, so if you're taking these medications, find out if you should also take a calcium supplement.

248 Managing Male Menopause

You never heard of male menopause? It's a term used to describe the emotional reactions men sometimes have in response to mid-life transitions. Between the ages of 40 and 60, some men begin to feel edgy and dissatisfied, overwhelmed by their obligations, and pessimistic about their futures. Typical symptoms include:

▶ Insomnia

▶ Sexual problems

▶ Increased dissatisfaction with work, marriage, and family life

▶ Preoccupation with the past, or worries about illness and death

▶ Abuse of alcohol, drugs, or both

▶ Impulsive behavior, or taking unnecessary or dangerous risks

These feelings and behaviors are often triggered by changes like children moving away from home, or other typical midlife events.

To cope with midlife change:

▶ Don't make radical or impulsive changes, like trading in an economical sedan for a luxury European sports car, or suddenly deciding you want a divorce.

▶ Don't use alcohol, drugs, or casual sex to escape or lessen the impact of change.

▶ Do share your fears and concerns with your family, and seek professional counseling if your troubles seem to be more than you can handle.

▶ Do cultivate skills and interests you'd enjoy but never took the time to pursue.

249 Don't Be Too Macho for Your Own Good

Men typically suffer more serious illnesses and die at a younger age than women. You wouldn't know it by looking at the average doctor's waiting room, though. Men don't report as many symptoms as women do, and they let a problem go further before they seek medical help.

If you have a tendency to ignore or downplay physical or emotional problems, or exhibit other kinds of self-destructive, "macho" behavior, make a conscious effort to change. Here's how:

▶ Pay attention to pain and discomfort. If you're sick or injured, see a doctor.

▶ Take safety precautions at work, home, or when you drive. (See chapter 14, Be Smart, Be Safe.)

▶ Balance work and play.
▶ Don't stifle feelings of compassion and sensitivity.
▶ Learn to express your feelings without losing your temper.
▶ Don't feel compelled to compete all the time.
▶ If you experience emotional problems, consult a professional counselor.

CHAPTER

11

A Happier,
Healthier
Sex Life

Sex certainly seems to have gotten complicated since we learned about spores and zygotes back in fifth-grade science class. Birth control options go beyond condoms, the rhythm method, and abstinence. And syphilis and gonorrhea are no longer the only sexually transmitted diseases (STDs) to worry about. The list of possible infections has grown to include herpes, chlamydia, genital warts, hemophilus vaginalis, non-gonococcal urethritis, cystitis, candidiasis, trichomoniasis, and AIDS, an often fatal and highly misunderstood disease. On top of all that are the usual worries about sexual attractiveness, performance, and satisfaction.

Some days, it seems as though sex has nothing but negative possibilities. Nevertheless, sex is still a normal, healthy, and welcome part of life. You can control or prevent disease, unwanted pregnancy, or other undesirable consequences of sex.

This chapter will help take the fear and worry out of sex. You'll learn to deal with problems like premature ejaculation and lack of sexual desire. And you'll learn how to spot the early symptoms of AIDS, syphilis, gonorrhea, chlamydia, herpes, and other STDs so you can seek treatment as soon as possible.

You'll also learn how to cope with special circumstances, like how to make sex safer after a heart attack and how to locate a trustworthy therapist if you can't resolve sexual problems on your own. (Certain male sexual problems, including impotence and infertility, are discussed in chapter 10, Men's Health Problems.)

250 Know Your Birth Control Options

Below is a summary of various birth control methods. Protection from HIV and STDs should also be considered. Discuss these options with your doctor.

Cervical Cap. Covers the cervix; prevents sperm from reaching egg. Needs a prescription and proper fitting by a doctor. Can be kept in place up to 3 days. Slight risk of infection when left in place for several weeks. Not to be used by those with a history of abnormal Pap smears. Should not be used during menstrual period. Failure rate %* for ideal use is 6%; for average use is 18%.

Condom (Female). Shaped like a male condom, but larger. Is placed inside the vagina like a lining. Made of polyurethane which is thinner and stronger than latex. Effective protection against STDs and HIV (especially when used with a male condom). Available over-the-counter. Can take time and patience to use correctly. Can twist if not inserted properly. Costs more than male condoms. Failure rate %* for ideal use is 5%; for average use is 25%.

Condom (Male). Thin pliable sheath worn over erect penis; prevents sperm from entering vagina. Latex brands are most effective. They protect against gonorrhea, syphilis and HIV. Slight risk of breakage. Easily damaged with improper storage. Deteriorate when exposed to ultraviolet light, heat, or moisture. Not good choice if allergic to latex. Failure rate %* for idea use is 2%; for average use is 16%.

Depo-Provera. A female prescription contraceptive given by injection every 3 months. Blocks ovulation. Highly effective in preventing pregnancy. May reduce risk of endometrial cancer. Provides no protection for STDs or HIV. May cause irregular periods, weight gain, fatigue, and headaches. Once stopped, it can take 4-18 months for a women to become fertile again. Failure rate %* for ideal use is 0.3%; for average use is 0.4%.

Diaphragm. Thin, soft, rubber cap that covers the cervix; prevents sperm from reaching egg. Needs doctor's prescription. Can be used over and over again. Helps protect against some STDs when used with spermicides. Requires proper fitting. May dislodge during intercourse. May increase chance of getting bladder infections. Should not be used during menstrual period. Failure rate %* for ideal use is 6%; for average use is 18%.

Spermicides (Foams, Jellies, Creams, Suppositories). Spermicides inserted into the vagina; kill sperm before entering the uterus. Available over-the-counter. More reliable when used with barrier methods (condoms, diaphragms). Protects against some STDs. May cause irritation. Must be applied within 10 minutes of intercourse. Failure rate %* for ideal use is 3%; for average use is 30%.

Intrauterine Device (IUD). Smaller copper device inserted into vagina; prevents pregnancy by interfering with sperm transport and fertilization. Needs to be inserted by a doctor. Remains in place at all times. Does not prevent STDs or HIV. May cause heavy menstrual flow. May become dislodged. Risk of infection and perforation of the uterus. Not recommended for those who have a history of pelvic inflammatory disease. Failure rate %* for ideal use is .8%; for average use is 4%.

Norplant. Six thin capsules (the size of match sticks) are placed under the skin of a woman's upper arm. Keeps a woman from making hormones needed for ovulation. Needs a doctor's prescription, insertion, and removal. One time insertion effective for up to six years. Can be removed at any time. Fertility returns soon after removal of implants. Does not prevent STDs or HIV. May cause irregular menstrual bleeding during the first 6 months after implants are put in. Failure rate %* for ideal use is .04%; for average use is .05%.

Pill (Oral Contraceptives). Prevent the release of eggs (ovulation). Needs a doctor's prescription. May reduce a woman's chance for: uterine and ovarian cancers, pelvic inflammatory disease (PID). Promotes regular periods, lighter menstrual flow. Does not prevent STDs or HIV. Must be taken as prescribed. May increase the risk of blood clots. Failure rate %* for ideal use is .1%; for average use is 6%.

Sterilization (Female). Tubal Ligation (having "tubes tied") - Surgery to burn, cut, or tie off the fallopian tubes. This prevents eggs from being fertilized. Permanent form of birth control. Should be used only when no more children are desired. Usually requires general anesthesia. Does not prevent STDs or HIV. Costs more than a vasectomy. Failure rate %* is .0003%.

Sterilization (Male): Vasectomy. The tubes through which the sperm travels from the testes are cut. Can be done with a surgical cut or a puncture tool (as outpatient with local anesthesia). Less costly than tubal ligation. Does not take effect right away. Sperm can still be present for 20 ejaculations. Vasectomies can be reversed with surgery, but this is not always successful. Does not prevent STDs or HIV. Failure rate %* for ideal use is .1%; for average use is .2%

(Note: In addition, natural family planning and total abstinence from sexual encounters are two other ways to prevent pregnancy. Using no method of birth control has about 90% chance of pregnancy in one year.)

SOURCE: HealthyLife® Women's Self-Care Guide, 3rd Edition, American Institute for Preventive Medicine, Farmington Hills, MI, 1996
*Failure Rate % - Percent failure rate is based on percentage of women who get pregnant, but do not intend to in the first year of use.
Ideal Use - is the percentage of pregnancies that occur among couples who use the method correctly for every time they have sexual intercourse.
Average Use - combines figures for ideal use with pregnancies that occur among couples who do not use the birth control method(s) correctly or every time when they have sexual intercourse.

251 The Too-Tired -for-Sex Syndrome

"Inhibited sexual desire" is the number one sexual problem in the United States today, doctors report. People in their late twenties, thirties, and forties complain that they have little or no interest in sex. Job demands, family responsibilities, lack of time, stress, and fatigue leave many too tired for sex.

Not surprisingly, couples who both work outside the home and also have children are most susceptible to low sexual desire. By the time they hop (or rather, crawl) into bed at night, sex seems like too much bother.

Here are some things a couple can do to rekindle their desire for sex.

▶ Make a point to spend at least 15 minutes of uninterrupted time together each day. If you can't meet face to face, call each other on the telephone.

▶ Remember to express your affection for each other every day.

▶ Plan to spend part of a day alone together at least once a week. Make a date to take a walk in the park, go out for dinner, or share other activities you both enjoy.

▶ Schedule a weekend away together every two months or so.

▶ Go to bed together, at the same time. Tell yourself that what you haven't accomplished by 11:00 P.M. can wait until the next day.

▶ Relax by giving each other a massage or taking a shower together.

▶ Keep the television out of the bedroom. Watching TV can be sexual suicide.

▶ Don't worry if your sexual encounters occasionally fail. Fatigue and stress are known to cause temporary impotence, a decrease in vaginal lubrication, or the inability to have an orgasm. Don't let yourselves become preoccupied with performance; just take pleasure in being together. Enjoy hugging, kissing, and caressing.

If attempts to relax and spend more quality time together don't perk up your sex life, consult your doctor. Alcohol, medication, and various other factors can put a damper on desire or performance.

252 Stop Premature Ejaculation

Few sexual problems are as frustrating as premature ejaculation. Men with this problem release semen before penetrating the vagina or immediately afterward. Ejaculating too soon is embarrassing and unsatisfying for both partners. If the problem occurs often, resentment and frustration build.

With patience and cooperation, couples can overcome this difficulty. The following can help stop premature ejaculation.

The squeeze technique. If a man feels he's about to ejaculate prematurely, he firmly pinches the penis directly below the head, using the thumb and first two fingers of one hand, and squeezes for 3 to 4 seconds. (This technique was developed by William H. Masters, M.D., and Virgina E. Johnson, founders of the Reproductive Biology Research Foundation.)

The start/stop method. The couple should abstain from sex for two weeks. The man then concentrates on the sensations in his penis as his partner touches his genitals and brings him to an erection. The man asks his partner to stop just before ejaculation. After a few minutes, his partner continues to arouse him, then stops again. This sequence is repeated twice more, with ejaculation occurring the fourth time. Then each time the couple has sex, foreplay is prolonged.

253 Improving Poor Sexual Response

The term *frigid* may be out of date, but many women today occasionally have problems with vaginal dryness, uncomfortable or painful intercourse, or other effects of poor sexual response. As with male sexual problems, couples can practice certain techniques to remedy sexual unresponsiveness in a woman. A few simple methods follow.

1. For the first week, limit lovemaking to cuddling, kissing, and nuzzling. Don't touch the genitals or breasts.

2. During the second week, the man should gently touch his partner's vaginal area during lovemaking but stop before she reaches orgasm, to increase vaginal lubrication.

3. During the third week, repeat the first two phases, then proceed with intercourse. If the vagina isn't adequately lubricated, apply a water-soluble lubricant such as K-Y Jelly to the penis to facilitate penetration. (Penetration may also be easier if the woman is on top.)

If a tight vaginal opening still makes penetration painful or impossible, the following exercise may help.

1. The woman should gently place the tip of her partner's little finger against her vagina and gently push his finger into her vagina. If this feels uncomfortable, she should stop and wait a few minutes.

2. The couple should continue this exercise until the man can insert two fingers in his partner's vagina without causing pain or

discomfort. (It may take several attempts over a period of weeks for this technique to work.)

If a woman remains sexually unresponsive despite these measures, professional therapy may be worth considering. (See Tip 265.)

254 Basic Facts about Sexually Transmitted Diseases (STDs)

There's only one way to guarantee you'll never get a sexually transmitted disease: Never have sex. Limiting your sexual activity to one person your entire life is a close second, provided your partner is also monogamous. A third line of defense includes avoiding sex with people at risk for carrying STDs, avoiding certain sexual practices (see Tip 261), and using a condom for protection.

But first, here are some basic facts about STDs.

Signs and symptoms. Each STD has its own set of symptoms, but a discharge from the penis or vagina, pain when urinating (in males), and open sores or blisters in the genital area are typical of most STDs. In some cases, the early stages of an STD produce no detectable symptoms. And you can have more than one STD at the same time. Gonorrhea and chlamydia, for example, are often contracted simultaneously.

How STDs spread. STDs are transmitted through intimate sexual contact.

Fast response counts. If you suspect you have an STD, see a doctor as soon as possible. Your sexual partner(s) should also be contacted and treated, if necessary.

Outlook for cure. Some STDs can be treated and cured with antibiotics. Others such as genital herpes and acquired immune deficiency syndrome (AIDS) can be treated, but can't be cured at this time.

Possible complications. Depending on the infection, STDs can cause serious, long-term problems like infertility, central nervous system disorders, or in the case of AIDS, death.

No "shots" for prevention. At present, no vaccines exist to prevent STDs.

Repeat episodes. Once you've had an STD, you can get it again. You don't develop an immunity once you've been exposed.

Parents don't have to know. A minor does not need parental consent to receive treatment for an STD.

255 Getting Rid of Genital Warts

Genital warts are soft, moist, painless, pink or brownish skin growths that crop up on the penis, lips of the vagina, anal area, and sometimes the cervix (the necklike passageway between the uterus and vagina). Symptoms may include bleeding during a bowel movement, if the anal area is involved, or painful urination, if the urethral area (the narrow canal leading to and from the bladder) is affected.

Genital warts are caused by a virus that's transferred from one person to another during sex. Fortunately, treatment of genital warts is fairly simple.

The doctor may freeze the warts with liquid nitrogen (cryosurgery), cauterize them (burn them off with an electrically heated needle), or remove them with lasers or other minor surgery.

Some doctors treat warts with podophyllin, a drug derived from a plant, but this medication can't be applied to the vagina or cervix, or applied during pregnancy.

256 Beating Trichomoniasis

Unlike most sexually transmitted diseases, trichomoniasis is caused by a parasite rather than by bacteria or a virus. In women, typical symptoms include vaginal itching and burning, a greenish yellow vaginal discharge with an offensive, fishy odor, and burning or pain when urinating. In men, symptoms include mild itching and irritation of the penis, pain during intercourse, discomfort when urinating, and discharge from the foreskin (in uncircumcised men). Men who have trichomoniasis usually don't experience any symptoms, however, and may unknowingly infect their sexual partners.

Trichomoniasis is diagnosed by examining a drop of vaginal fluid or penile discharge under a microscope or by growing a culture.

If you're being treated for trichomoniasis, follow these simple guidelines.

➤ Take medication as prescribed. The medication metronidazole (brand name Flagyl) is usually taken orally. (If you're a woman, don't take this drug during the first three months of pregnancy.)

➤ Avoid drinking alcohol for 24 hours before or after taking the metronidazole. The combination causes vomiting, dizziness, and headaches.

▶ Women should douche with a solution of diluted providine iodine or a mild vinegar-and-water solution. (Don't use as a substitute for metronidazole, however.) Ask your doctor what proportions he or she recommends, how often you should douche, and for how long.

▶ To soothe irritated skin around the penis or vagina, wash the genital area with mild, unscented soap and water at least once a day.

If you have trichomoniasis, your partner should be treated simultaneously. Otherwise, you'll continue to reinfect each other.

257 The Subtle Signs of Chlamydia

Chlamydia is now the most common nonviral sexually transmitted disease in the United States. In men, symptoms include burning when urinating and a whitish discharge from the tip of the penis. In women, symptoms include slight vaginal discharge and a frequent need to urinate. But symptoms are often so mild they go unnoticed. And if left untreated, chlamydia can cause a variety of serious problems, including infection and inflammation of the prostate and surrounding structures in men; pelvic inflammatory disease (PID), and infertility in women. Since the symptoms of chlamydia aren't always obvious, doctors recommend that sexually active people who are not involved in a long-term, monogamous relationship be tested periodically. You should be aware, though, that the most reliable test for chlamydia is a tissue culture that is expensive and not widely available. For that reason, many doctors use a simpler slide test instead.

Anyone who has chlamydia should be treated with oral antibiotics such as tetracycline, erythromycin, or azithromycin. Doctors will treat the infected sexual partner even if he or she doesn't show any symptoms.

258 Simple Steps against Herpes

Genital herpes is caused by the herpes simplex (type I or type II) virus. Type II is most often the culprit. Symptoms include sores with blisters on the genital area and anus. If infected for the first time, you may experience flu-like symptoms such as swollen glands, fever, and body aches, but subsequent attacks are almost always much milder and much shorter in duration.

So far, no cure for genital herpes exists. You can, however, take the following steps to decrease discomfort during an outbreak.

▶ Bathe the affected genital area twice a day with mild soap and water or use sitz baths to soak the affected area.

▶ Take a mild pain reliever.

▶ Ask your doctor about taking the antiviral drug acyclovir (brand name Zovirax).

To avoid spreading the virus to your eyes, don't touch your eyes during an outbreak. Also, avoid sexual intercourse when the herpes virus is active. Even condoms may not prevent the virus from infecting your partner during its active stage.

259 Telltale Signs of Syphilis

Syphilis is sometimes called "pox" or "bad blood". It is caused by a certain bacterium. Left untreated, syphilis is one of the most serious sexually transmitted diseases, leading to heart failure, blindness, insanity, or death. Syphilis can progress slowly, through three stages, over a period of many years. When detected early, however, syphilis can be cured. Be alert for the following symptoms.

Primary Stage. A large, painless ulcer-like sore known as a chancre occurs two to six weeks after infection and generally appears around the area of sexual contact. The chancre disappears within a few weeks.

Secondary Stage. Within a month after the end of the primary stage, a widespread skin rash may appear, cropping up on the palms of the hands, soles of the feet, and sometimes around the mouth and nose. Swollen lymph nodes, fever, and flu-like symptoms may also occur, and small patches of hair may fall out of the scalp, beard, eyelashes, and eyebrows.

Latent Stage. Once syphilis reaches this stage, it may go unnoticed for years, quietly damaging the heart, central nervous system, muscles, and various other organs, and tissues. The resulting effects are often fatal.

If you've been exposed to syphilis or have its symptoms, see a doctor or consult your county health department. For syphilis in its early stages, treatment consists of penicillin. If the disease has progressed further, you'll require three consecutive weekly injections. (If you're allergic to penicillin, you'll receive an alternative antibiotic, taken orally for two to four weeks.) You should have a blood test 3, 6, and 12 months after treatment, to be sure the disease is completely cured.

Once treatment is complete, you're no longer contagious. But you can get syphilis again if you have sexual contact with an infected partner.

260 If You Think You Have Gonorrhea, Do This

The signs of gonorrhea show up within two to five days after sexual contact with an infected person. In men, symptoms include pain at the tip of the penis, pain and burning during urination, and a thick, yellow, cloudy penile discharge that gradually increases. In women, symptoms include mild itching and burning around the vagina, a thick yellowish green vaginal discharge, burning on urination, and severe lower abdominal pain (within a week or so after their menstrual periods).

If ignored, gonorrhea can cause widespread infection and/or infertility. But gonorrhea can be cured with injections of penicillin. (If you've been infected with a type of gonorrhea that's resistant to penicillin, your doctor will have to use another antibiotic.)

To treat gonorrhea successfully, you should heed the following:

▶ Take prescribed medications.

▶ To avoid reinfection, be sure that your sexual partner is also treated.

▶ Have follow-up cultures to determine if the treatment was effective.

261 Protect Yourself against HIV/AIDS

Acquired immune deficiency syndrome (AIDS) is caused by the human immunodeficiency virus (HIV) that destroys the immune system, leaving the person unable to fight certain types of infection or cancer. HIV also attacks the central nervous system, causing mental and neurological problems. The virus is carried in bodily fluids (semen, vaginal secretions, and blood).

Certain activities are likely to promote contracting HIV. High-risk activities include:

▶ Unprotected* anal, oral and/or vaginal sex except within a monogamous relationship in which neither partner is infected with HIV.

▶ Unprotected* sex with many partners or with a partner who has had many partners.

▶ Unprotected sex when drunk or high.

▶ Sharing needles and/or "the works" when injecting any kind of drug.

▶ Pregnancy and delivery if the mother is infected with HIV (this puts the child at risk).

▶ Having had blood transfusions especially before 1985, unless tested negative for HIV.

HIV cannot be transmitted through casual contact (like kissing) or any airborne method of transmission.

Take these steps to avoid contracting HIV.

▶ Unless you are in a long-term, monogamous relationship, use male latex condoms during sexual intercourse. Animal (not human studies) suggest that spermicide with Nonoxynol-9 may inactivate HIV, so use it with a condom, not alone.

▶ Don't have unprotected sex with more than one person, especially with anyone whom you know or suspect has had multiple sex partners or engaged in high-risk behaviors. (If you have had sex with someone you suspect is HIV positive or has AIDS, see your doctor.)

▶ Don't share needles and/or "the works" when injecting any kind of drug.

▶ Avoid sexual activities that could tear the vagina or rectum (such as anal intercourse).

▶ If possible, donate your own blood for planned surgery.

Early symptoms of HIV/AIDS include fatigue, loss of appetite, diarrhea, weight loss, persistent dry cough, and night sweats. But symptoms may not show up for eight to eleven years after a person is infected with the virus.

Screening tests for HIV are available through doctors' offices, clinics, and health departments.

*Unprotected means without correctly used condoms or other latex barriers from start to finish for every sex act.

You can also find out your HIV status using an over-the-counter home collection test kit and counseling service such as Confide or Home Access. Results are kept anonymous and confidential.

262 What Condoms Can and Can't Do

Once a taboo topic of conversation among mixed company, condoms are now promoted in television and magazine ads. Although traditionally purchased by men, women are buying condoms now, too, and encouraging their partners to wear them. Although many people use condoms as a form of contraception, for others, condoms are used to help protect against sexually transmitted diseases.

When used correctly, condoms may protect both partners against gonorrhea, syphilis, and HIV, according to medical reports. Condoms are less effective for preventing the spread of genital warts and herpes, however, because the viruses responsible for those diseases are small enough to pass through the pores of a condom.

To increase the effectiveness of condoms as protection against pregnancy and STDs, follow these guidelines.

▶ Use condoms that are recently purchased.

▶ Choose condoms made of latex, not of animal membranes. Latex condoms are more durable than natural condoms and are less likely to break.

▶ Avoid condoms advertised as "ultrathin." They don't hold up well.

▶ Don't store condoms in a wallet, since they can be easily damaged

▶ Don't expose condoms to the sun or store them under hot and humid conditions. Condoms deteriorate when exposed to ultraviolet light, heat, or moisture.

▶ Apply the condom over an erect penis before sexual contact. It should be rolled down over the shaft of the penis to the base, leaving a space at the tip for semen to collect.

▶ Hold the condom against the base of the erect penis after ejaculation, until after withdrawal.

▶ Don't use petroleum or oil-based lubricants such as baby oil, petroleum jelly, or vegetable oil to make penetration easier when wearing a condom. They can cause the condom to weaken and tear. Instead, use a water-soluble lubricant like K-Y jelly (sold in drugstores).

▶ If a condom should break, immediately insert a spermicide containing Nonoxynol-9 into the vagina.

263 How to Talk to Teens about Sex

According to recent surveys, eight out of ten boys and seven out of ten girls have had intercourse by the time they reach the age of 19. Parents who know or suspect their teenager is sexually active commonly react in one of two ways. They either ignore the issue or get angry. Neither approach is likely to change matters or protect your child against the consequences of sex. The following guidelines can help parents deal with the situation calmly and intelligently.

▶ Tell your son or daughter why you're concerned. Don't be judgmental.

▶ Explain that you understand that the feelings of sexual desire and excitement are strong, but that sexual activity could result in serious consequences, like pregnancy, disease, or emotional problems.

▶ Since you can't be sure that your teenager will avoid intercourse, discuss birth control openly.

▶ Teach your teenager about the symptoms, consequences, and treatment of sexually transmitted diseases, and explain methods of protection.

264 Saying "Yes" to Sex after a Heart Attack

Many couples avoid sex after one partner suffers a heart attack, for fear of causing another. But that's unlikely to happen. As it does during any type of physical exertion, the heart does beat more rapidly during sex, but not dangerously so. The exertion of intercourse is roughly equivalent to the effort of climbing a flight of stairs. So if someone who's recovered from a heart attack can comfortably climb two flights of stairs or walk briskly around the block, sex probably poses little risk.

If you or your partner has had a heart attack, ask your doctor when you can resume sex, what signs and symptoms to be alert for, and what to do should sex trigger symptoms of a heart attack.

If you've had a heart attack, the following guidelines can minimize potential problems associated with sex.

▶ Plan on a time and place for sex where you won't be interrupted. (You may find it's better to have sex in the morning, when you're less likely to be tired, than later in the day or at night.)

▶ Avoid fatty foods, alcohol, and caffeine; they put extra demands on your heart.

▶ Wait approximately 3 hours after eating a meal before engaging in sexual activity.

▶ Take the bottom position to avoid supporting the weight of your body with your arms.

▶ If your doctor so advises, take a nitroglycerine tablet before engaging in sex.

265 Selecting a Sex Therapist

Some sexual problems aren't easy to solve, and a professional therapist may be of help. When considering a sex therapist, use the same type of criteria you'd use when selecting any other health professional. Here are some useful guidelines.

▶ Ask your gynecologist or urologist to recommend someone he or she feels is competent and trustworthy.

▶ Ask to see the therapist's credentials. The therapist should be certified by the American Association of Sex Educators, Counselors and Therapists (AASECT), which requires extensive training.

▶ Be sure that the therapist has expertise in the problem you're experiencing. Some therapists specialize in treating people with particular problems, like low sexual desire, impotence, incest, or sexual abuse.

▶ If you don't feel a therapist is helping you, don't hesitate to discontinue therapy and consult someone else.

Be aware of unethical practices. A sex therapist should:

▶ Never show shock or surprise with the client's problem or the subject matter being discussed.

▶ Never give a physical exam to a client unless the therapist is also a physician. Sex therapists who don't have a medical degree are not trained to diagnose and treat physical problems.

▶ Never ask their clients to engage in any form of sex with the therapist or in the therapist's presence.

CHAPTER

12

Better Health over 55

Right now, about one out of every eight Americans is over the age of 65. By the year 2025, every fourth citizen will be 65 or older. Also, the 75-plus group is now the fastest-growing age segment of the U.S. population.

Former president Ronald Reagan once said, "Each succeeding generation of older Americans is proving to be more vigorous and self-sufficient than were its forebears of comparable age."

In other words, Americans are living longer, healthier lives. The tips in this chapter will help you cope with some of the health problems that often occur as we grow older—and avoid problems that aren't as inevitable as many think.

266 Debunking the Myth of Senility

Don't think that you're getting senile just because you forget someone's name or can't remember where you parked your car. Everyone forgets occasionally. The truth is, most people do not become senile.

Senility (or senile dementia) is a state of confusion and forgetfulness triggered by mental decline. Almost 100 different conditions mimic the symptoms of senility. (Alzheimer's disease is the most common. See Tip

50 in chapter 2, Major Medical Conditions: Prevention, Detection, and Treatment.) Poor nutrition, hormone disorders, and use of certain medications can also cause confusion and forgetfulness. Even then, senility is misdiagnosed up to 20 percent of the time. So don't assume that you or anyone else is senile without a thorough medical exam.

267 Six Ways to Build Better Brainpower

Research shows that older adults who lead active, stimulating lives keep their brains fit and healthy, too. Your mind needs "exercise," just like the rest of your body.

Some mind-stimulating tips include:

▶ Learn something new—or try something different—every day. Studies show that curiosity keeps people mentally sharp.

▶ Play mind-stretching games such as Scrabble, chess, and cards.

▶ Do the crossword puzzle in the daily newspaper.

▶ Read books and magazine articles about subjects of interest to you.

▶ Attend lectures, plays, and exhibits, and watch educational television.

▶ Use memory aids, such as appointment calendars, "to do" lists, and Post-it notes.

Also, concentrate on what people say, repeat what you want to remember out loud, and associate an action with an object (like leaving your tote bag near the door so you remember to take it with you when you leave).

268 Guard against Macular Degeneration

Macular degeneration is a leading cause of blindness for those over 55 years of age. The central part of the retina (the macula) deteriorates, leading to loss of central, or "straight ahead" vision. One or both eyes may be affected.

If you're 50 or older, you should have an eye exam every 1 to 2 years to check for macular degeneration.

▶ Ask your ophthalmologist about home testing for signs of further degeneration. A simple home screening device is available from most ophthalmologists.

▶ Talk with your doctor about laser treatments, which may be effective for 10 to 20 percent of those with macular degeneration that's detected early.

269 Help for Hearing Loss

Do people seem to mumble a lot lately? Do you have trouble hearing in church or theaters? Do you lose the thread of conversation at the dinner table or at family gatherings? Does your family repeatedly ask you to turn down the volume on the TV or radio?

These are signs of gradual, age-related hearing loss called presbycusis. High-pitched sounds are especially difficult to discern. Another way to detect this problem is to hold a watch to your ear. If you can't hear it ticking, see an otolaryngologist (a physician who treats disorders of the ear, nose, and throat) or an otologist (a physician who specializes in ear disorders).

You should also get help if one or both ears ring continuously, or if loud noises cause pain in your ears.

Hearing loss from presbycusis cannot be restored, but hearing aids, along with the following self-help methods, are helpful.

▶ Ask people to speak clearly, distinctly, and in a normal tone.

▶ Look at people when they are talking to you. Watch their expressions to help you understand what they are saying. Ask them to face you.

▶ Try to limit background noise when having a conversation.

▶ In a church or theater, sit up front.

▶ To rely on sight instead of sound, install a buzzer, flasher, or amplifier on your telephone, door chime, and alarm clock.

Also, an audiologist (hearing therapist) may be able to show you other techniques for "training" yourself to hear better.

270 Enhance Your Sense of Taste

Adding a lot of salt to foods, eating more sweets, and finding meals less enjoyable are signs that your sense of taste is fading. As you age, you may lose up to 50 percent of your taste buds. But you don't have to resign yourself to a diet that tastes dull and bland. You can take the following steps to perk up your sense of taste.

▶ Eat fresh foods instead of canned or processed items. Fresh-cooked foods are more flavorful and have more texture, which adds to the enjoyment of food.

▶ Pep up your vegetables with flavor enhancers like savory herbs, lemon juice, slivered almonds, and sliced onions instead of extra salt.

▶ Marinate meats and fish in salad dressings or fruit juices before cooking.

▶ Include tart foods and beverages like salt-free pickles, oranges, and lemonade in your meals.

▶ Think visually. Colorful foods, garnishes, and an attractive table setting make meals more appetizing.

▶ Bring chilled foods to room temperature before serving. Flavors are more pronounced when food is warm.

271 Guard against Denture Trouble

Forget the image of dentures sitting in a glass of water next to the bed! Dentures require active care, not just a nightly soak. Improper denture care leads to bad breath, unsightly stains, diseased gums, and damage to the dentures. Daily dental hygiene should include these measures.

▶ Brush your tongue and gums with a soft brush to keep your breath fresh and your gums healthy.

▶ Brush your dentures at least once a day with denture-cleaning products.

▶ Rinse your mouth with a mild salt-water solution (1 teaspoon of ordinary table salt in ½ cup warm water) after meals and before going to bed.

▶ Don't leave your dentures where they can be lost or accidentally damaged.

How you eat can also protect your dentures, so take these precautions.

▶ Cut your food into bite-size pieces.

▶ Chew your food slowly and avoid biting down hard.

▶ Dentures make your mouth less sensitive to both heat and cold. So check the temperature of food and beverages before eating or drinking to avoid burning yourself.

See your dentist if you have any of the following problems.

▶ Gums that bleed or hurt after brushing.

▶ White or red spots in your mouth that don't clear up within two weeks.

▶ Dentures that become damaged. (Don't try to repair dentures yourself.)

▶ Difficulty talking, eating, and chewing when wearing your dentures.

▶ Dentures that slip and don't fit well.

To help keep your dentures fitting properly, see your dentist at least once a year.

272 Make the Most of Mealtime

Mealtime is something to look forward to. But for some older adults, especially men living alone, preparing meals can be both awkward and troublesome. This can lead to the "tea and toast" syndrome of skipped or unbalanced meals. Hit-or-miss eating habits can, in turn, lead to loss of energy and malnutrition. Coupled with the fact that older adults often need more calcium than other folks (for strong bones), more fiber (to prevent constipation), and adequate supplies of other important dietary components, poor meal habits can directly affect your health.

Here are a few hints to make preparing meals and eating meals more pleasant and convenient.

▶ Make a list before you shop for food. Include fish, poultry, lean meats, nonfat dairy products, whole-grain breads and cereals, fresh fruits and vegetables.

▶ When you shop for meat or produce, ask a store clerk to cut or repackage large quantities into smaller, single- or double-serving portions.

▶ Take advantage of salad bars in supermarkets. They're a convenient way to incorporate fresh vegetables into your diet.

▶ Buy some back-up supplies of nutritious foods—like tuna canned in water or low-salt soups—for days when you don't have the time or inclination to cook a full meal from scratch.

▶ Read labels, and avoid foods high in fat, salt, and sugar. These ingredients contribute to many of the chronic health problems that strike people after age 40.

▶ Prepare double portions of main dishes, so you can reheat leftovers a day or two later.

▶ Share shopping, meal preparation, and meals with a friend or neighbor.

273 A Diet for Lifetime Health

Studies show that some older adults are deficient in vitamins B_6, B_{12}, C, and folate (a B vitamin). To guard against vitamin deficiencies, plan a diet that includes food sources of these nutrients.

▶ Whole-grain breads and cereals, as well as organ meats and fish, are high in B_6.

▶ Milk, eggs, and meat are excellent sources of B_{12}.

▶ Carrots, broccoli, and almost all green, leafy vegetables are high in folate.

▶ Citrus fruits, tomatoes, cantaloupe, and strawberries are rich in vitamin C.

Studies also suggest that older adults require more protein and calcium in their daily diets than many people consume. Low-fat dairy products are rich sources of calcium. Two servings a day of 2 to 3 ounces of meat, chicken, or fish provide the protein you need. Other, less concentrated sources of protein include cooked dried beans, peanut butter, nuts, and eggs. (For more details on the nutrient content of foods, see chapter 4, Eating for Better Health.)

274 Tips for Good Digestion

Around the age of 40, people begin to notice that they can't tolerate certain foods as well as they used to. As you get older, your stomach produces a smaller volume of digestive enzymes and other secretions, and your body may not digest or absorb foods as easily as it did when you were younger.

If you are prone to digestive problems, follow these tips.

▶ See a dentist if you are having trouble with your teeth or dentures. Poorly fitting dentures, sensitive teeth, and diseased gums can make chewing difficult.

▶ Eat smaller, lighter meals, spaced throughout the day, instead of heavy meals. As a person ages, the blood supply to the small intestine declines, hindering the absorption of nutrients from a sudden, large delivery of food.

▶ To prevent gas and bloating, don't gulp liquids or talk while chewing food.

▶ Limit the amount of gas-producing foods you eat. Cabbage, onions, and cooked dried beans are common offenders.

▶ Eliminate milk products from your diet if they cause bloating, intestinal gas, or diarrhea, but be sure to supplement your diet with calcium. (You may be able to tolerate small amounts of milk or milk products if you treat them with Lactaid, a digestive aid sold in many health food stores. See Tip 113 in chapter 4, Eating for Better Health.)

▶ Avoid wearing tight clothing around your waist at mealtime.

▶ Don't lie down for at least 2 hours after you've finished a meal, and don't eat right before bedtime.

275 How to Prevent Bowel Problems

By the time people reach their forties, fifties, or sixties, they will usually experience some form of bowel trouble such as diverticulosis, irritable bowel, and constipation.

To prevent various kinds of bowel trouble, practice these healthful habits.

▶ Eat a diet high in fiber. (Oat bran, wheat bran, beans, fruit, and vegetables are good sources of fiber.)

▶ Avoid routine use of laxatives, since they disrupt the normal rhythm of the bowel. To ease elimination, take a high-fiber preparation like Metamucil instead.

▶ Drink six to eight 8-ounce glasses of water a day.

▶ Avoid straining when passing stool.

You should see your doctor if you notice blood in the stool, experience severe abdominal pain, pass pencil-thin stools, or note a significant change in your bowel habits.

276 Help for Bladder Control

Many people are inconvenienced and embarrassed by urinary incontinence—they leak urine when they laugh, cough, sneeze, or lift heavy objects.

Incontinence can be caused when muscles used to control the bladder weaken due to childbirth or prostate surgery. Neurological complications caused by injury or stroke, or neurologic disease (like multiple sclerosis) can also weaken bladder control. So can diabetes. But the most common cause of urinary incontinence in the older population is what doctors call urge incontinence or bladder instability: Frequent, involuntary bladder contractions release small amounts of urine.

If urinary incontinence is a problem for you, see a urologist, a doctor who specializes in problems and diseases of the urinary system. Medications, biofeedback bladder training, exercise, or surgery can improve or cure urinary incontinence.

To help manage urinary incontinence:

▶ Empty your bladder at least every 2 hours.

▶ Avoid highly spiced foods, which irritate the bladder.

▶ Avoid caffeine and alcohol at least 4 hours before bedtime.

▶ Practice Kegel exercises to improve bladder control. (These are also described in Tip 232 in chapter 9, Women's Health Problems.) To feel the muscles to be exercised, practice stopping the flow of urine. Then practice the following three exercises.

— Squeeze these muscles for 3 seconds, then relax the muscles for 3 seconds. Do this ten times, three times a day.

— Squeeze and relax the muscles as quickly as possible. Repeat ten times, three times a day.

— For women only: Imagine pulling up a tampon in the vagina. Hold for 3 seconds. Then bear down as if having a bowel movement, holding for 3 seconds.

▶ If you wear sanitary pads or incontinence pads, change them often to prevent odor and infection.

277 How to Care for Mature Skin

As your skin ages, the sebaceous glands produce less oil, and the skin loses elasticity. The result is dry, wrinkled skin—unless you take steps to prevent (or minimize) those effects.

Here's what to do to stay one step ahead of Mother Nature.

▶ Shower or bathe with a mild soap or transparent glycerin soaps to prevent dry, flaky skin. Don't use deodorant soaps on your face—they're too harsh for sensitive facial skin.

▶ Avoid alcohol-based astringents, toners, or after-shave lotions, which dry the skin.

▶ Apply a moisturizing lotion immediately after showering or bathing. (Dry skin makes wrinkles more noticeable, so using a moisturizer makes wrinkles less noticeable.)

▶ Use a room or furnace humidifier during the winter months, to further prevent dry skin.

▶ When washing dishes or working with strong detergents, protect your hands with rubber gloves.

▶ Apply sunscreen lotion with a sun protection factor (SPF) of 15 or higher whenever you go outdoors.

If you're thinking about having a face lift, chemical peel, or collagen injection for wrinkles, contact your local medical society for the names of board-certified surgeons or dermatologists with experience in the procedure you're considering.

278 Don't Be Duped by Antiwrinkle Creams

Don't be misled by over-the-counter skin care products that claim to get rid of wrinkles. There's no such thing. The closest thing to a wrinkle-removing cream is retinoic acid, a synthetic form of vitamin A. Applied to the skin surface, retinoic acid increases blood flow and stimulates skin cells called fibroblasts to produce new collagen (a protein that keeps skin smooth). This process can help to eliminate tiny wrinkles and make deep wrinkles less noticeable. Retinoic acid also speeds up the rate that your skin's cells move to the surface and die off to be replaced with new cells, so your skin looks younger.

Retinoic acid is available by prescription only under the trade name Retin-A. Regular vitamin A has no effect on wrinkles, whether it's taken orally or applied directly to the skin.

279 What to Do about Liver Spots

Years spent soaking up the sun can result in circular patches of light brown pigmentation, called liver spots or age spots, on your face, arms, neck, and the back of your hands. Liver spots have nothing to do with the liver, though; they're "superfreckles"—areas of dark pigment triggered by overexposure to the sun.

Here's what you can do to minimize liver spots.

▶ Apply a concealer (cover-up cream) that matches your skin tone.

▶ Always apply a sunscreen lotion with a sun protection factor (SPF) of 15 or higher 30 to 45 minutes before you go outdoors.

▶ Apply an over-the-counter bleaching cream to the discolored areas. (Don't expect overnight results, though. These products take months to work and lighten spots only slightly.)

If these tactics don't help, consult a dermatologist. He or she may recommend one of the following medical treatments for liver spots.

▶ A prescription bleaching cream

▶ A prescription peeling cream, like Retin-A

▶ Chemical peels (a mild acid is applied with a cotton swab to each patch of pigment)

▶ Dermabrasion (the skin is numbed, then rubbed with a high-speed electrical device)

These treatments all produce some discomfort and sometimes leave a permanent white spot where the skin has been treated, however.

280 Help for People Who Snore and Twitch

Does your bed partner snore or toss and turn during the night? Does he or she periodically twitch like a mackerel out of water for no reason at all? Are you faced with two alternatives: Sleeping in the guest room or not sleeping at all?

Older adults—especially men—tend to develop two kinds of sleep disturbances. One is sleep apnea: Breathing stops for short periods of time and is followed by loud snoring. The other is nocturnal myoclonus, or restless legs—frequent jerking motions that sometimes awaken both the jerker and the person who shares the bed.

Sleeping with the head of the bed elevated can make breathing easier and discourage snoring. Since being overweight and drinking alcohol seem to aggravate both sleep apnea and myoclonus, losing excess pounds and avoiding alcohol can help. Sleeping pills, too, can aggravate sleep apnea, so people who have this problem should use other ways to get a good night's sleep. (See Tip 4 in chapter 1, Fast Relief for Everyday Health Problems.)

You may suffer one or both of these sleep disturbances and not even know it unless your partner complains—and you should take the complaints seriously.

Sleep apnea may seem like nothing more than a nuisance, but it can be life-threatening if left untreated. So if you or your partner has this problem, see a doctor.

281 Four Ingredients for a Happy Retirement

Retirement involves major changes in your income, lifestyle, social life, and self-image. Not surprisingly, retirement can be very stressful—or blissful.

Advance planning is a key ingredient for a happy retirement. A survey conducted by researchers at the University of Michigan found that 75 percent of those who had planned for retirement enjoyed it.

Here are some specific ways you can make retirement less stressful and more satisfying.

Get a part-time job.   For some people, gradual retirement is easier to handle than being employed one day and unemployed the next. To smooth the transition, you may want to either work part-time at your present job for a few months or get a part-time job at another firm when you leave.

Practice living on a retirement budget before you retire.   And start saving for retirement as far ahead of time as possible. Don't expect Social Security to cover all your expenses.

Take care of yourself while you're young.   You can help to preserve your health by eating a low-fat diet, not smoking, drinking moderately (if at all), learning to manage stress, getting regular checkups, and being physically active.

Cultivate hobbies and other outside interests. Fitness activities, community work, or academic studies can fill the void left by not having to report to work every day. To prevent boredom, consider a variety of activities—indoor and outdoor, mental and physical, group and individually oriented. And start thinking about projects you'd like to work on well before retirement, so you don't stall out when the time comes.

282 Stress Relief for Caregivers

If you're the primary caregiver for a spouse, parent, or other relative, you face a tough challenge. Here's what you can do to make the workload easier.

▶ Set up the sickroom on the main floor, so you don't have to continually go up and down stairs.

▶ Purchase or rent equipment that will make caregiving easier. Examples include an electric hospital bed, an over-bed table, and a walker or wheelchair.

▶ Keep clean bed linens, towels, washcloths, hand lotion, drinking cups, and other supplies in or near the sickroom.

▶ Develop a daily schedule and stick to it.

To reduce the stress of your ongoing responsibility:

▶ Delegate some tasks to family and friends.

▶ Investigate community services that provide transportation, deliver meals, and provide other kinds of help.

▶ Enlist the services of a home health care agency. The social service or discharge planning department of your hospital, Social Security Administration, local agency on aging, county public health department, or your physician can refer you to an agency in your area.

▶ Plan to get out of the house to shop or socialize at least one day a week.

▶ Find out if the cost of hiring help to care for someone at home is covered by your medical insurance provider, Medicaid, or Medicare. The Veterans Administration may be able to provide financial assistance for veterans' medical or nursing care.

CHAPTER

13

The Healthy Traveler

Each year 30 million Americans travel abroad, and those who don't usually take some sort of family vacation within the United States. Unfortunately, when people hit the road, the road sometimes hits back.

Whether you're traveling for business or pleasure, nothing can spoil a trip faster than injury or illness. According to the National Institutes of Health, that's exactly what happens to one out of three travelers. Some problems, like sunburn, jet lag, motion sickness, and tired feet, are minor. Others, like the flu, malaria, yellow fever, or traveler's diarrhea, can be life-threatening.

With some advance planning, almost all of these medical problems can be avoided, however. This chapter will help you plan safer, more enjoyable trips.

283 Your Prevacation Checklist

You'll enjoy your trip much more if you don't have to worry about how things are going back home while you're away. Taking care of this checklist of pretravel tasks will give you peace of mind while you're gone.

▶ Take care of any maintenance problems before you leave to prevent serious damage while you're gone.

▶ Leave a house key with a neighbor, family member, or friend. Ask them to check your house both inside and out while you're gone.

▶ If you're going to be away for a month or more, contact your creditors and ask about arranging for your bills to be paid on schedule.

▶ Leave a copy of your itinerary and the name of your airline and flight numbers with family or friends, so they can track you down in the event of an emergency.

See Tip 312 in chapter 14, Be Smart, Be Safe, for more advice about precautions you should take before you leave home.

284 Immunizations: Your Best Shot against Infectious Disease

Polio, yellow fever, cholera, malaria, typhoid, and hepatitis are no longer problems in the United States and most developed countries. But outbreaks are common in certain rural or undeveloped parts of the world. Here's what to do if you plan to travel outside the United States.

▶ Be sure you've been immunized against diphtheria, pertussis (whooping cough), tetanus, polio, measles, rubella, and mumps. Most people are routinely immunized against these diseases in childhood. You should have a booster shot for tetanus every ten years, however.

▶ Ask your doctor if he or she recommends medicine to prevent malaria or immunizations against influenza, pneumonia, or hepatitis.

▶ Contact your local health department to determine if you need to receive additional immunizations for your trip. Vaccination requirements for specific countries are also listed in the booklet, *Health Information for International Travel,* available from the Superintendent of Documents, U.S. Government Printing Office, Washington, DC 20402.

▶ Direct travel to most foreign countries from the United States generally does not require you to have immunizations. The primary exception to this is travel to 17 countries in Africa. Call your local health department to be certain.

▶ Ask your doctor to record your immunizations on a yellow form called the International Certificate of Vaccinations. Required immunizations must be validated by the health department or by vaccinating physicians who have an official "Uniform Stamp." The international certificate of vaccination is available from your health department or by sending $2 to the Superintendent of Documents, U.S. Government Printing Office, Washington, DC 20402. Write the code number 017-001-04405 on the envelope.

285 Don't Forget Your Medication

Running out of your high blood pressure medicine or other prescription drugs at home probably isn't a big problem: You can just call your doctor or go to the drugstore for a refill. If you use up your medicine when you're traveling, however, you're stuck. To avoid running out of vital medications, take these steps.

▶ Ask your doctor or pharmacist for enough medication to last the duration of your trip.

▶ Carry medication with you in a small bag. Never pack medicine in checked luggage, in case it gets lost or delayed.

▶ If you take liquid medications, ask the pharmacist to put it in a plastic container instead of a glass bottle to avoid breakage.

▶ To avoid having your medicine confiscated by Customs agents, keep all medicine in its original container, with contents clearly labeled.

▶ Keep your medications away from humidity, direct sunlight, and hot temperatures, which can reduce the potency.

▶ Insulin-dependent diabetics should check with their doctors about adjusting their dosage schedules to local time when traveling to a different time zone.

286 Pack a Traveler's First-Aid Kit

You can handle many minor medical emergencies that crop up as you travel—*if* you have the right supplies at hand. Use the following list as a guideline for packing your own first-aid kit.

▶ Rubbing alcohol

▶ Hydrogen peroxide

▶ Antibacterial cream or spray

▶ Adhesive strips

▶ Gauze pads and cotton swabs

▶ Elastic bandages

▶ Mild pain relievers such as aspirin, acetaminophen, or ibuprofen

▶ Antacids

▶ Cough and cold remedies

▶ Diarrhea medication

▶ Broad-spectrum antibiotic (requires a doctor's prescription)

To conserve space in your baggage, purchase supplies in trial-size containers. If you're going to travel by airplane, avoid aerosol products—they can explode if subjected to drastic changes in air pressure.

You should also carry your medical insurance card and the name, address, and phone number of your physician.

287 Check Your Health Insurance Coverage

Don't assume that your medical insurance policy covers medical care you receive outside the United States. To protect yourself against unforeseen—and perhaps costly—medical charges, take these steps.

▶ Check with your insurance carrier to see if you're covered when abroad, or if they offer health insurance for travelers.

▶ If your insurance doesn't fully cover you away from home, you may be able to purchase traveler's health insurance through a major credit card company.

▶ If you're traveling with a package tour that offers a health insurance option, consider purchasing it. Some plans also cover the cost of returning home in case of an emergency.

▶ Find out if your policy places any restrictions on coverage. Some insurance companies do not cover chronic illness, complications during the third trimester of pregnancy, or sports-related injuries.

288 Taking the Stress out of Travel

Even if you're jetting to a sunny clime on your dream vacation, travel can be stressful. Any change in routine, scenery, eating habits, or time zones can take its toll on your well-being.

Here are some things you can do to minimize travel stress.

▶ Begin to prepare for your trip well in advance of your departure date. Make a list of things to do each day.

▶ Finish packing your bags at least one full day before you leave. Devote the rest of the day to quiet activities such as reading, napping, taking a leisurely bath, or listening to soothing music.

▶ Allow plenty of time to reach your destination or catch your flight. It's better to have time to spare than to rush.

▶ Once you reach your destination, don't overschedule every day with endless hours of shopping, sightseeing, sports, and partying. Allow for some "downtime."

▶ Don't overeat, especially at night.

▶ Get enough sleep. Otherwise, you'll come home pooped instead of renewed and refreshed.

▶ Get some exercise.

▶ Schedule your return so you have a day or so to "decompress" before you return to work.

289 How to Prevent Jet Lag

Jet travel makes it possible to reach the far corners of the world in a matter of hours. Yet crossing several time zones disrupts your body's natural rhythm of eating and sleeping. The result is a combination of fatigue, disorientation, indigestion, headaches, and insomnia, collectively called jet lag. Traveling from east to west is more of a problem than traveling west to east. Traveling north or south doesn't cause jet lag because you don't change time zones.

Ways to prevent jet lag include the following:

▶ Three nights before you leave, change your bedtime. If you're traveling east, go to bed 1 hour earlier for each time zone you will cross. If you're traveling west, go to bed 1 hour later for each time zone you will cross.

▶ Follow the anti–jet lag diet developed by Charles F. Ehret, Ph.D., of the Argonne National Laboratory in Argonne, Illinois. (If you have any restricted diet, consult your doctor before making changes, however.)

— Three days before your trip, eat foods high in protein, like turkey, chicken, or nonfat cottage cheese for breakfast and lunch. Eat foods high in carbohydrates, like pasta, for dinner. On the next day, eat light meals consisting of fruit, broth-based soups, salads, and dry toast. On the third day, follow the same diet as the first day.

— Limit your intake of caffeine-containing beverages such as coffee, tea, and some soft drinks between the hours of 3:00 and 5:00 P.M. all three days.

— If you're traveling west, fast until noon on the day of departure. Coffee or other caffeine-containing beverage is permissible in the early morning.

— If you're traveling east, fast the entire day of your departure. Drink caffeine-containing beverages between 6:00 and 11:00 P.M. only, if at all.

— When you arrive at your destination, eat a high-protein breakfast and lunch and a high-carbohydrate dinner.

▶ During the flight, avoid sleeping pills, alcohol, and caffeine. Drink plenty of water or juices to avoid dehydration. The air in the aircraft is very dry.

▶ If you arrive at your destination during the day, plan to spend some time outdoors. Try to expose yourself to as many hours of daylight as the number of time zones you crossed.

▶ Don't go to bed until evening.

290 Fitness in Flight

Sitting in a narrow, crowded airplane seat for hours causes cramped and achy muscles, swollen feet, and fatigue. And anyone who has a problem with circulation in his or her legs runs a risk of thrombophlebitis when sitting for long periods of time. Fortunately, there are ways to prevent the typical aches and pains travelers frequently experience during long flights. One is to charter your own plane and stretch out in comfort.

If you're like most people, however, a private plane is probably beyond your means. Instead, you can try to reduce stiffness with the following exercises.

► Tense your feet for 5 seconds, then relax them. Repeat with each muscle group, including your calves, thighs, buttocks, shoulders, neck, forearms, and hands.

► Drop your head forward. Then slowly move it to your right, and continue rotating your head, to the back, to the left, and to the front again. Repeat four times. Then reverse direction, and repeat five times.

► Raise both shoulders, then move them back, down, and forward in a circular motion.

► Reaching toward the ceiling, stretch your right arm. Then repeat with your left arm.

To promote circulation in your legs:

► Flex and extend your feet, pointing your toes up and down.

► Try to get up and walk at least once every 2 hours, if possible. You should also make an effort to breathe slowly and deeply. Aircraft air is lower in oxygen than outdoor air, and deep breathing helps you to get enough oxygen into your blood and avoid fatigue or sluggishness.

291 Plane Travel for Those with Special Health Problems

Physical limitations or medical problems don't necessarily have to keep you homebound.

► If you have an artificial joint or pacemaker, carry a card from your physician saying so, and present the card before going through the airport metal detector.

► If you're on a restricted diet, contact the airline at least 24 hours in advance of your trip to make arrangements for your meals or tell the airline representative who books your flight. Most airlines offer low-sodium, low-cholesterol, diabetic, and other special meals.

▶ If you need a wheelchair, contact the airline 48 hours before your trip. Airlines can provide wheelchairs narrow enough to negotiate the aisle of a plane.

▶ If you depend on a seeing-eye dog, call the airline to find out if your dog can accompany you.

292 Prevent In-Flight Ear Pops

If you're riding in a plane, your ears might feel full during takeoff and landing, then suddenly "pop." Ear pops result from pressure changes in the middle ear as a plane changes altitude. You may feel pain or only mild discomfort. And if you have a head cold, ear pops can promote an ear infection.

It's rarely convenient to cancel or postpone your flight because of ear trouble. It is highly recommended, however, that you don't fly if you have an acute ear infection, a severe head cold, or sinusitis. Consult your physician regarding this. If you still decide to fly, here are some ways to keep your ears from popping.

▶ Swallow frequently, yawn, or gently blow through your nose while pinching the nostrils shut, to equalize pressure within your ears. (Don't do this if you have a head cold, as it will promote an ear infection.)

▶ If you have a mild head cold, use a nasal spray to keep the nasal passages open. Oral decongestant medications are also effective.

Infants and young children tend to develop ear pain when traveling by plane, too. To prevent discomfort and ear infections in your children:

▶ Have your infant suck on a pacifier or bottle during the takeoff and landing. (Nursing a baby helps, too.)

▶ Ask your doctor about giving children a mild decongestant and antihistamine 1 hour before takeoff and 1 hour before landing.

293 How to Prevent Motion Sickness

Motion sickness is like a hangover you don't deserve. Symptoms include fatigue, dizziness, nausea, vomiting, pallor, and sweating. Experts think this misery results because your eyes and inner ear receive conflicting messages when you travel by car, boat, or plane. The inner ear, which is responsible for your sense of balance, tells your body it's moving in one direction, while your eyes tell you you're moving in another. So closing your eyes can reduce the conflict.

The following steps can also help prevent motion sickness. Aboard ship:

▶ Spend as much time as you can on deck in the fresh air.

▶ If you're going to be spending the night (or nights) on a boat, try to get a cabin near the middle of the craft, close to the waterline, where there's less pitching and rolling.

On a plane:

▶ Request a seat over the wings. Avoid sitting in the tail section; it's the bumpiest.

▶ Open the overhead vents and direct air at your face.

On land transportation:

▶ Fix your gaze on the scenery straight ahead, not to the side.

▶ Sit near an open window, for fresh air, unless you're traveling through a heavily polluted area.

▶ If you're traveling by car, offer to drive. The person at the wheel never gets motion sickness.

In addition, the following steps are helpful no matter what your means of conveyance.

▶ Get plenty of rest before setting out. Fatigue makes you more vulnerable to motion sickness.

▶ Avoid drinking alcohol before or during travel, and don't overindulge the night before.

▶ Take an over-the-counter motion sickness medication (such as Dramamine) approximately 30 minutes before travel begins. Read the package for cautions and other important informaton.

▶ If over-the-counter medications don't bring relief, ask your doctor about a prescription medication containing scopolamine, available as a patch that's usually worn behind your ear.

▶ Don't read while traveling and don't try to focus on any other stationary object. Aboard a ship, lie down on your back and close your eyes.

▶ If any of your traveling companions get sick, move as far away from them as possible; otherwise, you may get sick, too.

Some people report that taking tablets of powdered gingerroot relieves their motion sickness. Others find relief by pressing on an acupressure point about midway on the inside of the wrist, where the hand and forearm meet.

If preventive measures fail and you feel sick anyway, you can try the following:

▶ Breathe in slowly and deeply.

▶ Remove yourself from smoke and food odors, and get some fresh air.

▶ To reduce tension and anxiety, concentrate on relaxing all your muscles, as though you're a limp rag doll, and visualize a peaceful scene.

▶ To settle a queasy stomach, eat dry crackers.

294 Eat, Drink, and Be Wary

It's been said that travel expands the mind and loosens the bowels. One-third of visitors to developing countries suffer from travel sickness, or turista, a disagreeable combination of diarrhea, cramps, fatigue, and sometimes fever and nausea. Food and water contaminated with bacteria are usually to blame. Here's what to do.

▶ If you plan to travel outside the United States, check with the local tourist board to find out if the water is safe for foreign visitors to drink. Often, natives who are used to the local water can drink it with no ill effects, but outsiders experience nausea or diarrhea (or both).

▶ If you know or suspect the water is unsafe, drink and brush your teeth with bottled water that has a sealed cap. The same goes for making ice cubes, washing fruits and vegetables, or cooking.

▶ Carry an immersion coil so you can boil your water. Boil the water for at least 10 minutes, and allow it to cool before you use it.

▶ If you can't boil your water, use purifying tablets such as Halazone or Potable Aqua tablets, which you can buy at most drugstores and many sporting goods stores.

▶ Order drinks without ice cubes.

▶ Don't eat raw fruits or vegetables (including salad). The exception: fresh fruit you peel yourself.

▶ Don't order undercooked meat. Beef, pork, chicken, and fish should be cooked thoroughly.

▶ Don't eat raw or undercooked shellfish, which can carry hepatitis.

▶ Avoid smorgasbords and buffet meals, where food is often left out for long periods of time, giving disease-causing microbes plenty of time to flourish.

▶ Avoid unpasteurized milk and cheeses in countries outside the United States and western Europe.

▶ If your choice of safe foods is severely limited, take a daily multiple vitamin and mineral capsule to supply the nutrients you may be missing out on.

Ask your doctor about taking Pepto-Bismol as a preventive measure. You can take 2 ounces four times a day (or two chewable tablets four times a day), beginning the day of travel and continuing until two days after returning home. (Don't take Pepto-Bismol if you're allergic to aspirin or if you'll be traveling for more than two weeks, though.)

295 What to Do If Turista Strikes

If you avoid risky food and water and still come down with traveler's sickness, do this:

▶ To prevent dehydration, drink plenty of bottled caffeine-free soft drinks and fruit juice.

▶ To guard against the loss of important minerals, drink Gatorade or Gastrolyte, Pediolyte, or other rehydration formulas available at drugstores. Or do the following:

— Drink one 8-ounce glass of fruit juice to which you've added a teaspoon of either honey, corn syrup, or sugar, and a pinch of salt.

— Next, drink one 8-ounce glass of purified water containing ¼ teaspoon of baking soda.

▶ Avoid solid foods until the diarrhea stops.

▶ Avoid milk and dairy products, high-fiber foods, and greasy foods until diarrhea has stopped for a couple of days.

▶ Take up to 8 ounces of Pepto-Bismol at a rate of 1 ounce or two tablets every 30 minutes. Disregard this advice if you have bloody stools or fever, however. In that case, see a doctor.

▶ Don't take over-the-counter diarrhea medications like Enterovioform or Mesaform available in foreign countries. According to the Food and Drug Administration, these medicines aren't safe.

▶ See a doctor if diarrhea continues for more than three days, if you have blood in your stool, or if diarrhea is accompanied by fever. You may need an antibiotic.

296 Footwear and Foot Care for Travelers

Hours of shopping and sightseeing can leave your feet tired, aching, and sore. Here's what to do to save yourself the agony of sore feet, blisters, and other foot problems.

To prepare your feet for the rigors of travel, do each of these exercises several times a day.

▶ Take off your shoes and socks, and pick up a pencil with your toes as you sit.

▶ Rotate your feet in a circular motion in one direction, then in the other.

▶ Point your toes to the ceiling, then to the floor.

▶ Stand, and roll up on your toes and hold for a count of 25.

▶ If you have foot problems and plan to travel, see your podiatrist. He or she may be able to remove corns, for example, or take care of other problems that might cause discomfort if you're going to be on your feet a lot.

▶ Pack comfortable shoes that you've already worn several times. Walking or jogging shoes are best. Avoid high heels, dress oxfords, or other fashion footwear that don't adequately support your feet.

▶ Take along two pairs of walking shoes, and alternate footwear every other day.

▶ Wear cotton socks, not nylon. (And don't go sockless.)

► If your ankles and feet tend to swell, wear support stockings. Support hose are available for both men and women.

If those suggestions fail to prevent achy feet or blisters, try these remedies.

► Soak your feet in a tub of cool water to which you've added 1 cup of Epsom salts for every gallon of water.

► Wash and thoroughly dry your feet every day. Then apply a powder to help absorb perspiration.

► Gently massage your feet with a moisturizing lotion. Begin at your toes and work up to your ankles. Massaging the feet can also help to relieve foot cramps.

► Don't pop blisters. Instead, cushion them with a corn pad or bunion pad.

297 Travel Hints for Retirees on the Go

Some of the most avid travelers are in their fifties, sixties, and seventies. Yet people in this age group are susceptible to certain health problems. To minimize your risk of health trouble away from home, take these precautions.

► Before confirming your reservations, be sure the itinerary is not too demanding for you or your traveling companion.

► Visit your doctor and dentist before your trip. Schedule your appointments far enough in advance to allow time to take care of any health problems that need to be resolved before departure.

► If you're being treated for an ongoing medical condition, carry copies of your medical records when you travel in case you become ill.

► Get adequate sleep before and during your trip. Fatigue aggravates existing medical conditions and reduces resistance to illness.

► Pace yourself, and take time to rest once or twice a day.

► Medicare recipients who need supplemental travel health insurance for travel outside the United States should contact the American Association of Retired Persons (AARP) Insurance Division at 1-800-523-5800 for further information.

298 Safe Travel for Pregnant Women

Expecting to travel before your baby is due? Follow these guidelines.

▶ Check with your physician to make sure travel is permissible. Travel during pregnancy is least risky during the fourth to sixth months.

▶ If you're planning to travel by airplane or train, ask for an aisle seat so you can get to the lavatory more easily.

▶ Don't exert yourself to the point of fatigue.

▶ If you experience motion sickness, get some fresh air or eat soda crackers. Don't take motion sickness medication.

▶ If you're traveling by car, wear a safety belt. It should fit snugly across your chest and hips, not over your stomach.

299 The ABCs of Traveling with Children

Traveling with children can be very trying—you try to keep them from getting tired, bored, hungry, sick, or lost. Here are a few strategies to help you succeed.

▶ Make sure your child has had all immunizations required or recommended for travel (see Tip 284).

▶ When your trip takes you through several time zones, gradually adjust your child's sleeping schedule before the trip, as described in Tip 289 on preventing jet lag.

▶ Have each child wear an identification tag that includes his or her name, plus your name and home address and where you'll be staying. In airports, add the name of your airline, flights, and departure times. And tell your child what to do if he or she gets lost.

▶ Take along a child-strength painkiller, motion sickness medication, cold preparations, an antibiotic, syrup of ipecac (an antidote for poisoning), and Pedalyte (a medicine that replaces essential body minerals lost due to vomiting and diarrhea).

▶ Dress your child in loose, comfortable travel clothing and shoes.

▶ On long automobile trips, stop every 2 hours and walk around with your child. When flying or traveling by train, take your child for a walk around the coach or cabin.

▶ Help prevent your child from getting motion sickness by following the guidelines given in Tip 293. Children between the ages of 2 and 12 are more prone to motion sickness than toddlers or teens.

▶ If your child will be flying unaccompanied by an adult, make arrangements for an adult to escort them on and off the plane. Most major airlines can arrange this.

▶ Avoid introducing a young child to a lot of unfamiliar foods away from home. His or her digestive system is more sensitive than an adult's.

▶ When traveling in developing countries, repeatedly remind your child about food and beverage safety.

300 How to Locate a Physician away from Home

The best made travel plans can't guarantee against illness or injuries. Although travelers don't like thinking about the possibility of a medical emergency, a little forethought can save you a lot of misery or aggravation. Knowing what to do and who to contact should you need medical help especially when traveling abroad, reduces anxiety and avoids wasting time when minutes count.

Specialized travel medical clinics exist in some areas. Consult the following for names of physicians you can contact, if need be, in the area you plan to visit.

▶ International Association for Medical Assistance to Travelers (IAMAT), 417 Center Street, Lewiston, NY 14092 (716) 754-4883.

▶ Overseas Citizens Emergency Center, 1425 K Street NW, Washington, DC 20005 (202) 647-5225.

▶ The American Embassy or American, British, or Canadian consul or consulate in the country you're visiting.

▶ The Red Cross. (Check a phone directory or directory assistance for the phone number and location of the chapter nearest you, or to locate a chapter where you intend to travel.)

Also, check appendix B for the addresses and phone numbers of national organizations for people with kidney disease, diabetes, heart conditions, or other diseases. These organizations may be able to provide information on medical aid for people with special health problems who travel overseas.

You can probably manage many minor medical problems without assistance from a doctor. The following symptoms call for medical attention, however.

▶ Fever over 101°F for more than two days

▶ Severe vomiting and diarrhea

▶ Abdominal or chest pains

▶ Difficulty breathing

▶ Fainting

▶ Slurred speech

▶ Feelings of disorientation

▶ Severe weakness

CHAPTER

14

Be Smart,
Be Safe

Each year, about 44,000 people die in car accidents. Another three million are injured in the "safety" of their own homes, and 27,000 die in home accidents. Add to that the number of fires, burglaries, and other misfortunes that can disrupt daily life, and the picture gets pretty grim.

While a certain amount of misfortune is simply a matter of bad luck, carelessness or oversight is responsible for many accidental injuries. Conversely, proper safety precautions can go a long way to prevent unnecessary injury.

Mark Twain once said, "It's better to be careful a hundred times than to get killed once." This chapter may not provide a hundred ways to be careful, but it comes pretty close. Most of the tips take only minutes to put into practice, but they can prevent heartbreaking property loss, spare you months of pain, or perhaps even save your life.

301 The Twenty Most Dangerous Household Hazards

You'd think that things like knives and ladders would top the list of dangerous household objects, but they're outranked by seemingly harmless items like tables and chairs. (Did you know, for instance, that each year thousands of children are injured falling out of bunk beds?)

The following is a list of the objects, activities, or backyard games that most often cause accidental injury, as reported by hospital emergency rooms. Note these potentially hazardous items or activities well, and approach each with caution.

- Stairs
- Floors or flooring materials
- Basketball
- Bicycles
- Knives
- Baseball
- Football
- Beds
- Doors
- Tables
- Chairs
- Ceiling and walls
- Household cabinets, racks, and shelves
- Nails, screws, tacks, or bolts
- Household containers and packaging
- Skating
- Windows
- Bathtubs and showers
- Soccer
- Ladders

302 Audit Your Home for Safety

Most accidents happen at home. If you think your house is "home, safe home," take a look around. At first glance it may look orderly, but certain common trouble spots can lead to cuts, falls, burns, or other injuries. The following room-by-room checklist can alert you to accidents waiting to happen.

Kitchen

_____ Cleaners and dangerous chemicals should be stored out of children's reach.

_____ Scissors, knives, ice picks, and other sharp tools should be stored separately from other utensils and out of the reach of children.

_____ Towels, curtains, and other flammable materials should hang a safe distance from heat sources like the stove.

_____ Kitchen fans and stove ventilation exhausts should be clean and in good working order.

_____ Electrical cords should run a safe distance from the sink or range.

_____ Electrical outlets should not be overloaded.

_____ A sturdy stepstool should be available to help reach high cabinets.

_____ Vinyl floors should be cleaned with nonskid wax.

_____ A nonskid floor mat should be in place in front of the sink.

_____ The kitchen should be well-lit.

Bedroom

_____ Electrical cords should be tucked away from foot traffic and in good working order.

_____ Electrical outlets should not be overloaded.

_____ Electric blankets should not be covered by bedspreads or other blankets when in use.

_____ Carpeting should be secured to the floor.

_____ A night-light should be situated between the bed and the bathroom or hallway.

_____ The bedroom telephone should be easy to reach, even from the floor, if necessary.

_____ Ashtrays, irons, electric hair curlers, and other potential fire hazards should be located away from bedding, curtains, or other flammable material.

_____ Smoke detectors should be located near entrances to rooms.

Bathroom

_____ Floor mats should have nonskid backing.

_____ Rubber mats or adhesive-backed strips should be in place in the bathtub or shower stall.

_____ A support bar should be securely installed in the bathtub or shower stall.

_____ Hair dryers, electric shavers, or other electric appliances should be kept away from water and unplugged when not in use.

_____ A light switch should be located near the bathroom entrance or entrances.

Halls and Stairs

_____ Halls and stairs should be well-lit, with a light switch at each end of a stairway.

_____ If a staircase is dimly lit, the top and bottom steps should be marked with reflective tape.

_____ Sturdy hand rails should be securely installed on both sides of each stairway.

_____ Floor covering on stairs and in halls should be skidproof or carpeted and not creased or frayed.

_____ Stairways should be clear of shoes, books, toys, tools, or other clutter.

_____ When young children are in the house, gates should block access to stairways.

Basement and Garage

_____ To avoid confusion and misuse, all chemicals and cleaners should be kept in their original containers.

_____ Hazardous chemicals should be kept under lock and key or out of reach of children.

_____ Sharp or otherwise potentially hazardous tools should be in good working order.

_____ Gasoline and other flammable materials should be stored in airtight containers and away from heat sources (outside the home, if possible).

___ Buy a radon test kit from your state department of health or department of environmental protection, or contact the National Radon Hotline at 1-800-767-7236 for information on radon testing. (Radon is an invisible gas that causes health problems if it builds up in homes and can't escape.) If your home has high radon levels, hire a reliable radon expert to help you reduce levels of this gas in your home.

Elsewhere around the House

___ Outdoor porches and walkways should be kept clear of ice in winter weather.

___ Window screens should be securely fastened, especially if small children are around.

Take steps to remedy unsafe situations as soon as possible.

308 Easy Ways to Childproof Your Home

Is your home safe for curious children?

To see your home from a toddler's point of view, get down on your hands and knees and crawl around.

Look for conditions that can lead to burns, falls, electric shock, entrapment, or poisoning. Then take steps to prevent harm. Some suggestions:

▶ Cover all toddler-height electrical outlets with plastic outlet covers, available at hardware stores and home-improvement stores.

▶ Install childproof locks on cabinets where household cleaners and chemicals are stored.

▶ To prevent scalding burns, lower the thermostat on the water heater to 120°F or lower.

▶ Store medicines and alcohol in high, out-of-reach places. Never leave them on a countertop.

▶ Toddlers should eat and drink from plastic dishes and cups only.

▶ Don't place a child's crib or bed next to a window. An active or curious toddler could accidentally fall out.

▶ Keep all sharp objects like scissors, knives, or pins out of a toddler's reach.

▶ To prevent suffocation, dispose of all plastic bags, or keep them out of reach of children.

▶ Don't leave objects small enough to be swallowed within reach of children.

304 Use Ladders Safely

At least 93,000 people a year end up in hospital emergency rooms with injuries sustained on ladders. Here are some safety tips to keep you from being one of them.

▶ Make sure your ladder is long enough for you to reach the job without standing on the top three steps or overextending your body.

▶ Check the ladder for cracks or weak spots before you use it. Metal ladders should have nonskid steps and footings. (Don't paint a ladder; you'll hide defects.)

▶ Make sure the soles of your shoes or boots are dry and have enough tread to prevent slipping.

▶ Always steady a ladder on firm ground or a flat board.

▶ Never place a ladder in front of a door that someone may open.

▶ Wear tools on a belt or keep them in your pocket so you can keep your hands free when climbing up or down a ladder.

▶ To avoid losing your balance while standing on a ladder, don't lean too far back or to the side.

▶ Don't use a ladder outdoors on a very windy day.

▶ To avoid electrocution, don't use metal ladders near power lines.

305 Keep This First-Aid Kit Handy

It takes just one emergency to alert people to the need for a first-aid kit. Better yet, make it two—keep one at home and the other in your car. Include the following items, available in most drugstores.

▶ Ace bandage

▶ Adhesive bandages (assorted sizes)

▶ Adhesive tape

▶ Antibacterial ointment

▶ Antihistamine

▶ Calamine lotion

▶ Epinephrine (particularly if someone in the family has an allergy to bee stings)

▶ Eyewash cup

▶ Hydrogen peroxide

▶ Instant chemical cold pack

▶ Oral thermometer

▶ Rubbing alcohol

▶ Safety pins

▶ Scissors

▶ Sterile gauze dressings (pads and a roll)

▶ Syrup of ipecac (for some poisonings)

▶ Triangular cloth (for immobilizing a broken arm or other broken bone)

▶ Tweezers

▶ Up-to-date edition of the American Red Cross first-aid manual or other reliable first-aid book

Keep everything together in a sturdy box. (Fishing tackle boxes work well.) Clearly label the kit "First Aid." Don't store the first-aid kit in the bathroom or other humid area. A high shelf in a hall closet, where young children can't reach, is best.

Before using any over-the-counter ointments or other first-aid medicines, read the directions—and follow them to the letter.

306 Install Smoke Detectors—And Be Sure They Work

Smoke detectors save lives. But if a smoke detector is placed in the wrong spot or not maintained, it may be useless in a fire.

To install and maintain smoke detectors:

▶ Install at least one smoke detector on each level of your house. Best locations are in hallways and just outside bedroom doors.

▶ As an added safety measure, install two types of smoke detectors. The photoelectric cell variety detects smoldering fires, and the ionization type detects hot, flaming fires.

▶ Check for a UL (Underwriters Laboratory) emblem on the label to be sure the detectors you buy meet industry standards. And make sure they each come with a warranty, in case they're defective.

▶ Affix detectors on the ceiling or high on an interior wall, because smoke and heat rise.

▶ Once a month, check the detectors to make sure the batteries still work. Most detectors have a test button. If you push the button and hear a beep, the batteries are good. If you hear a chirping sound, the batteries need to be replaced. (To be safe, you should replace the batteries annually, whether the malfunction signal goes off or not. To help you remember, choose an annual holiday, like New Year's Day, as replacement time.)

▶ To make sure the sensing chamber works, you should also test the device with a lit match or candle.

▶ Be sure the alarm rings loudly enough to alert your family.

▶ Most smoke detectors last three to five years. Replace as needed.

307 Know How to Use a Fire Extinguisher

Every home should have at least one fire extinguisher. Extinguishers should be mounted in plain sight and be simple for all family members (except small children, of course) to use in an emergency. Show the babysitter how it works, too.

▶ Buy a multipurpose extinguisher rated 2A10BC or higher. The letters indicate the type of fire the extinguisher will douse. "A" units are for combustible materials like paper or wood, "B" units are for flammable liquids like gasoline, and "C" units are for electrical fires. The numbers relate to the size of the fire. The higher the number, the greater the capacity to extinguish that fire.

▶ Check for a UL (Underwriters Laboratory) or FM (Fire Mutual) code. They tell you the product is effective, safe, and reliable.

▶ Be sure the directions are simple to understand.

▶ Mount the fire extinguisher securely, in plain sight.

▶ Be sure you understand how the firing mechanism works. Check to see whether you need to push a button or pull a lever. Don't activate the extinguisher, though. Once you do, it must be serviced and recharged, even if you only use it for a few seconds and the gauge indicates it's full.

▶ Check the pressure indicator once a month to be sure the extinguisher works.

To use a fire extinguisher, remember the acronym PASS.

Pull the pin

Aim the nozzle or barrel at the base of the fire, not at the flames

Squeeze the handle

Sweep back and forth at the base of the fire

308 Kitchen Safety

Kitchen fires are responsible for four out of five household fires. To prevent such a catastrophe, take these precautions.

▶ Pay attention to what you're doing. When you're at the stove, don't try to do other chores or talk on the phone.

▶ If you have to leave the stove or kitchen for even a few minutes, turn the burner down or off.

▶ If you leave the house, check to see that the stove, toaster oven, coffeepot, and other kitchen appliances are turned off.

▶ Remove flammable items like potholders, paper towels, and dishcloths from the stove area.

▶ Don't wear loose clothing or clothing with long, loose sleeves when you cook. (Or at least roll up your sleeves.)

▶ Turn pot handles to the center of the range, to avoid knocking them over accidentally.

▶ If you deep-fry food, don't fill pans to the brim with oil.

Here's what to do if you're faced with a fire despite these precautions.

▶ Keep a pot cover handy to smother flames in the event a pot of food catches fire. Covering the pot cuts off the oxygen. If a pot cover isn't handy, use a cookie sheet, acrylic cutting board, or other flat, nonflammable item larger than the burning pot. Once the fire is out, don't remove the cover until the pot has cooled down completely. Exposing the source of the fire to oxygen could reignite it.

▶ Don't try to douse a grease fire with water; the fire may spread.

▶ Don't try to move or carry a pot of grease that's in flames. You could easily burn yourself or spread the fire.

Most important, you should keep a fire extinguisher in the kitchen and know how to use it. (See the previous tip.)

309 What to Do If Your Clothing Catches Fire

Few things are more terrifying than having your clothes catch fire. Teach your children and everyone else in your family this simple, lifesaving technique, known as stop, drop, and roll.

Stop. Your natural inclination may be to run. But motion only fans the flames.

Drop. Get to the ground, cover your face with your hands, and keep your face as far from the flames as possible. (If a blanket, rug, or coat is handy, use it to smother the flames. But doing so should never delay stop, drop, and roll.)

Roll. Roll back and forth, again and again, until the flames go out.

310 Only You Can Prevent Christmas Tree Fires

Every Christmas season, many families tragically lose their homes because of Christmas tree fires. Here's how to prevent them.

To choose a tree:

▶ Pick the freshest tree you can find. Hold the tree by the trunk and tap it against the ground. If needles drop profusely, look for another tree.

▶ Keep the tree outdoors with the trunk in water as long as possible. Once you bring the tree into a heated building, it will dry out more quickly.

▶ Indoors, keep the trunk in water. Check the water level daily, and refill when needed.

▶ Don't stand the tree near a fireplace, wood stove, heat register, or electrical wires.

To decorate the tree:

▶ Purchase only tree lights bearing a UL label from Underwriters Laboratory, which shows they meet safety standards.

▶ Check for broken bulbs, worn-out insulation, and damaged sockets. Replace or repair as necessary.

▶ Never attach electrical lights to an artificial, metal tree.

▶ Don't overload extension cords.

▶ Discourage children from touching a decorated tree—it may tip over.

▶ To discourage pets from attacking the tree, avoid shiny decorations, and don't place tinsel or ornaments on the lower branches.

311 How to Save Your Life in a House Fire

Knowing how to react fast in a house fire can save your life and the lives of those you love. Here are some guidelines to follow.

▶ Keep the phone number of your local fire department clearly posted near all telephones in the house. (Try to memorize the number, in case you have to use a neighbor's phone.)

▶ Establish a prearranged plan for family members to follow in case of fire. Conduct fire drills using your escape route.

▶ If you live in a two-story house, purchase and install an emergency escape ladder and practice using it.

▶ If a fire breaks out, don't stop to collect personal possessions. Get people out of the house.

▶ If you can't get to within 10 to 12 feet of a fire, you can assume it's too big to handle on your own. Call the fire department immediately. (Call them for small fires, too.)

▶ If you try to put out the fire, make sure you can get to an exit. Don't back yourself into a corner.

▶ Smother a fire thoroughly and keep it covered so it doesn't reignite. The fire department will determine if the fire has been contained or if it has spread.

▶ If you fail to extinguish the fire and smoke is accumulating, get out of the house quickly. Poisonous gases and smoke are often more dangerous than flames. (Smoke rises, so remember to "stay low and go." Crawl if you must. And if you can, place a wet towel over your face to filter out smoke and fumes.)

312 Burglarproof Your Home

Since most home burglaries are the work of amateurs, a house that's easy to get into is more likely to be hit. Take these steps to prevent your house from being an easy mark.

▶ Inspect the locks on all exterior doors. Some locks can be opened easily with a screwdriver or plastic credit card. If your locks aren't secure, replace them with single cylinder deadbolt locks. Bolts should be at least 1 inch long and anchored into strike plates which in turn are anchored by 3- or 4-inch screws.

▶ Install outside lighting around the house. And keep bushes in front of windows trimmed, to make it difficult for a burglar to hide when attempting to break in.

▶ Consider installing an alarm system.

▶ Engrave your driver's license number on your stereo, television, and other valuables. This identification marking makes it harder to sell items and makes tracing them easier.

▶ Join a neighborhood watch group.

▶ Contact your local police department for further advice for making your home safe.

If you're going to be away from home for several days:

▶ Notify trustworthy neighbors and ask them to watch your house. Leave a key with them and ask them to periodically check the house.

▶ Discontinue delivery of mail and newspapers.

▶ Ask someone to mow the lawn or shovel your walks while you're gone so the house looks occupied.

▶ Use automatic light timers, preset to keep the house well-lit during the evening. And leave a radio preset to a 24-hour-a-day news or talk station.

▶ Let the police know you'll be gone and ask them to periodically check for signs of attempted entry or other suspicious activity.

313 In Case of Accidental Poisoning, Act Fast

To prevent accidental poisoning:

▶ Always read warning labels on pesticides, household cleaners, and other products that could be poisonous. Follow instructions for use and storage.

▶ Flush unused medications down the toilet and rinse the containers before discarding them.

▶ Have the phone number of your local poison control center prominently posted near the telephone. It's also a good idea to post the numbers of the nearest hospital emergency room, ambulance service, and your physician.

▶ Keep a 1-ounce bottle of syrup of ipecac handy, in case the poison control center or your physician tells you to use it to induce vomiting.

If your child accidentally swallows or inhales poison, or spills poison on the skin or eyes, don't panic. Instead:

▶ Call the poison control center (or hospital or physician). Explain the problem and identify the cause.

▶ Remain calm and quickly follow the instructions you're given. Most accidental poisonings can be handled at home.

314 Master the "Hug of Life"

The "hug of life" is an appropriate name for the Heimlich maneuver. If someone can't talk and grasps his or her throat, the person is probably choking, and you may be able to dislodge the object with the Heimlich maneuver. Here's how:

1. Without delay, stand behind the person who's choking.

2. Wrap your arms around the person between the navel and the rib cage. Make a fist with one hand. The thumb of that hand should rest against the person's upper abdomen.

3. Ask the person to keep his or her head upright and facing forward.

4. Grab your fist with the opposite hand and push against the abdomen, delivering four quick, upward thrusts. (Simply squeezing the abdomen won't work.) Forceful thrusts should release air from the lungs to the windpipe and expel the food or other foreign object.

If your first attempt fails, repeat the maneuver, several times if necessary. You should try to extract the object with your fingers as a last resort only, because reaching for the object may push it farther down the throat.

You can use the Heimlich manuever on a choking victim whether he or she is conscious or not. Don't use the Heimlich maneuver if the victim is able to speak or whisper, however, or if he or she can cough. The windpipe may be only partially blocked, and forceful coughing may free the lodged item in a minute or so. But if the object remains stuck and the person is visibly weakening, perform the manuever.

Don't use the Heimlich manuever on a child younger than a year old. Instead, support the child's head in your hand while he or she lies face down over your forearm, and deliver four blows to the back, between the shoulder blades.

If you're choking, you can perform the Heimlich maneuver on yourself by placing one fist over the other and giving a quick upward thrust to your abdomen. If this fails, thrust yourself against the back of a chair, keeping your fist on your upper abdomen.

Note: The Heimlich maneuver can also be used to revive near drowning victims. (See Tip 316.)

315 Learn the ABCs of CPR

Knowing how to perform cardiopulmonary resuscitation (CPR) can mean the difference between life and death. CPR can restore the flow of oxygen to the brain if the heart has stopped beating due to heart attack, drowning, electrical shock, suffocation, drug overdose, or when someone has stopped breathing for some other reason.

To perform CPR correctly, you need expert training. It takes just 3 hours to learn, and anyone strong enough to compress the sternum 1½ inches is capable of performing CPR. The essential steps can be remembered as ABC:

Airway. Tilt the victim's head back to clear the airway.

Breathing. Pinch the nose closed and perform mouth-to-mouth rescue breathing.

Circulation. Using both hands, compress the chest at a point over the sternum (about midpoint in the front of the rib cage) to compress the heart and deliver blood to the body until the heart can resume beating on its own.

Call your local chapter of the Red Cross or the American Heart Association or your local hospital to find out where you can learn CPR.

316 Procedures for Near Drowning

CPR is standard treatment for near drowning. But if CPR doesn't seem to work, the airways may be obstructed. The rescuer may then use the Heimlich maneuver to expel water and help the victim breathe, according to the American Heart Association.

Here's how to apply the Heimlich maneuver in near-drowning situations.

1. Place the unconscious victim on his or her back and turn the face to one side so water can drain from the mouth. If you suspect the airway is blocked, however, don't turn the head, because it will prevent expulsion of the object.

2. Kneel astride the victim's hips, facing toward the head.

3. Place the heel of one hand on the victim's abdomen, slightly above the navel and below the rib cage. Place the other hand on top of the lower hand.

4. Press into the victim's abdomen with quick, upward thrusts. Repeat until water no longer flows from the victim's mouth.

The victim should see a physician immediately after rescue. If the victim doesn't regain consciousness, proceed with CPR and call for emergency medical assistance.

SOURCE: Henry Heimlich, M.D., and Edward Patrick, M.D., "Using the Heimlich Maneuver to Save Near Drowning Victims," *Postgraduate Medicine* (August, 1988).

317 Six Things You Should Never Do in Your Car

Driving takes total concentration. If you try to do other things when you're at the wheel, you risk having an accident.

▶ Adjust your child's safety belt before you start out, not while you're in traffic.

▶ Don't peer into the rearview mirror to comb your hair or touch up your makeup.

▶ Don't drive with one hand holding the wheel and the other holding a hamburger. If you're hungry, stop and eat.

▶ If a bee or flying insect dive-bombs you or your passengers, pull off the road and get rid of the winged invader. Don't swat at the bug while maneuvering through traffic.

► Don't try to drive and read a road map at the same time. If you're lost or need to get your bearings, pull off the road and look at a map, or have a passenger help you follow directions.

► If your children start to misbehave, don't turn around to discipline them. Pull off the road and settle the problem, and teach your children how dangerous it is to misbehave in a car.

Note: You *should always* wear a safety belt and heed the warning for air bags given by your car manufacturer. Doing so can make the difference between surviving a car crash intact or not surviving at all, between walking away with just a scratch or never walking again.

318 Keep a Survival Kit in Your Car

No car should be without a survival kit of items that you might need in the event you're in an accident, run out of gas, have a breakdown, or get stuck. Items to include:

► First-aid kit (itemized in Tip 305)

► Flares

► White cloth, for distress signal

► Flashlight with spare batteries

► Snow shovel

► Knife or other basic tools

► Empty gas can, for purchasing gas

► Small fire extinguisher

► Paper and pencil

► Blanket

► Change, for phone calls and tolls

► Food and water, for long trips through unpopulated areas

► Whistle

319 How to Steer Clear of Drunken Drivers

People who drive under the influence of alcohol are responsible for half of all auto accidents. If you can spot a drunken driver and stay out of his or her way, you may be able to avoid an accident. Watch out for drivers who:

▶ Drive too fast or too slow

▶ Make jerky starts or stop abruptly

▶ Overshoot stop signs

▶ Ignore traffic signals

▶ Follow cars too closely

▶ Pass other cars too quickly or too slowly

▶ Change lanes frequently

▶ Drive without their lights on after sundown

▶ Drive with their windows rolled down in cold or wet weather

▶ Are obviously partying and having a good time with their passengers when they should be paying attention to the road

320 Traffic Tips for Tots

Young children often don't realize busy streets or highways are dangerous. You have to either look out for them yourself or, if your children are old enough, teach them to get around safely. Here are some pointers.

▶ Never leave children unguarded or out of your sight near parked or moving cars.

▶ Never summon children from across the street; go over and get them.

▶ Always hold a child's hand when you cross the street together.

▶ When exiting a parked car, allow your child to exit on the curb side.

321 Take the Hazard out of Halloween

Dressing up to go trick-or-treating is a traditional childhood ritual. But wandering the streets in the dark dressed in bizarre costumes and knocking on strangers' doors to ask for food can pose hazards. To be sure your children have a Halloween that's fun *and* safe, take these precautions.

▶ Choose white or bright costumes, preferably of flame-retardant fabric and marked with reflective tape.

▶ Be sure a costume is short enough so that your child won't trip.

▶ Don't let your trick-or-treaters wear masks, which can interfere with their vision. Instead, apply makeup to their faces.

▶ Trick-or-treaters should carry flashlights, not candles.

▶ Small children should be accompanied by an adult.

▶ Avoid trick-or-treating at homes on dark streets or in unfamiliar neighborhoods.

▶ Check all treats before your children eat them. Don't let children eat candy or other treats that aren't commercially wrapped or look as though they've been tampered with.

▶ Keep carved, candlelit pumpkins out of reach of young children. And be sure to set your jack-o'-lantern on a nonflammable surface.

322 After-Dark Joggers, Heed This Advice

If you walk, run, or jog after sundown, the following tips help motorists spot you.

▶ Attach reflective tape to the front and back of your clothes.

▶ Carry a lit flashlight.

▶ Don't use the road; stay on the shoulder, or preferably the sidewalk.

▶ Move against (facing) traffic if you must use the shoulder.

▶ Be aware of your surroundings and plan to jump to safety if a vehicle veers toward you.

323 Pedaling Safely with Your Toddler

It's easy to equip a bicycle with a child safety seat so your toddler can ride with you. To ensure the safety of your pint-size passenger:

▶ Be sure the seat is properly installed. If you aren't sure how to install it correctly, consider having someone at a bicycle repair shop do it.

▶ A plastic cover should shield the back wheel, so the child's clothing doesn't get caught in the spokes.

▶ The back of the seat should be high enough to support and protect the child's back and neck, and it should be marked with reflective tape if you ride after dark.

▶ A passenger restraint (safety belt) should fasten over the child's shoulder.

▶ The seat should have a footrest, and the child's legs should not hang free.

Test the bicycle seat by riding without the youngster to be sure it's securely fastened. When you take your child riding, be sure he or she is wearing a helmet. (See the following tip.)

324 Never Cycle without a Helmet (and Other Tips for Safer Biking)

Wearing a helmet is the single most important thing you can do to prevent serious injury from bicycle accidents. In one recent year, more than 125,000 cyclists suffered head injuries, most of which could have been prevented if they'd been wearing helmets. Other injury-preventive measures include wearing gloves, choosing the right size bike, and riding on well-maintained roads (discussed later in this tip). But wearing a helmet is still critical.

Not just any old helmet will do, however. Look for the following features.

▶ Outer layer or shell is bright yellow, white, orange, or red (so motorists can see you more easily), and is constructed of hard plastic or polycarbonate

▶ Waterproof finish

▶ Stiff polystyrene lining

▶ Securely attached nylon strap and fastener

▶ Label signifying that the American Standards Institute or the Snell Memorial Foundation has certified the helmet as safe

Whatever your cycling style, don't sacrifice safety for thrills. To be sure your equipment is safe and reliable:

▶ Choose a bike that's right for your size. When seated, you should be able to put one foot on the ground without leaning the bike to one side or the other.

▶ Brakes should be in good working order—that is, enabling you to stop within 15 feet while riding at 10 miles per hour.

▶ Check tires for worn spots, punctures, or other signs of wear. Fix or repair, as needed.

▶ By law, all bicycles must have red reflectors, visible for 500 feet, on the sides, rear, and pedals.

▶ The bicycle should have headlights.

▶ Rearview mirrors are optional, but helpful.

Additional tips every bicyclist should bear in mind:

▶ Obey all traffic laws, just as you would if you were driving a car. (Ride with traffic, not against it; observe traffic signs and signals; stay to the right; maintain a safe following distance between you and the vehicle ahead of you; and use hand signals for turning.)

▶ Look behind you before turning or changing lanes.

▶ Consider walking your bike across intersections not governed by traffic signals, especially if traffic is heavy.

▶ Whenever possible, choose routes over smooth pavement.

▶ Drive defensively, anticipating the actions of motorists, pedestrians, and other bikers.

▶ Keep your eyes on the road. Watch for potholes, parked cars, and children or animals entering your path.

▶ Pay attention. Don't listen to a portable radio or tape player while riding.

▶ Don't B.W.I.—bike while intoxicated. It's just as risky as driving under the influence of alcohol or drugs.

The above rules apply whether you're biking for exercise, sport, or transportation.

325 Accident-Free Boating

If you enjoy sailing, motorboating, rowing, canoeing, or kayaking, "safety first" can make boating accident-free. Keep in mind the following:

▶ Learn how to navigate and maintain your watercraft. The whole family should take a boating safety class.

▶ Be sure your boat is equipped with safety and rescue gear. By law, you must have a personal flotation device (life jacket) for each person on board. And it's a good idea for passengers of all ages, swimmers and nonswimmers alike, to wear them. Many adults who can swim are knocked unconscious, then fall overboard and drown because they're not wearing a flotation device.

▶ Don't overload your boat. Know the passenger limit and stick to it.

▶ Know your limits. Exposure to bright sunlight, heat, boat motion, vibration from a motor, and noise can leave you stressed and fatigued. After 4 hours on the water, your reaction time is considerably slower than when you start out. So allow plenty of time for maneuvers, keep your distance from other crafts, and head for shore before you get tired.

▶ Pay attention to the weather. Head back to shore—or don't go out—if a storm threatens.

▶ Don't drink and navigate. Drinking alcohol while boating reduces reaction time, dulls vision, and impairs judgment. As with autos, half of all boating accidents are alcohol-related. If you must drink, wait until the boat is docked.

▶ Tell someone on shore where you're headed and when you expect to return. If you're delayed due to a storm or breakdown, they can send someone to rescue you.

▶ If you're towing a water-skier, the law requires that someone in the boat observes the person in tow.

▶ If your boat capsizes, stay with it. Don't try to swim to shore—you may overestimate your swimming skills.

3.26 Lawn Mower Safety

Getting sliced by a lawn mower blade and being hit by rocks or other propelled objects are the two most common lawn mower–related injuries. (Mower blades rotate at nearly 200 miles per hour, and seemingly harmless sticks and stones often become dangerous missiles when picked up and hurled at that speed.)

To mow grass safely:

▶ Before you start to mow, clear the lawn of sticks, stones, toys, garden hoses, and so forth.

▶ Don't use electric mowers on wet grass.

▶ Wear heavy-duty shoes and long pants to protect your legs.

▶ Wear safety goggles to protect your eyes.

► Wear ear protectors (like those worn on shooting ranges) to protect your hearing.

► Push the mower, never pull it (if you have a push mower).

► Mow across a slope, not up or down, so the mower doesn't slide or fall on top of you.

► Look several feet ahead when mowing.

► Turn off the engine if you have to check the blade, or clean or adjust the mower.

► Never fuel a lawn mower when the engine is hot. Spilled fuel or fumes can result in an explosion or fire. Instead, allow the engine to cool before refueling.

► Never allow children to operate a power mower, and keep small children far away from a mower that's in use.

327 A Safer Way to Shovel Snow

Many people underestimate just how strenuous shoveling snow can be. They know this activity puts many at risk for back injury or heart attack, but think, "It won't happen to me" and shovel anyway.

It's pretty obvious why shoveling can strain your back—you're bending at the waist to lift a load. And shoveling can trigger a heart attack in three ways. The increase in activity requires your heart to work harder. Also, without realizing it, you may hold your breath as you lift, which can trigger a sudden rise in heart rate and blood pressure. And cold weather causes blood vessels to constrict, so the heart has to pump more blood. If you have heart disease, you've got the makings of a heart attack.

If you have a history of back problems or heart problems, don't shovel snow, period. Have someone else do it. If you're over age 40 and overweight, if you have high blood pressure, if you smoke, or if you lead a sedentary life, check with your doctor before lifting a shovel.

The following hints can help make a tough job easier, even if you're not at special risk for back or heart problems.

► Dress properly. Protect your head and hands from the cold, and don't bundle up so much that you overheat or can't move freely.

► To prevent back strain, keep your knees slightly bent and both feet planted firmly on the ground or pavement.

► Consider removing snow with a snowblower or plow instead of a shovel—it's far less stressful and gets the job done quickly.

Dental Health: Beautiful Teeth for Life

Sharks. Earthquakes. Dental visits. All strike fear in our hearts. There's nothing wrong with a healthy fear of sharks. And it can't hurt to avoid vacationing along the San Andreas Fault. But if you put off going to the dentist—or avoid it altogether—your teeth could be in for big trouble: Cavities; infections; gum disease; loose, wobbly teeth; and other serious dental problems can be avoided with regular professional dental care.

What's more, you can minimize these problems—and prevent uncomfortable, expensive dental work—if you take care of your teeth on a daily basis. You already know you should brush and floss. But did you know that some mouthwashes can help prevent serious gum disease and keep your teeth from falling out? Or that eating certain foods, like cheese or peanut butter, can help protect your teeth against cavity-forming bacteria?

This chapter tells you about a few simple no-fuss techniques you can use to keep your teeth and gums strong for a long, long time—and keep you *out* of the dentist's chair.

328 All about Brushing and Flossing

Whiter teeth, fresher breath, fewer cavities. Who could ask for more from toothpaste? Yet some modern dentifrices make additional claims. Here's a short guide to ingredients and product claims to help you decide which toothpaste is best for your teeth.

Fluoride. Children and adults alike should use a toothpaste that contains fluoride, to prevent cavities. The American Dental Association recommends Colgate with MFP, Crest (Mint and Regular), and McLeans fluoride toothpastes. Look for the American Dental Association (ADA) seal on the package.

Note: Many dentists prescribe fluoride supplements for people whose household drinking water contains little or no fluoride. If your drinking water is low in fluoride, you might want to ask your dentist about this option.

Desensitizing toothpaste. Sensodyne, Protect, Denquel, and Promise toothpastes are specially formulated for people whose teeth are sensitive to touch or temperature changes.

Plaque control. Plaque is a sticky, bacteria-laden goo that clings to the surface of your teeth. Unless plaque is removed every 24 to 36 hours, it can turn into a cementlike substance called tartar. And tartar destroys your gums. Plaque- and tartar-control formula toothpastes, used along with flossing and regular dental visits, can help to prevent plaque buildup. Mouthwash can help, too (see the following tip).

Stain removers. Avoid using tooth polishes and so-called smoker's toothpastes. These products contain high levels of abrasives that wear away tooth enamel.

Don't Forget to Floss

Waxed. Unwaxed. Fine. Regular. Plain or fancy, all dental floss does the job: It removes bacteria and plaque from between your teeth and above and below the gum line—areas your toothbrush can't reach. It also removes particles of food lodged between your teeth.

Floss carefully at least once a day to help keep plaque from building up. (If plaque hardens into cementlike deposits called tartar, your teeth can start to decay or wobble due to loss of bone.) Here's how to floss.

1. Cut a piece of floss about 1½ feet long. Wrap the ends of the floss about your middle fingers.

2. Hold the floss tightly between your thumb and index finger,

exposing about 1 inch of floss. Gently guide the floss between your teeth, being careful not to snap it into the gums.

3.   With the floss at the gum line, curve it into a C shape against one tooth and gently scrape the side of the tooth with the floss. Repeat on each of your teeth, top and bottom, using a fresh section of floss for each tooth.

4.   After you've flossed, rinse your mouth with water or mouthwash to remove all debris. Your gums may be tender and bleed for the first week. That's normal. But if the bleeding continues, see your dentist.

Here are some additional hints.

▶   If you find flossing awkward and messy, try using a dental floss holder sold in drugstores. Instead of wrapping the floss around your fingers, you insert the floss in a small, plastic forklike holder.

▶   To help you remember to floss daily, without fail, floss before or after some other daily habit, like shaving, removing your contact lenses, or applying makeup.

329 The Right Way to Use Mouthwash

Be it red, green, blue, or amber, consumers spend millions of dollars a year on mouthwash. Many mouthwashes are strictly cosmetic—they leave your mouth smelling fresh and feeling tingly for a few minutes but don't appreciably affect oral health. If you want to fight plaque, look for mouthwash containing cetylpridinium chloride or domiphen bromide, ingredients that dissolve this troublesome film of bacterial goo. If you want to fight cavities (especially cavities that form between teeth, where your toothbrush can't reach), look for mouthwash that contains fluoride.

To get the best results from your mouthwash, follow this routine.

▶   Brush first, then rinse (unless the product label instructs otherwise).

▶   Swish mouthwash around in your mouth for a full minute, then spit it out. (Don't swallow mouthwash.)

▶   Rinse with mouthwash once a day, preferably at bedtime.

▶   Don't eat or drink anything for 30 minutes after rinsing.

330 Sticky Snacks Spell Trouble

Sticky, chewy foods—like cough drops, hard candies, and sugary pastries—cling to the surface of your teeth, where they mix with bacteria in the mouth and produce acids that gradually wear away tooth enamel. Granola bars, many dried fruits, and foods or cereals sweetened with honey, maple syrup, corn syrup, or molasses are particularly troublesome. But starchy foods like bread, crackers, potato chips, or pretzels— which are turned into sugar by saliva—can also be a problem.

To minimize this difficulty:

▶ If you eat fruit and other foods high in sugars, eat them with meals. Other, nonsugary foods will help to buffer their acid-forming effect on teeth.

▶ Don't eat sweets, fruit, or starchy foods before bedtime. Saliva production slows down overnight, enabling cavity-causing bacteria to feed on food particles more easily. And brushing doesn't effectively prevent the problem.

▶ Avoid sugar-sweetened gum and beverages.

▶ Snack on "detergent foods" like bagel slices or carrots. They help to clean the tooth surfaces as you chew.

331 Foods That Fight Cavities

Now you know how sticky sweets promote tooth decay. What you may not realize is that some foods *prevent* tooth decay. Research studies show that certain foods, like cheese and peanut butter, counteract the acids in the mouth that wear down the tooth enamel. (Be careful to buy plain, all-natural peanut butter, without added sugar of any kind.) Other tooth-saving foods include:

▶ Nuts and seeds

▶ Meat, fish, poultry, and eggs

▶ Olives and dill pickles

▶ Milk, plain yogurt, and cheese

332 Seal Out Tooth Decay

Even if you brush, floss, rinse with fluoride, and never eat a sticky sweet, decay-causing bacteria can invade the tiny pits and crevices in your molars, or chewing teeth. To head off that kind of decay, researchers have developed sealants—special plastic coatings that form an impervious barrier between bacteria and the chewing surfaces of your teeth, where fluoride is less effective.

Approximately 90 percent of the cavities in school-age children occur in crevices in the back teeth, so sealants are best applied when the permanent molars first emerge. (The American Dental Association reports a significant decrease in cavities in children who have sealants applied to their teeth.) But that doesn't mean sealants aren't useful or appropriate for adults who have cavity-prone teeth. So ask your dentist or dental hygienist about sealants the next time you have a dental checkup.

The procedure is simple, pain-free, and won't interfere with later dental work. Sealed teeth may need to be touched up periodically, though.

333 Take a Good Look at Your Gums

Plaque buildup, crooked teeth, illness, poorly fitting dentures, trapped food particles, and certain medications can irritate or destroy your gums. With good oral hygiene, however, you can prevent gum (periodontal) disease. If caught in the early stages, gum disease is easily treated. If ignored, the gums and supporting tissues wither, and your teeth may loosen and fall out.

Knowing the signs and symptoms of periodontal disease is important for early treatment. Pay attention to the following:

▶ Swollen red gums that bleed easily (a condition called gingivitis)

▶ Teeth that are exposed at the gum line (a sign that gums have pulled away from the teeth)

▶ Permanent teeth that are loose or separating from each other

▶ Bad breath and a foul taste in the mouth

▶ Pus around the gums and teeth

334 Safety Tips for Your Teeth

Your teeth are vulnerable to nicks, chips, stains, and strains. To protect your teeth from damage and injury, take these precautions.

▶ Don't chew ice, pens, or pencils.

► Don't use your teeth to open paper clips or otherwise function as tools.

► If you smoke a pipe, don't bite down on the stem.

► If you grind your teeth at night, ask your dentist if you should be fitted for a bite plate to prevent tooth grinding.

► If you play contact sports like football or hockey, wear a protective mouth guard.

► Always wear a seat belt when riding in a car.

► Avoid sucking on lemons or chewing aspirin or vitamin C tablets. The acid wears away tooth enamel.

335 What to Do for Toothaches and Other Dental Emergencies

Any swelling, pain, or bleeding in the mouth or jaw are often signs of serious trouble. A toothache, fractured jaw, broken or knocked out tooth constitutes a dental emergency. You should see a dentist as soon as possible. Follow these guidelines until you get help.

For a toothache:

► To reduce discomfort, take aspirin or other mild pain reliever.

► Never place a crushed aspirin on the tooth. Aspirin burns the gums and destroys tooth enamel.

► See a dentist even if the pain subsides.

For an abscess (infection with pain and swelling), take a mild pain reliever, like regular-strength aspirin or acetaminophen, and contact your dentist immediately so he or she can prescribe an antibiotic for you.

For a broken, loose, or missing tooth:

► To reduce swelling, apply a cold compress to the area.

► Save any broken tooth fragments, and take them to the dentist.

If your tooth has been knocked out:

► Rinse the tooth with clear water.

► If possible (and if you're alert), gently put it back in the socket or hold it under your tongue. Otherwise, put the tooth in a glass of milk.

► Try to get to a dentist within 30 minutes of the accident.

For a fractured jaw:

▶ To secure the jaw, close your mouth and secure the jaw with a necktie, towel, or scarf tied around your head and chin.

▶ To reduce pain and swelling, hold an ice pack against the fractured bone.

▶ Go to a dentist or hospital emergency room immediately.

336 Ways to Relieve Dental Anxiety

If you dread going to the dentist, ask about anxiety-reducing techniques you can use to help stay calm and relaxed. Some effective strategies follow.

▶ Tell your dentist how you feel. Some dentists are trained in systematic desensitization, a technique to help anxious patients overcome fear of dental procedures.

▶ Ask if you can listen to soothing music or relaxation tapes played on a stereo headset. Some dentists provide cassettes and headsets as part of their service.

▶ If your dentist is skilled at hypnosis, consider being hypnotized.

▶ If your anxiety is more than you can handle, see a psychotherapist who specializes in treating dental anxiety and other phobias.

Have a routine cleaning and checkup every six months. Preventive care will minimize the need for more painful and lengthy treatment.

337 Treating TMJ

Temporomandibular joint (TMJ) syndrome occurs when the muscles, joints, and ligaments of the jaw move out of alignment. Resulting symptoms include earaches, headaches, pain in the jaw area radiating to the face or the neck and shoulders, ringing in the ears, or pain when opening and closing the mouth. Symptoms of TMJ frequently mimic other conditions, so the problem is often misdiagnosed.

TMJ has a number of possible causes.

▶ Bruxism (grinding your teeth in your sleep)

▶ Sleeping in a way that misaligns the jaw or creates tension in the neck

▶ Stress-induced muscle tension in the neck and shoulder

▶ Incorrect or uneven bite

If you think you may have TMJ, see your dentist. He or she may prescribe anti-inflammatory medication. Or you may need braces to correct your bite or a bite plate to wear when you're asleep. Some doctors recommend surgery to correct TMJ, but you should get more than one opinion before consenting to a surgical remedy.

If you have TMJ, you may be able to minimize symptoms in the following ways.

▶ Don't chew gum.

▶ Try not to open your jaw wide (including yawning or taking big bites out of triple-decker or submarine sandwiches or other difficult-to-eat foods).

▶ Massage the jaw area several times a day, first with your mouth open, then with your mouth closed.

▶ To help reduce muscle spasms that can cause pain, apply moist heat to the jaw area. (A washcloth soaked in warm water makes a convenient hot compress.)

▶ If stress is a factor, consider biofeedback and relaxation training. (See chapter 6, Success over Stress.)

338 Don't Pull That Tooth

At one time, dentists had no choice but to extract an infected tooth. Pulling an infected tooth solved one problem but led to others—poor appearance, change in bite, difficulty chewing food, and less support for adjacent teeth. But tooth extraction is rarely necessary now, thanks to a procedure known as root canal. The dentist (or more likely a specialist known as an endodontist) removes the injured and diseased dental pulp (the inner core that contains nerves, blood vessels, and other tooth tissues) but leaves the tooth intact.

If you're told you need root canal therapy, be sure to let your dentist or endodontist know if you have a heart murmur, history of rheumatic heart disease, or mitral valve prolapse. If so, you may need to take an antibiotic before undergoing this procedure.

339 Bonding for a Beautiful Smile

Bonding can correct certain dental problems effectively and inexpensively. By bonding plastic or porcelain to the tooth, a dentist can:

▶ Cover discoloration

▶ Close small gaps between teeth

▶ Repair fractured and chipped teeth

▶ Protect exposed roots caused by receding gums

▶ Seal out decay-causing bacteria on back teeth

If you've had your teeth bonded, take these steps to prevent chips, stains, or other problems.

▶ Don't chew ice or bite down on hard foods or candy.

▶ Avoid smoking, drinking coffee or tea, or eating blueberries or other foods that easily stain.

▶ Have the bonded teeth checked every three to five years. They may need to be touched up or done over.

340 When to Consider Crowns

Crowns can restore teeth that are broken, chipped, missing, or damaged by decay or disease. A crown is a tooth-shaped porcelain cap that fits over the natural tooth. Crowns improve your appearance, but they also protect your teeth and prolong their useful life.

Ask your dentist about crowns if you have any of the following dental problems.

▶ Badly decayed and damaged teeth

▶ Stained, chipped, or cracked teeth

▶ Noticeable spaces or gaps between teeth

▶ Teeth loosened by periodontal (gum) disease

▶ Teeth that have undergone root canal therapy

341 Brace Yourself for Adult Orthodontics

Each year, over four million people—many of them adults—are fitted for braces. If you have any of the following dental problems, you may be a likely candidate for braces.

▶ Crowded or crooked teeth

▶ Buckteeth or other problems with misaligned teeth

▶ Lower teeth that protrude

▶ Poor bite

▶ Wide spaces between teeth

It takes about two years for braces to realign teeth. In the meantime, you can avoid damage to the braces and decrease the risk of tooth decay and gum disease by practicing the following:

▶ Don't chew gum.

▶ Don't eat nuts or sticky candy or bite down hard on candy or ice.

▶ Don't bite into whole apples, pears, or other crunchy fruit. Instead, cut them into bite-size pieces.

▶ Don't eat corn from the cob.

▶ After eating, brush your teeth with a fluoride toothpaste. Some orthodontists also recommend cleaning your teeth with a water irrigation appliance after you brush.

▶ To guard against decay, rinse your mouth daily with a fluoride mouthwash.

▶ If sores develop in your mouth, or if your gums become red or swollen or bleed easily, contact your orthodontist for advice.

▶ If a wire from the braces becomes loose, don't try to repair it yourself. See your orthodontist.

CHAPTER

16

All about Medical Care

By following the tips in the previous chapters of this book, you can probably prevent many health problems. Despite your best efforts, however, sooner or later you will need medical advice and care. The tips in this chapter will help you get the best medical care available. You'll be better able to communicate with your physician, learn about medication and tests, understand your treatment options, and learn what to expect if you're hospitalized or need surgery.

~~342~~ Symptoms Your Doctor Should Know About

Common sense tells us to avoid visits to the doctor when they are not really necessary. Yet there are important symptoms for which a doctor should be consulted. The following are some symptoms to check out without delay.

▶ Headaches with blurred vision or nausea

▶ Easy bruising

▶ Bleeding gums

▶ Persistent thirst

▶ Chronic cough

▶ Persistent sore throat or trouble swallowing

▶ Coughing or vomiting blood

▶ Chest pressure, shortness of breath

▶ Chest pain that radiates to the neck, shoulder, or arm

▶ Breast lumps

▶ Any unexplained lump or swelling

▶ Change in a mole

▶ Unexplained itching

▶ Recurring chills, sweating, or fever

▶ Convulsions

▶ Insomnia or fatigue

▶ Unexplained severe weight loss or gain

▶ Abdominal pain 2 to 3 hours after meals

▶ Severe depression

▶ Loss of motor function, numbness

▶ Irregular menstrual bleeding

▶ Rectal bleeding or black, tarry stools

▶ Unrelieved diarrhea or constipation

▶ Frequent or painful urination

343 See Your "Primary" Doctor Before You See A Specialist

Internists, family doctors, and pediatricians are examples of primary care doctors. They give general medical care. If you are a member of a Health Maintenance Organization (HMO), your primary care doctor is the doctor you select from the HMO plan to be the "gatekeeper" of all your medical needs. This person could be a family doctor, internist, obstetrician/gynecologist, etc. Whether or not you belong to an HMO, call or see your primary care doctor before you see a specialist. If your primary care doctor cannot take care of your health problem, he or she will refer you to a specialist.

Doctors and Their Specialties.

The most common doctors and a description of their specialties are listed below.

Allergist. Diagnoses and treats allergies

Anesthesiologist. Administers anesthetics that are used during surgery

Cardiologist. Diagnoses and treats diseases of the heart and blood vessels

Dermatologist. Diagnoses and treats diseases and problems of the skin

Emergency Medicine. Specializes in rapid recognition and treatment of trauma or acute illness

Endocrinologist. Diagnoses disorders of the internal glands such as the thyroid and adrenal glands

Family Practitioner. Provides total health care of the individual and the family. Scope is not limited by age, sex, or organ system

Gastroenterologist. Diagnoses and treats disorders of the digestive tract: stomach, bowels, liver, gallbladder, and related organs

Gynecologist. Diagnoses and treats disorders of the female reproductive system

Internist. Diagnoses and treats diseases especially those of adults

Nephrologist. Diagnoses and treats diseases and problems of the kidneys

Neurologist. Diagnoses and treats disorders of the nervous system

Obstetrician. Provides care and treatment of females during pregnancy, labor and delivery, and six weeks after delivery

Oncologist. Diagnoses and treats all types of cancer and other types of benign and malignant tumors

Ophthalmologist. Diagnoses, monitors, and treats vision problems and other disorders of the eye and prescribes prescription lenses

Orthopedist. Diagnoses and treats skeletal injuries and diseases of the bones and muscles

Otolaryngologist. Diagnoses and treats disorders that affect the ears, respiratory, and upper alimentary systems (in general, the head and neck)

Pathologist. Examines and diagnoses organs, tissues, and body fluids

Pediatrician. Diagnoses and treats the physical, emotional, and social problems of children

Physiatrist. Provides physical and rehabilitative treatment of muscle and bone disorders

Psychiatrist. Treats and prevents mental, emotional, and/or behavioral disorders

Radiologist. Uses x-rays and radiant energy for diagnosis and treatment of disease

Urologist. Diagnoses and treats diseases of the urinary or urogenital tract

344 How to Make the Most of a Doctor Visit

When a doctor knows how to really communicate well with a patient, it can make a big difference in how that patient responds. But communication is a two-way process. Listening as well as speaking to one another is something both doctor and patient must work on together. Being honest and open with each other is also important.

What Your Doctor Should Know about You

Aside from a general health history, it is important that your doctor ask certain questions about the following:

► Dietary habits (Are you a frequent junk-food eater? Are you especially fond of cheesecake, sour cream, or other fatty foods?)

► Your occupation (Do you work in a high-stress job? Are you exposed to nickel, nuclear power radiation, or other toxic substances?)

► Sleep habits (Do you frequently awaken before dawn or have problems getting to sleep?)

► Family problems (Are you currently going through a divorce?)

► Lifestyle (Do you get any exercise?)

► Stress (Do you work in a noisy environment?)

► Health attitude (Are you serious about quitting smoking?)

► History of family illness (Does heart disease, high blood pressure, diabetes, kidney problems, or cancer run in your family?)

► Major life events (Have you recently retired from work?)

► Living arrangements (Do you live alone?)

Quizzing Your Doctor

Because a doctor's time is valuable, patients often feel rushed or uneasy taking it up. And when you're sick, there is a tendency to feel vulnerable and passive. But by heeding these suggestions, you can still make the most of your doctor-patient communications.

► Repeat back in your own words what the doctor has told you. Use simple phrases like "Do I hear you say that . . . ?" or "My understanding of the problem is . . ."

▶ Plan ahead of time what you will say to your doctor about your problem. Your observations about a health problem can be invaluable in making a diagnosis.

▶ Take notes on what is wrong and what you need to do.

▶ If you are confused by medical terms, ask for simple definitions. There is no need to be embarrassed by this.

▶ When a medication is prescribed, ask about its possible side effects, its effectiveness, and how long it must be taken.

▶ If your doctor discusses surgery, ask about alternatives, risks, and a second opinion.

▶ Be frank with the doctor if any part of the office visit is annoying, such as lengthy waiting time or discourteous staff. Be tactful, but honest.

▶ Don't be afraid to voice your fears or apprehensions about what you've heard. The doctor may be able to clarify any misconceptions.

▶ Discuss any self-care practices you've used that have relieved symptoms.

▶ Find out the best time for the doctor to receive your phone calls should any questions arise.

345 Rate Your Doctor

In order to feel good about your medical care, you should feel good about your doctor, too. Use this checklist when evaluating your physician.

▶ Is your doctor "board certified" or "board eligible"? Board certified means that he or she has two or more years of training in a specialty after medical school graduation and has passed a national examination certifying competence in the specialty. Board eligible means that the training has been completed, but not the exam. Please note, however, that credentials do not guarantee competency.

▶ Does your doctor listen to you and answer all your questions about the causes and treatment of your medical problems, or is he or she vague, impatient, or unwilling to answer?

▶ Are you comfortable with your doctor? Can you openly discuss your feelings and talk about personal concerns, including sexual and emotional problems?

▶ Does your doctor take a thorough history, asking about past physical and emotional problems, family medical history, drugs you are taking, and other matters affecting your health?

▶ Does your doctor address the root causes of your medical problems or simply prescribe drugs to treat the symptoms?

▶ Does your doctor have an associate to whom you can turn should he or she be unavailable?

▶ Do you feel at ease asking your doctor questions that may sound "silly"?

▶ Does your doctor explain the nature of your condition in simple language?

▶ Is the office staff cordial and attentive to you?

▶ Does your doctor return your telephone calls the same day?

▶ Are you generally seen promptly, or are you kept waiting for a long time when you have an appointment?

▶ Does the doctor have hospital privileges at a respected hospital?

346 The Importance of an Emergency Room Companion

Should you require treatment in an emergency room, ask a relative or a friend to accompany you to serve as your "clear head." He or she can keep track of what procedures are being done and what kind of treatment you're getting, and speak on your behalf if treatment seems too slow in coming.

Having a reassuring companion nearby can also help reduce the stress of an emergency room visit. Your companion should also know about any medications that you are currently taking. Try to bring these medications with you. Most important, your companion can take you home if any medicine given would preclude you from driving.

After you are treated, your companion should help you find out:

▶ What follow-up care is necessary?

▶ What is the name of the emergency room doctor who treated you?

▶ Are there special considerations for the next 24 to 48 hours?

▶ Should your private physician be notified?

▶ Do you have a prescription that must be filled immediately?

347 The ID Card That Can Save Your Life

Heart attacks, car accidents, and other emergencies that leave you unconscious or in a state of shock make it impossible to communicate with health professionals. This is why carrying some sort of medical identification is so important. Three options to consider:

Medic Alert tags. These medical tags alert others to the fact that you have a medical condition that might deserve immediate attention. The tags are given for such conditions as epilepsy or diabetes. To obtain one, contact the MedicAlert Foundation International, 2323 Colorado Ave., Turlock, CA 95380, 1-800-344-3226.

Microfilm ID cards. Many hospitals give their patients special cards that contain a small piece of film called microfiche. The film contains extensive medical history information that you provide when the card is issued. During an emergency, the card is read with the use of a microfilm machine.

Nonmedical ID cards. Medical information can be written on a card that is provided by a variety of health organizations or one that is "homemade." Because there is no official record of this information, health professionals may be reluctant to use some of it.

Medical ID cards should include the following information.

▶ Name

▶ Address

▶ Phone number

▶ Person to call in an emergency

▶ Physician's name and phone number

▶ Blood type

▶ Allergies

▶ Medical conditions

▶ Required medication

▶ Pharmacy name and phone number

▶ Poison control phone number

348 Deciphering Prescriptions and Drug Labels

Doctors and pharmacists communicate in a kind of shorthand—including some abbreviations of Latin terms—to convey instructions for filling prescriptions. Here are some commonly used prescription abbreviations, and how they translate on drug labels. (When your doctor writes a prescription, it will contain five basic pieces of information: the name of the drug prescribed; dosage; whether it's in liquid, capsule, or tablet form; how many you will receive; and the number of refills, if any, permitted. If you still don't understand what's on your prescription or drug label, ask your pharmacist to explain it.)

ad lib: Freely, as needed

a.c.:   Before meals

b.i.d.:   Twice a day

caps: Capsule

gtt: Drops

h.s.:   At bedtime

P.O.:   Orally

p.c.:   After meals

p.r.n.:   As needed

q.4.h.:   Every 4 hours

q.i.d.:   Four times a day

q.d.:   Daily

q.o.d.:   Every other day

t.i.d.:   Three times a day

Ut dict.; UD.:   As directed

SOURCE: *FDA Consumer*, vol. 11, no. 17 (Dec./Jan. 1976–77).

349 Questions You Should Ask about Medications Prescribed for You

Anyone taking prescription medicine needs—and should ask for—the following information.

▶   What is the drug's name?

▶   How does it work?

▶ How long before it takes effect?

▶ What will it do for me?

▶ How long will it be effective?

▶ When should I take it?

▶ Are there possible side effects, both short- and long-term?

▶ Should I take it with meals?

▶ How long should I take the medicine?

▶ Is there a generic equivalent?

▶ Will it interfere or interact with another drug I'm taking and cause problems?

▶ May I stop taking it if I start to feel better?

350 The Seven Golden Rules of Prescription Medicine

Popping that pill into your mouth or spooning down that elixir may be hazardous to your health if you don't observe basic rules.

1. Report adverse reactions, especially unexpected side effects, to your physician. Not everyone responds to medication in the same manner.

2. Because two or more drugs taken within a 24-hour period may interact negatively, tell your doctor if you are taking more than one kind of drug. One drug may slow down or speed up the effect of the other.

3. Ask your pharmacist about food and drug interactions. Some foods may affect the rate at which a medication works, or they can prevent it from working at all. Some combinations can have even more dangerous consequences. When prescription drugs used to treat depression (MAO inhibitors) are consumed with cheese and other foods containing tyramine, for example, dangerously elevated blood pressure levels may result.

4. Don't drink alcohol while on a medication if you don't know its effect. Regular alcohol use can speed up the metabolism of certain drugs, reducing their intended effectiveness. When alcohol is present in the system, other drugs such as sedatives can become deadly.

5. If you are having laboratory tests performed, be sure to inform the physician of all drugs, including nutritional supplements, you have been taking. Certain test results can be influenced. If you have administered a medical self-test, ask your pharmacist about possible drug influence.

6. Always ask your physician if a generic equivalent would be okay to use. Generic drugs are usually less expensive than the brand name item, and may be equally effective. There are certain situations in which a specific brand of medication may be required in order to ensure a consistent dosage. This is particularly important with medications for the heart, lung, and for hormonal disorders.

7. Tell your doctor if:

— You've ever experienced an allergic reaction, and to what.

— You are pregnant or breastfeeding.

— Another doctor is also treating you.

— You have diabetes or kidney or liver disease.

— You're regularly taking vitamins, birth control pills, insulin, or other drugs.

— You use alcohol or tobacco.

SOURCE: *FDA Consumer,* HHS Publication No. (FDA) 84-3124 (June 1982).

351 How to Take Painkillers Safely

About 40 million Americans suffer from some form of chronic or severe pain. Many will seek relief with painkilling drugs or analgesics. Painkillers treat the symptom of pain rather than the root cause.

Simple analgesics. This type of painkiller, such as aspirin or acetaminophen, provides relief from pain at the site of the injury or inflammation. (Aspirin decreases inflammation in addition to its analgesic effect.) These are not habit forming and they maintain effectiveness even after repeated use.

Narcotic analgesics. Analgesics such as codeine or morphine provide relief by acting on the central nervous system, rather than by decreasing inflammation. The cause of the pain does not disappear, but it is easier to endure. These drugs also cause sedation. As the body builds up a tolerance to the narcotic, dosages may need to be increased. When discontinued, withdrawal symptoms can occur.

To minimize unwanted effects of painkillers:

▶ Take painkillers with a full glass of milk or water. It will speed entry into the digestive system and minimize stomach upset.

▶ Remember that all drugs have side effects. Find out early what to expect by asking the pharmacist for the drug package insert or asking your physician.

▶ Take only the weakest form and the smallest dosage that will provide relief.

▶ Don't wait until the pain is too severe to begin your medication. Delay makes it more difficult for the painkiller to be effective, and you may need a stronger dose.

▶ If pain keeps you from sleeping, never take a sleeping pill along with painkillers. Use analgesics only for the pain itself.

▶ If you are a cigarette smoker, painkillers may be metabolized at a different rate so tell your doctor if you smoke.

▶ Before considering switching painkillers because of side effects, ask your doctor if he or she can reduce your dosage.

▶ If you are taking a narcotic type of painkiller, check with your physician about alternating it with aspirin or an acetaminophen analgesic. This will help reduce the possibility of developing a tolerance.

▶ Don't think of painkillers as your only weapon against pain. There are other techniques—such as relaxation training (see chapter 6, Success over Stress) or cold compresses—that your physician can help you with.

352 Over-the-Counter Drugs: Reducing the Risks of Self-Prescription

Over-the-counter (OTC) drugs are widely advertised in magazines and on TV and are consumed by millions of people. Generally less potent than prescription drugs, they can be taken without the authorization of a doctor. But before purchasing an over-the-counter remedy, ask yourself:

▶ Am I trying to cover up symptoms that need to be evaluated by a doctor?

▶ Will continued use cause new problems (dependency on laxatives or sleeping pills, for example)?

▶ Are there unwanted side effects from these drugs (for example, increased blood pressure, dizziness, headaches, rashes)?

▶ Do I already have a similar product at home?

Often, reading the package labels—or looking up the name of the drug in the *Physician's Desk Reference for Nonprescription Drugs,* can help you answer these questions.

Keep in mind, too, that when taken in large quantities, an OTC drug might equal the dose of a medicine that is available only by prescription.

If there is any uncertainty in your mind whether or not a particular OTC medication will help or harm you, call and check with your doctor before you purchase it.

353 Aspirin Dos and Don'ts

It's not hard to guess what the most widely used drug in America is. It's aspirin, with over 20 billion tablets swallowed yearly. You can also take it in chewing gum, capsules, or suppositories. If you want more powerful relief, consider those labeled "extra strength," as they contain a higher dose of the aspirin.

Because aspirin is really an acid (acetylsalicylic acid), it can be irritating to the stomach. For this reason, aspirin can be purchased in buffered form. This means it has been combined with an antacid-like magnesium carbonate. Enteric-coated aspirin—that is, tablets or capsules which have been treated with a special coating to prevent its release and absorption until the pill reaches the intestines—is even less irritating to the stomach. Taking plain aspirin with food will also help avoid stomach irritation.

Aspirin should be avoided under certain circumstances.

▶ During pregnancy, especially in the first and last trimesters. It can prolong labor and cause delivery problems. Avoid aspirin unless your doctor deems it necessary.

▶ Taken prior to surgery, aspirin can produce bleeding difficulties.

▶ If diabetics take aspirin regularly, their urine sugar tests may be affected with misleading results.

▶ Parents should not give aspirin to children under 19 who have or are recovering from the chicken pox or flu. There is a definite relationship between aspirin used during these illnesses and Reye's syndrome, a nervous system disease that can be fatal. (See Tip 73 in chapter 2, Major Medical Conditions: Prevention, Detection, and Treatment.)

▶ If you take aspirin regularly or in high doses, drinking alcoholic beverages may increase stomach irritation.

▶ People with asthma, kidney problems, gout, ulcers, or bleeding conditions should always check with a doctor before taking aspirin, which can aggravate these conditions.

▶ Always consult a doctor when considering aspirin in combination with prescription drugs like anticoagulants, oral diabetes medication, anti-gout drugs, and arthritis medications.

354 Overhaul Your Medicine Cabinet

Who knows what mysterious bottles lurk on the shelves of your bathroom medicine cabinet! If it's been more than a year since you last housecleaned your cabinet, it's certainly time to take inventory. Here's how:

▶ Take out the entire contents of the medicine cabinet and get some clear idea of what you really need to keep.

▶ Check expiration dates. Throw out all outdated medicine. If you're uncertain about a particular item, call your pharmacist and ask what the shelf life is.

▶ Are all medications in original containers and labeled clearly? If not, into the trash they go. It's dangerous to store medicines in anything but their original containers. Some medicines come in tinted glass, for example, because exposure to light may cause them to deteriorate.

▶ Discard old tubes of cream that have become hardened or cracked. Throw out any liquid medicines that now appear cloudy or filmy.

▶ If there are children in the house, every medication is a potential poison. Discard all unnecessary medications by flushing them down the toilet, and keep all others locked in a high cabinet, well out of their reach.

▶ Keep a container of syrup of ipecac handy in case of accidental poisoning.

355 When—And How Often—To Have a Cholesterol Test (and Other Routine Tests)

Is it time for a mammogram or blood pressure reading? Most people have only a very general sense of when routine medical tests are needed. They tend to rely on a reminder from their physicians. But what if you don't have a personal physician and haven't seen one for years? The following table will help in anticipating when important medical tests should be done.

Here is what the tests will check.

Blood Pressure Test – Checks 2 kinds of pressure within the blood vessels. The higher number (systolic blood pressure) gauges the pressure when your heart is pumping and the lower number (diastolic blood pressure) represents the pressure between heartbeats. High blood pressure is a symptomless disease that can lead to a heart attack and/or a stroke.

Vision. Checks for marked changes or degeneration of eye functioning

Pap Test. Is used to detect the early signs of cervical cancer, uterine cancer and herpes

Mammography. An X-ray to detect breast tumors or problems

Professional Breast Exam. A physician or nurse examines the breasts for signs of abnormalities

Digital Rectal Exam. Checks for early signs of colorectal and/or prostate abnormalities including cancer

Stool Blood Test. Checks for early signs of colorectal abnormalities, including cancer

Sigmoidoscopy. Checks for early signs of colorectal abnormalities and cancer

Cholesterol Blood Test. Checks the levels of fatty deposits (cholesterol) in the blood. High cholesterol levels are linked to heart disease.

Glaucoma Screening. Checks for increased pressure within the eye. Glaucoma can result in blindness if not treated.

Guidelines for Routine Tests

AGES		20-29	30-39	40-49	50 and older
Physical Exam		▓ (2-3 years)	▓ (2-3 years)	▓ (2-3 years)	▥ (1-2 years)
Blood Pressure		▥ (1-2 years)	▥ (1-2 years)	▥ (1-2 years)	▥ (1-2 years)
Vision		▨ (3-5 years)	▨ (3-5 years)	▨ (3-5 years)	▓ (2-3 years)
Pap Test[1]	**W**	▓ (2-3 years)	▓ (2-3 years)	▓ (2-3 years)	▓ (2-3 years)
Mammography[2]	**O**				■ (every year)
Breast Self-Examination	**M** **E**	Monthly	Monthly	Monthly	Monthly
Professional Breast Examination	**N**			■ (every year)	■ (every year)
Testicular Self-Exam (Men)		Discuss With Your Doctor			
Digital Rectal Exam				Discuss With Your Doctor	
Stool Blood Test					■ (every year)
Sigmoidoscopy					▨ (3-5 years)
Cholesterol Blood Test[3]		▨ (3-5 years)	▨ (3-5 years)	▨ (3-5 years)	▨ (3-5 years)
Glaucoma Screening[4]					▓ (2-3 years)
Regular Dental Checkup		■ (every year)	■ (every year)	■ (every year)	■ (every year)

■ Every year ▥ Every 1–2 years ▓ Every 2–3 years ▨ Every 3–5 years

Note: These guidelines apply only to healthy people who do not have symptoms of illnesses. Consult your doctor for a schedule of routine medical tests and exams that is best for you. Also, check with your insurance company to see if and when tests are covered.

1. Pap tests should start at age 18, or under age 18 if sexual activity has begun. They should be given every year until tests are normal 3 years in a row. Thereafter, pap tests should be given at least every 3 years. *Note:* The American College of Obstetricians and Gynecologists recommends an annual pap test.
2. As recommended by The National Cancer Institute.
3. The National Cholesterol Education Program (NCEP) recommends a blood cholesterol test at least once every 5 years, and that high-density lipoprotein (HDL) be part of the initial cholesterol testing.
4. Glaucoma screening is recommended earlier for African Americans. It should be done every 2 to 3 years between the ages of 40 and 49.

SOURCE FOR TEXT AND TABLE: *Health at Home*™, American Institute for Preventive Medicine, Farmington Hills, Michigan, 1997.

Know Your Cholesterol Levels

Average doesn't necessarily mean healthy, especially when you're talking about cholesterol, a fat-related substance found in the blood. Too much cholesterol can build up and form artery-clogging plaques, slowing blood to a trickle and ending in a heart attack that could be fatal.

According to a panel of experts convened by the National Heart, Lung, and Blood Institute, cholesterol should be 200 milligrams per deciliter or lower. Yet the average cholesterol level for men in the United States is 211, and for women, it's 215. So if your doctor tells you your cholesterol is "normal" or "average," ask for the exact numbers, and if it's elevated, take steps to reduce it. (Cholesterol levels of 200 to 240 milligrams per deciliter put adults at moderate risk for heart disease; levels of 240 or higher constitute a high risk.)

Better yet, ask for a blood test that measures not only your total cholesterol but also your triglycerides (another kind of blood fat), HDL (high-density lipoprotein) cholesterol, a protective kind of fat, and LDL (low-density lipoprotein) cholesterol. Ideally, your triglyceride level should be 160 milligrams per deciliter or lower.

The more HDL, the better, and the less LDL, the better. An HDL below 35 is cause for concern; so is an LDL over 130. Also, the ratio of total cholesterol to HDL cholesterol ideally should be 4.0 or less. (To calculate your ratio, divide the total cholesterol number by the HDL number.) A ratio less than 4.0 is low risk; more than 6.0 is high risk.

Most people can improve their cholesterol and triglyceride readings by eating less dietary fat, not smoking, getting more exercise, avoiding overweight, consuming a limited amount of alcohol and sweets, and eating certain kinds of food high in fiber. (For more details on a heart-healthy diet, see chapter 4, Eating for Better Health.)

356 Ask "Is This X-Ray Really Necessary?"

Most of the time x-rays are necessary, but it's up to the patient to question them anyway. You must stay alert to the possibility of being exposed to harmful levels of radiation through unnecessary x-rays, both medical and dental. The risks of overexposure can include sterility, birth defects, and the development of cancer in certain sensitive tissues.

If you're pregnant, or even suspect you might be, further precautions become even more imperative. Dental x-rays might be postponed or, if a medical x-ray is needed, a lead shield should cover the abdominal and pelvic area. Ask your doctor if an ultrasound examination might substitute.

If you have switched to another doctor or dentist, it's not always necessary to start fresh with new x-rays. Have your previous x-ray records sent to the new office.

357 A Word to the Wise about Home Medical Tests

Medical self-testing kits are convenient, relatively inexpensive, and readily available. They can be used without a visit to the doctor. It's no wonder that Americans are purchasing them in increasing numbers, spending $500 million or more annually. Home tests offer consumers a sense of self-reliance that can complement, though not take the place of, the advice of their physicians.

While hundreds of different medical self-testing kits exist, they generally can be grouped into three categories.

➤ Those that diagnose when symptoms are present. These include the popular self-testing kits for pregnancy.

➤ Those that diagnose when no symptoms are present. These include kits that test for blood in the stool, which could indicate colon cancer, or kits that help couples conceive by testing for the time of ovulation.

➤ Those that monitor an ongoing condition. These include glucose testing for diabetes and blood pressure screening for hypertensives.

The U.S. Public Health Service and the Food and Drug Administration (FDA) offer the following suggestions for safe and effective use of self-testing kits. (Each of these precautions does not necessarily apply to all tests.)

➤ For test kits that contain chemicals, note the expiration date. Beyond that date, chemicals may lose potency and affect results. Don't buy or use a test kit after the expiration date.

▶ Check whether the product needs protection from heat or cold. If so, don't leave it in the car trunk or by a sunny window on the trip home. At home, follow storage directions.

▶ Study the package insert. First, read it through to get a general idea of how to perform the test. Then, go back and review the instructions and diagrams carefully so that you fully understand each step.

▶ Be sure you understand what the test is *intended* to do and what its limitations may be. Remember, the tests are not 100 percent accurate.

▶ If the test results rely on color comparison and you're color blind, be sure someone who *can* discern color helps you interpret the results.

▶ Note special precautions, such as avoiding physical activity or certain foods and drugs before testing.

▶ Follow instructions exactly, including the specimen collection process, if that is a part of the test. Sequence is important. Don't skip a step.

▶ When collecting a urine specimen—unless you use a container from a kit—first wash the container thoroughly and rinse out all soap traces, preferably with distilled water.

▶ When a step is timed, be precise. Use a stopwatch, or at least a watch with a second hand.

▶ Note what you should do if the results are positive, negative, or unclear.

▶ If something isn't clear, don't guess. Consult a pharmacist or other health professional, or check the insert for a toll-free "800" number to call for additional information.

▶ Keep accurate records of results.

▶ As with medications, keep test kits that contain chemicals out of the reach of children. Promptly discard used test materials as directed.

Any malfunction of a self-test should be reported to the manufacturer or to the FDA through the agency's reporting system at the U.S. Pharmacopeia. To report a problem to the pharmacopeia, write to USP, Problem Reporting Program, 12601 Twinbrook Parkway, Rockville, MD 20852. The report also may be called in toll-free at 1-800-638-6725 (in

Maryland, call collect at 301-881-0256).
SOURCE: *FDA Consumer*, HHS Publication (FDA) 86-4206 (February 1986).

358 How to Avoid Hospital Germs

Florence Nightingale once said, "The first requirement of a hospital is that it should do no harm." Unfortunately, that goal has still not been totally achieved. There is a good deal of research that shows spending time in a hospital can make you sick—for several reasons.

▶ There are a number of viruses and bacteria brought into hospitals by patients, employees, and visitors.

▶ The hospital rounds made by the staff can transmit viruses and bacteria from one patient to another.

▶ Hospital procedures like injections and I.V. therapy penetrate the skin, bypassing the body's first line of defense against disease.

In fact, some 300,000 patients develop nosocomial (hospital-linked) pneumonia each year. Nosocomial infections are estimated to account for 15 percent of hospital charges. Here's what you can do to protect yourself.

▶ Try to be as well-rested and as well-nourished as possible before you're admitted to the hospital.

▶ If a hospital roommate becomes infected with pneumonia, ask to have your room changed.

359 A Dozen Rights Every Patient Should Expect

What rights and privileges can you expect from a hospital when you become a patient? According to the American Hospital Association (AHA), there are specific standards of care that all patients are entitled to. The AHA has developed a voluntary code—the Patient's Bill of Rights—that presents guidelines for both staff and patients.

1. You have the right to considerate and respectful care.

2. You have the right to obtain from your physician complete, current information concerning your diagnosis, treatment, and

prognosis in terms you can reasonably be expected to understand.

3. You have the right to receive from your physician information necessary to give informed consent prior to the start of any procedure and/or treatment.

4. You have the right to refuse treatment to the extent permitted by law, and to be informed of the medical consequences of your action.

5. You have the right to privacy concerning your own medical care program.

6. You have the right to expect that all communications and records pertaining to your care should be treated as confidential.

7. You have the right to expect that within its capacity a hospital must make a reasonable response to your request for services.

8. You have the right to obtain information about any relationship of your hospital to other health care and educational institutions insofar as your care is concerned.

9. You have the right to be advised if the hospital proposes to engage in or perform human experimentation affecting your care or treatment.

10. You have the right to expect reasonable continuity of care.

11. You have the right to examine and receive an explanation of your bill regardless of the source of payment.

12. You have the right to know what hospital rules and regulations apply to your conduct as a patient.

360 Review Your Patient Chart

Guess what every patient in a hospital has? No, we're not speaking of those less-than-attractive hospital gowns or the plastic ID bracelets. The answer is a patient chart. Although the chart is legally the property of the hospital and generally kept at a nursing station, the patient should be aware of its content. Ask your doctor for an explanation. The chart may contain the following:

▶ Your medical history
▶ Hospital laboratory results

► Lists of medications (doses and schedules)

► Special treatments or therapy

► Dietary restrictions or recommendations (low-sodium diet, for example)

► Scheduled diagnostic procedures (such as x-rays)

► Surgical notes (length of operation, assisting medical staff, type of anesthesia administered, recovery notes)

If you suspect a problem or error—in how often you are being given medication, for instance—ask a nurse or your doctor to show you your chart and explain what is written there.

361 Know What Treatment You've Agreed To

Every patient should be aware of the policy of Informed Consent, an ethical standard in medicine that implies that you have been given an explanation and fully understand your treatment. You should be able to explain in your own words what your treatment is about. You should know what the likelihood is that the medical procedure will accomplish what it's supposed to. The benefits and the accompanying risks should always be identified clearly. You should also be notified if your treatment is experimental in nature.

The physician should review any alternatives that are available in lieu of surgery or other procedures. Informed Consent enables you to make a rational and educated decision about your treatment. It is also a tool that promotes greater understanding between you and your doctor and encourages joint decision making.

Three principles of Informed Consent that involve your responsibility as a patient are:

► You cannot demand services that go beyond what are considered "acceptable" practices of medicine or that violate professional ethics.

► You must recognize that you may be faced with some uncertainties or unpleasantness.

► You should, if competent, be responsible for your choices and not pass them along to others.

362 When to Refuse Tests or Surgery

An average of 40 medical tests per person are done each year in the United States. It's estimated that at least one-quarter of them are not needed. A study published in the *Journal of the American Medical Association* found that nearly 60 percent of the study's 2,800 presurgery tests were not warranted because there were no symptoms indicating that the tests should be done. Just 22 percent of the tests studied yielded results, and even these played a very small role in treatment. Yet medical tests make up about half of the typical patient's hospital charges, according to David Sobel, M.D., the director of patient education at Kaiser Permanente.

Be frank with your doctor and ask for an explanation of why a particular test is being done. You'll want to ask the following:

▶ Will the test results determine the treatment?

▶ Are there risks to the testing?

▶ Are there alternatives?

▶ Can outpatient testing be considered?

If your doctor recommends a hysterectomy, tonsillectomy, coronary bypass, or gallbladder removal, ask questions about alternatives. According to Eugene Rubin, M.D., of Stanford University, these procedures are among the surgeries performed excessively. Others that Dr. Rubin lists are:

▶ Dilatation and curettage (D and C)

▶ Cesarean sections

▶ Pacemaker insertion

▶ Joint surgery

Find out about the following:

▶ Alternatives that are not as radical as surgery.

▶ If it would be risky to postpone the surgery.

▶ If the surgery is not effective, what treatment you should try next.

SOURCE: Adapted from
Drs. David Sobel and Tom Ferguson, *The People's Book of Medical Tests* (New York: Summit Books, 1987).
Dr. Eugene Rubin, *Matters of Life & Death: Risks Versus Benefits In Health* (New York: Harper & Row, 1984).

363 When in Doubt, Get a Second Opinion

The very first thing you should do if a doctor suggests surgery is to get the opinion of a second doctor. Programs to encourage patients to pursue other options have been established all over the country in an effort to curtail the enormous amount of unnecessary surgery.

Ask your physician or someone else you trust to recommend a nonsurgeon or another surgeon not affiliated with the same hospital as your physician who will review your case and offer an opinion. Generally, you should not submit to surgery on the basis of one medical opinion alone.

The table below indicates the percentage of surgeries not recommended by the physician giving a second opinion.

Results of Second Surgical Opinions

Surgery	Percentage Not Recommended on Second Opinion
Bunionectomy	40
Knee surgery	40
Hysterectomy	35
Prostatectomy	35
Deviated nasal septum surgery	30
Breast surgery	25
Dilatation and curettage (D and C)	25
Varicose vein surgery	25
Cataract removal	23
Tonsillectomy	20
Cholecystectomy	10
Hernia repair	10

SOURCE: Eugene G. McCarthy, *Second Opinion: Elective Surgery* (Boston: Auburn House, 1981).

Always check with your insurance company to see if the cost of a second opinion will be covered. Most policies include this feature. Both Medicare and Medicaid cover second surgical opinions.

The U.S. Health Care Financing Administration, a governmental agency, sponsors a toll-free number, 1-800-638-6833, and provides a list of local physicians to consult for a second opinion.

364 Reducing Presurgery Jitters

Knowing what to expect prior to surgery can reduce preoperation stress and make you feel more comfortable.

▶ The hospital will have you sign a surgical consent form. Take the time to read it over. Ask your doctor any questions you may have.

▶ Expect a visit from the anesthesiologist or the surgeon (or both). They will review the surgical plans with you. This includes the time and length of surgery, estimated recovery room time, and the type of anesthesia being used. The anesthesiologist will need to know about any previous surgeries, any medical conditions, and any allergies to medications. Ask him or her what time you can expect to return to your room.

▶ Eating in the hours prior to surgery can cause life-threatening vomiting during the operation, so there are usually a prescribed number of hours prior to surgery when no food should be eaten. If a meal is brought to you, don't eat it until you've double-checked with a nurse. It may be a mistake that could cause your surgery to be canceled. Your patient chart should read NPO or non per os (nothing by mouth).

▶ Depending on the nature of the operation, some surgical "preps" may be ordered. This may include a special liquids-only diet, cleaning and shaving of the surgical area, placing a catheter into the bladder, giving an enema, or putting drops into the eyes.

▶ A sleeping pill may be offered the night prior to surgery. Most people will feel anxious about the surgery and find the medication helpful. You are not required to accept it, however, and your patient chart should indicate your preference.

▶ Before surgery, give all valuables or possessions to a friend or relative. These would include jewelry, watches, and eyeglasses. If you wear contact lenses, remove them.

365 The Ins and Outs of Ambulatory Surgery

Can you have surgery without being admitted to a hospital? Yes, and it's recommended in many cases. Ambulatory surgery facilities or short-term centers, as they are sometimes called, are usually freestanding facilities that perform a select group of minor surgeries.

Procedures that best qualify for ambulatory centers:

▶ Do not require opening a primary body section like the chest or skull.

▶ Do not require blood transfusions.

▶ Require very little or no general anesthesia.

▶ Do not require specialized postoperative care.

▶ Do not require hours on the operating table.

▶ Pose little risk of complication or additional surgery.

The most common types of surgeries performed in an ambulatory care center include, hernia repair, some plastic surgeries, tubal ligation, dilatation and curettage (D and C), breast biopsy, tonsillectomy, cataract removal, adenoidectomy, orthopedic procedures (such as setting a broken bone), cystoscopy, varicose vein surgery, and glaucoma procedures.

There are several important advantages of ambulatory or outpatient surgery.

▶ Hospitalization poses the risks of exposure to infection (see Tip 358) and also may keep patients bedridden longer than is necessary. Ambulatory surgery gets you in and out quickly.

▶ The surgeries are scheduled by appointment for patient convenience and are not like hospital morning surgery schedules. The patient has a good deal of choice as to when the surgery will occur.

▶ Most people prefer recuperating at home in their own beds to staying in a hospital. Familiar surroundings and the comforts of home can be a more conducive environment in which to recuperate than the hectic schedules in many hospitals.

▶ Medical bills are much lower if you don't have to stay in a hospital overnight.

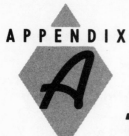

APPENDIX A

The Healthy
Habit Test

To find out just how healthy a lifestyle you lead, take this simple test. The results will help you determine which of your health habits, if any, need improvement—something the tips in this book can help you achieve.

Directions

Put a check beside each statement that applies to you, then tally your score on page 350.

 ## Alcohol Use

(If you do not drink, check all five items even though some items would not apply.)

_____ I drink less than two drinks a day.

_____ In the past year, I have not driven an automobile after having more than two drinks.

_____ When I'm under stress or depressed, I do not drink more.

_____ I do not do things when I'm drinking that I later regret.

_____ I have never experienced any problem because of my drinking.

◆ Tobacco Use

(If you have never smoked, check all five items even though the last two items would not apply.)

_____ I have never smoked cigarettes.

_____ I haven't smoked cigarettes in the past year.

_____ I do not use any other form of tobacco (pipes, cigars, chewing tobacco).

_____ I smoke only low-tar and low-nicotine cigarettes.

_____ I smoke less than one pack of cigarettes a day.

◆ Blood Pressure

_____ I have had my blood pressure checked within the past six months.

_____ I have never had high blood pressure.

_____ I do not currently have high blood pressure.

_____ I make a conscious effort to avoid salt in my diet.

_____ There is not a history of high blood pressure in my immediate family.

◆ Weight and Body Fat Levels

_____ According to height and weight charts, my weight is average for my height.

_____ I have not needed to go on a weight reduction diet in the past year.

_____ There is no place on my body that I can pinch an inch of fat.

_____ I am satisfied with the way my body looks.

_____ None of my family or friends or health care professionals have ever urged me to lose weight.

◆ Physical Fitness

_____ I do some form of vigorous exercise for at least 30 minutes a day three times a week or more.

_____ My resting pulse is 70 beats a minute or less.

_____ I don't get fatigued easily while doing physical work.

_____ I engage in some recreational sport such as tennis or swimming on a weekly basis.

_____ I would say that my level of physical fitness is higher than most of the people in my age group.

◆ Stress and Anxiety

_____ I find it easy to relax.

_____ I am able to cope with stressful events as well as or better than most people.

_____ I do not have trouble falling asleep or waking up.

_____ I rarely feel tense or anxious.

_____ I have no trouble completing tasks I have started.

◆ Automobile Safety

_____ I always use seat belts when I drive.

_____ I always use seat belts when I am a passenger.

_____ I have not had an automobile accident in the past three years.

_____ I have not had a speeding ticket or other moving violation for the past three years.

_____ I never ride with a driver who has had more than two drinks.

◆ Relationships

_____ I am satisfied with my social relationships.

_____ I have a lot of close friends.

_____ I am able to share my feelings with my spouse or other family members (or both).

_____ When I have a problem, I have other people with whom I can talk it over.

_____ Given a choice between doing things by myself or with others, I usually choose to do things with others.

◆ Rest and Sleep

_____ I almost always get between 7 and 9 hours of sleep a night.

_____ It rarely takes longer than 20 minutes for me to fall asleep.

_____ I wake up few, if any, times during the night.

_____ I feel rested and ready to go when I get up in the morning.

_____ Most days, I have a lot of energy.

◆ Life Satisfaction

_____ If I had my life to live over, I wouldn't make very many changes.

_____ I've accomplished most of the things that I've set out to do in life.

_____ I can't think of an area in my life that really disappoints me.

_____ I am a happy person.

_____ As compared to the people with whom I grew up, I feel I've done as well or better than most of them with my life.

Scoring

Record the number of checks (from 0 to 5) for each area. Then add up the numbers to determine your score.

Alcohol use	_____
Tobacco use	_____
Blood pressure	_____
Weight and body fat levels	_____
Physical fitness	_____
Stress and anxiety	_____
Automobile safety	_____
Relationships	_____
Rest and sleep	_____
Life satisfaction	_____
TOTAL	_____

Interpreting Your Score

▶ A score of 40 to 50 indicates a healthier-than-average lifestyle.

▶ A score of 25 to 39 indicates an average lifestyle.

▶ A score of 0 to 24 indicates a below-average lifestyle (and need for overall improvement).

▶ A score of less than 3 in any one area indicates a need for improvement in that particular area.

SOURCE: John Cavendish, Ed.D., assistant professor of health education, West Virginia University, Morgantown.

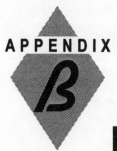

APPENDIX

Hotline
to Health

Free health information is just a phone call away. The toll-free numbers listed below cover everything from diabetes to dyslexia and Alzheimer's to AIDS. (The organizations are listed alphabetically by subject.)

Most organizations staff their phones from 9:00 A.M. to 5:00 P.M. local time, Monday through Friday. Call early in the day when the telephone lines are least busy.

To find a toll-free number not listed in this directory, call the toll-free information operator at 1-800-555-1212 and explain what kind of information you're looking for.

Inclusion in this directory does not indicate endorsement of the organization by the American Institute for Preventive Medicine.

Alcohol and Drug Abuse
Al-Anon Family Group Headquarters
(includes Alateen)
P.O. Box 862, Midtown Station
New York, NY 10018-0862
1-800-356-9996
Provides information and help to
family members and friends of
alcoholics.

Youth Power
(Formerly "Just Say No" International)
300 Lakeside Drive, Ste. 1340
Oakland, CA 94612
1-800-258-2766
Assists parents, children and schools in
setting up "Just Say No" clubs to
prevent drug abuse.

National Cocaine Hotline
c/o Phoenix House
164 West 74th Street
New York, NY 10023
1-800-COCAINE or 1-800-662-HELP
Answers questions, makes referrals to
local programs, and offers counseling
on cocaine use and other drug problems.

National Council on Alcoholism
12 W. 21st St.
New York, NY 10010
1-800-622-2255
Offers various kinds of information on
alcoholism.

Children's Diseases

Cystic Fibrosis Foundation
6931 Arlington Rd.
Bethesda, MD 20814
1-800-344-4823 or 1-800-CF-FIGHT
Provides information and local physician referrals for children with cystic fibrosis.

Juvenile Diabetes Foundation
International
120 Wall Street, 19th Floor
New York, NY 10005
1-800-223-1138
Provides information and answers questions about juvenile diabetes.

National Reye's Syndrome
Foundation
P.O. Box 829
Bryan, OH 43506
1-800-233-7393
Distributes information to the public and the medical community on Reye's syndrome.

General Health Information

American Academy of Family
Physicians
8880 Ward Pkwy.
Kansas City, MO 64114
1-800-274-2237
A national association of family doctors who govern and maintain high standards in such areas as patient and continuing education.

American Osteopathic Association
142 E. Ontario St.
Chicago, IL 60611
1-800-621-1773
Provides information on osteopathic medicine. Makes local referrals to osteopathic centers.

National Health Information Center
P.O. Box 1133
Washington, DC 20013-1133
1-800-336-4797
Provides information and referrals for consumers looking for various types of health information.

Health Problems

Acquired Immune Deficiency Syndrome (AIDS)

AIDS Information Hotline
U.S. Public Health Service
1-800-342-AIDS
1-800-344-7432 (in Spanish)
1-800-243-7889 (for hearing impaired)
Provides information on HIV/AIDS and makes local referrals for medical assistance.

Alzheimer's Disease

Alzheimer's Association
919 North Michigan Ave., Suite 1000
Chicago, IL 60611-1676
1-800-272-3900
Provides information to the public and health care professionals. Makes referrals to local chapters and support groups.

Anemia

Cooley's Anemia Foundation
129-09 26th Avenue
Flushing, NY 11354
1-800-221-3571
Provides information on patient care, support groups, and research on Cooley's anemia.

Cancer

Cancer Information Service (National Cancer Institute)
900 Rockville Pike
Bethesda, MD 20892
1-800-4-CANCER
Provides information on cancer to both the public and medical community.

Diabetes

American Diabetes Association
1660 Duke St.
Alexandria, VA 22314
1-800-232-3472
Provides health education information, supports research, and offers assistance in forming diabetes support groups.

Domestic Violence

National Domestic Violence Hotline
1-800-799-SAFE
Offers confidential crisis intervention, and referrals to local shelters, counseling, support groups and legal services to an abuse victim and his or her friends and family members.

Disabilities

National Rehabilitation Information Center
8455 Colesville Rd., Suite 935
Silver Spring, MD 20910
1-800-34-NARIC
Provides current information and referrals for people with disabilities.

Dyslexia

Orton Dyslexia
Chester Bldg., Suite 382 8600
LaSalle Rd.
Baltimore, MD 21204-6020
1-800-ABCD-123
Provides information, supports research, and makes referrals for people suffering from this learning disability.

Epilepsy

Epilepsy Foundation of America
4351 Garden City Dr., 4th Floor
Landover, MD 20785
1-800-332-1000
Provides information about epilepsy and makes referrals to local resources.

Headaches

National Headache Foundation
428 W. St. James Place
Chicago, IL 60614
1-800-843-2256
Provides information on headaches and their treatment. Also provides physician member list and headache clinic list.

Hearing and Speech problems

Better Hearing Institute-Hearing Help Line
P.O. Box 1840
Washington, DC 20013
1-800-327-9355
Offers information and help for hearing problems and prevention of deafness.

National Hearing Aid Helpline
20361 Middlebelt Rd.
Livonia, MI 48152
1-800-521-5247
Provides information on hearing loss and referrals to those in need of hearing aids. Serves both the general public and health professionals.

Heart Disease

American Heart Association
7272 Greenville Ave.
Dallas, TX 75231-4596
1-800-242-8721
Supports research and public education. Offers multiple services focusing on the prevention and treatment of heart disease.

National Heart Lung and Blood Institute (NHLBI)
P.O. Box 30105
Bethesda, MD 20824-0105
1-800-575-WELL
Provides information on asthma, heart disease, high blood pressure, and other conditions that affect the heart, lungs, and blood.

Kidney Diseases

American Kidney Fund
6110 Executive Blvd., Suite 1010
Rockville, MD 20852
1-800-638-8299
Provides information on kidney
disease and organ donations. Also
grants financial assistance to needy
kidney patients.

Liver Diseases

American Liver Foundation
1425 Pompton Ave.
Cedar Grove, NJ 07009
1-800-223-0179
Makes referrals to local self-help
support groups and offers educational
information for people with liver
ailments. Also publishes a newsletter
for physicians and the general public.

Lung Diseases

National Jewish Center for Immunol-
ogy and Respiratory Medicine-Lung
Line
1400 Jackson St.
Denver, CO 80206
1-800-222-LUNG
Answers questions and provides
information on respiratory problems,
including asthma, emphysema, and
chronic bronchitis.

Lupus

Lupus Foundation of America
4 Research Place, Suite 180
Rockville, MD 20850-3226
1-800-558-0121
Provides patient education, support
groups, and public and professional
services to people with lupus.

Parkinson's Disease

National Parkinson Foundation
1501 N.W. 9th Ave.
Bob Hope Rd.
Miami, FL 33136

1-800-327-4545
Answers questions, furnishes
information, and makes physician
referrals for people with Parkinson's
disease.

Sickle Cell Anemia

Association of America for Sickle
Cell Disease
200 Corporate Pointe, Suite 495
Culver City, CA 90230
1-800-421-8453
Prepares and distributes educational
materials, trains counselors, and
conducts educational programs for
the public and health care professionals. Also supports research and
conducts diagnostic screenings.

Visual Problems

American Council for the Blind
1155 15th Street, Suite 720
Washington, DC 20005
1-800-424-8666
Provides information and cassettes
and makes referrals to local agencies
and vision care professionals.

Prevent Blindness America
500 E. Remington Rd.
Schaumberg, IL 60173
1-800-221-3004
Sponsors research and glaucoma
screenings. Also offers educational
materials, consultations, and professional education programs.

Hospital and Hospice Care

Hill-Burton Hospital Free or Reduced
Cost Health Care Program
U.S. Public Health Service
5600 Fishers Ln., Room 1125
Rockville, MD 20857
1-800-638-0742
1-800-492-0359 for Maryland only
Furnishes information and referrals to
participating hospitals.

Insurance
Inspector General's Hotline
P.O. Box 17303
Baltimore, MD 21203-7303
1-800-368-5779
Handles Medicare and Social
Security fraud, abuse, and waste.

Medical Identification
MedicAlert Foundation International
2323 Colorado Avenue
Turlock, CA 95380
1-800-344-3226
Dispenses medical identification
bracelets, neck chains, or cards to
individuals who have chronic medical
conditions,

Mental Health
National Mental Health Association
1-800-969-NMHA
Provides information and referrals for
various mental health problems.

National Runaway Switchboard
3080 N. Lincoln Ave.
Chicago, IL 60657
1-800-621-4000
Makes referrals and provides
counseling to troubled and /or
runaway teenagers.

Nutrition
National Center for Nutrition and
Dietetics
American Dietetic Association
216 West Jackson Boulevard, Suite
800
Chicago, IL 60606
Consumer Nutrition Information
Hotline: 1-800-366-1655

Organ Donation
The Living Bank
P.O. Box 6725
Houston, TX 77265
1-800-528-2971

Registers people who wish to donate
their organs or tissues after death.
Offers printed materials, and
encourages public education for both
health care professionals and organ
donors.

Pregnancy
International Childbirth Education
Association (ICEA)
P.O. Box 20048
Minneapolis, MN 55420
1-800-624-4934
Furnishes information on pregnancy-
related concerns through their book
center.

ASPO-LAMAZE
1200 19th Street, N.W., Suite 300
Washington, DC 20036
1-800-368-4404
Provides information and makes local
referrals for childbirth preparation
classes and instruction in breathing
techniques used during delivery.

Safety
National Highway Traffic Safety
Administration
Auto Safety Hotline
400 7th St. SW
Washington, DC 20590
1-800-424-9393
Provides information on passenger
safety, auto recalls, and child safety
seats. Also handles consumer
questions about auto safety
regulations.

National Safety Council
1121 Spring Lake Drive
Itasca, IL 60143-3201
1-800-621-7619
Provides information on accident
prevention and general safety
guidelines.

U.S. Consumer Product Safety
Commission
Washington, DC 20207
1-800-638-2772
Takes calls from consumers with
product complaints. Also works to
protect consumers from injury in and
around their home caused by
products, including children's toys.

Senior Citizen Health
ElderCare Locator
1-800-677-1116
A public service of the National
Association of Area Agencies on
Aging. Provides access services for
information on local programs, legal
services, transport services, nursing
homes, Medicare, etc.

Healthy Older People
National Health Information Center
P.O. Box 1133
Washington, DC 20013-1133
1-800-336-4797
Supplies public education materials
on health promotion for older
Americans.

National Council on Aging
409 Third Street, S.W. Suite 200
Washington, DC 20024

1-800-424-9046
Provides information on aging and
makes referrals to local agencies.

Sports
Aerobics and Fitness Association of
America
15250 Ventura Blvd., Suite 310
Sherman Oaks, CA 91403
1-800-445-5950
Answers questions about safe
exercise practices and aerobic fitness
programs.

Surgery
American Society of Plastic and
Reconstructive Surgeons, Inc.
444 E. Algonquin Rd.
Arlington Heights, IL 60005
1-800-635-0635
Provides information on aesthetic and
reconstructive surgical procedures
and makes physician referrals.

Medicare Telephone Hotline
200 Independence Ave. SW
Washington, DC 20201
1-800-638-6833
Provides referrals to local surgeons
who can provide second opinions
regarding a recommended surgery.

SOURCE: Adapted from *HealthyLife® Toll-Free Hotlines to Health* and
Health at Home™, American Institute for Preventive Medicine, Farmington Hills,
Michigan, 1997.

To communicate with Don R. Powell, Ph.D., or for more information about
the American Institute for Preventive Medicine's programs, products and
services, contact:

American Institute for Preventive Medicine
30445 Northwestern Hwy, Suite 350
Farmington Hills, MI 48334-3102
Telephone: (248) 539-1800
Fax: (248) 539-1808
Don_Powell@ameritech.net

Index

Page references in *italic* indicate tables.